16 00

Other monographs in the series, *Major Problems in Clinical Pediatrics:*

Avery: *The Lungs and Its Disorders in the Newborn Infant*—Second Edition published in June 1968

Markowitz and Kuttner: *Rheumatic Fever*—published in May 1965

Cornblath and Schwartz: *Disorders of Carbohydrate Metabolism in Infancy*—published in February 1966

Oski and Naiman: *Hematologic Problems in the Newborn*—Second Edition published in March 1972

Rowe and Mehrizi: *The Neonate with Congenital Heart Disease*—published in June 1968

Brewer: *Juvenile Rheumatoid Arthritis*—published in January 1970

Smith: *Recognizable Patterns of Human Malformation*—published in February 1970

Lubchenco: *The Infant of Low Birth Weight*—to be published early 1973

Scriver and Rosenberg: *Disorders of Amino Acid Metabolism*—to be published early 1973

Solomon and Esterly: *Neonatal Dermatology*—to be published January 1973

INCREASED INTRACRANIAL PRESSURE IN CHILDREN

By

William E. Bell, M.D.
Professor, Departments of Pediatrics and
Neurology, Director, Section of Pediatric Neurology,
The University of Iowa College of Medicine,
Iowa City, Iowa

and

William F. McCormick, M.D.
Professor, Departments of Neurology and
Pathology, and Chief, Division of Neuropathology,
The University of Iowa College of Medicine,
Iowa City, Iowa

Volume VIII in the Series
MAJOR PROBLEMS IN CLINICAL PEDIATRICS
ALEXANDER J. SCHAFFER
Consulting Editor

W. B. Saunders Company · Philadelphia · London · Toronto · 1972

W. B. Saunders Company: West Washington Square
Philadelphia, Pa. 19105

12 Dyott Street
London, WC1A 1DB

833 Oxford Street
Toronto 18, Ontario

Increased Intracranial Pressure in Children   ISBN 0-7216-1683-6

© 1972 by W. B. Saunders Company. Copyright under the International Copyright Union. All rights reserved. This book is protected by copyright. No part of it may be reproduced, stored in a retrieval system, or transmitted in any form or by any means, electronic, mechanical, photocopying, recording, or otherwise, without written permission from the publisher. Made in the United States of America. Press of W. B. Saunders Company. Library of Congress catalog card number 75-186948.

Print No.:   9   8   7   6   5   4   3   2   1

Foreword

It gives us great pleasure to present this volume as the eighth in the series of Major Problems in Clinical Pediatrics. The subject is of utmost importance to pediatricians, and the team which has undertaken the task is supremely qualified for it.

Dr. Bell, a native of West Virginia, received his medical education at the university of that state and at the Medical College of Virginia. He then served his residency and fellowship years, in both pediatrics and neurology, at the University of Iowa, and has remained there. He is now Professor of Pediatrics and Neurology at that medical institution. He has taught constantly, lectured widely, and contributed many papers dealing with a variety of aspects of pediatric neurology, all of them scholarly and stimulating.

Dr. McCormick moved from Tennessee to Iowa in 1964, and there he is currently both Professor of Pathology and Professor of Neurology. He too has been author or co-author of many contributions to medical literature, a large proportion of which are concerned with neuropathology.

It is not surprising that the authors, adept in pediatrics, pathology and neurology, have succeeded in writing a complete, detailed, highly instructive volume on one aspect of pediatric neurology. I found the manuscript very readable and highly useful and look forward to further volumes on related topics from Doctors Bell and McCormick.

ALEXANDER J. SCHAFFER

Preface

Within the broad spectrum of diseases which may afflict the nervous systems of children, those accompanied by increased intracranial pressure present the most challenging and often the most perplexing problems to the attending physician. Such disorders are often potentially life-threatening, but the prompt and judicious use of appropriate diagnostic measures can frequently lead to the identification of a cause amenable to therapy which restores the child to good health.

When assessing the child who has a disorder accompanied by increased intracranial pressure, one hopes to assemble sufficient diagnostic information to permit precise identification of both the site and the nature of the pathologic condition without producing unnecessary adverse effects as a result of the investigative efforts. The potential hazards of some of the available diagnostic methods add appreciably to the clinical complexity of this group of childhood diseases.

The authors' goals have been to present information about most of the diseases which can produce intracranial hypertension, and to describe a reasonably logical and relatively safe way of proceeding toward diagnostic analysis. We wish to emphasize that our suggestions concerning diagnostic procedures and plans of therapeutic management are not necessarily the only acceptable ways that the problems in question can be managed. Although a detailed history and an extensive physical examination must always serve as the basic foundation of the clinical evaluation, there can be no "routine work-up" beyond these methods of inquiry. One cannot overemphasize the need for individualized logical analysis and selective judgment by the clinician at each step along the way toward diagnosis of the child who presents with symptoms and signs of increased intracranial pressure.

We wish to acknowledge the encouragement and support provided by Dr. A. L. Sahs and Dr. M. W. Van Allen during the preparation of this volume. Our appreciation is extended to Dr. Alexander J. Schaffer for agreeing to publish this volume in his excellent series and for his advice and suggestions. Mr. John J. Hanley of the W. B. Saunders Company has been of immeasurable help at each phase of the development of the manuscript and deserves credit for his editorial expertise. We also thank Miss Pat Norris for her tireless secretarial assistance and Dr. Sydney S. Schochet, Jr., for many hours of proofreading.

WILLIAM E. BELL
WILLIAM F. MCCORMICK

Contents

PART I
Increased Intracranial Pressure in Childhood

Chapter One
GENERAL COMMENTS 3

Chapter Two
HEADACHES IN CHILDHOOD 11

Chapter Three
LUMBAR PUNCTURE WITH INCREASED INTRACRANIAL PRESSURE 31

Chapter Four
ROENTGENOGRAPHIC SIGNS OF INCREASED INTRACRANIAL PRESSURE 34

Chapter Five
TRANSTENTORIAL AND CEREBELLAR HERNIATIONS 41

PART II
Causes of Increased Intracranial Pressure in Childhood

Chapter Six
GENERAL COMMENTS 49

Chapter Seven
CEREBRAL EDEMA 58

Chapter Eight
HYDROCEPHALUS 62

Chapter Nine
BENIGN INTRACRANIAL HYPERTENSION (PSEUDOTUMOR CEREBRI) 111

Chapter Ten
LEAD ENCEPHALOPATHY 116

Chapter Eleven
HEAD TRAUMA 123

Chapter Twelve
BRAIN ABSCESS 147

PART III
Intracranial Tumors in Childhood

Chapter Thirteen
GENERAL COMMENTS 157

Chapter Fourteen
CLINICAL SIGNS AND DIAGNOSTIC ASSESSMENT 169

Chapter Fifteen
POSTERIOR FOSSA TUMORS 184

Chapter Sixteen
TUMORS IN THE REGION OF THE PINEAL GLAND 198

Chapter Seventeen
PARAPITUITARY, PITUITARY AND HYPOTHALAMIC TUMORS 203

Chapter Eighteen
CEREBRAL HEMISPHERE TUMORS 224

Chapter Nineteen
CONGENITAL TUMORS 234

Chapter Twenty
MISCELLANEOUS TUMORS 239
INDEX 257

PART
I

Increased Intracranial Pressure in Childhood

Chapter One

GENERAL COMMENTS

Increased intracranial pressure in infancy and childhood occurs with a great variety of disorders. Recognition of the presence of increased pressure is extremely important because many of the causes are amenable to specific therapeutic measures. Awareness of an abnormal elevation of intracranial pressure is also necessary so that potentially harmful measures may be avoided. For example, it is generally unwise to administer enemas to children with increased pressure. Straining may markedly elevate the intracranial venous pressure, possibily precipitating tentorial herniation with brain stem compression and death. A tap water enema may result in expansion of the vascular volume because of water absorption from the rectum, producing further expansion of the intracranial contents with potential disaster. Narcotic drugs, such as meperidine and morphine, may also be hazardous in patients with increased intracranial pressure and must be used only with caution. Perhaps the potentially most dangerous problem with conditions accompanied by increased pressure concerns the events at the time of lumbar puncture, a consideration to be discussed later.

There is normally a delicate balance between the volume of the intracranial space and the volume of the contents occupying the intracranial space. After the fontanels have closed and the skull sutures have fused, the intracranial space is a rigid container incapable of significant adaptation to the development of mass lesions within the skull or enlargement of any of the contained structures. The intracranial contents include the meningeal compartments, the brain parenchyma, fluid within the ventricular and subarachnoid spaces, and blood vessels and their contents.

For pressure relationships to remain unaltered, enlargement of any one of these intracranial structures must be accompanied by a reduction in volume of one or more of the others. The margin of safety afforded by this adaptive mechanism is limited, and the usual response to primary enlargement of any of the intracranial compartments is the appearance of the various manifestations of increased intracranial pressure. Enlargement of the cerebral ventricles resulting from cerebral atrophy is clearly a different matter in most instances, because here the ventricular dilatation is a secondary phenomenon resulting from the more basic atrophic state of the brain.

The rigidity and lack of expansile change of the skull of older children and adults does not exist in infants and young children. The potential ability of the intracranial volume to increase in the infant as an adaptation to increasing pressure accounts for certain differences in the clinical manifestations at various ages. The anterior fontanel in the normal infant may remain patent until 15 to 20 months of age. Although this may serve only slightly as a mechanism for compensation for increasing pressure within the skull, it does provide a valuable clinical sign indicative of abnormal elevation of intracranial pressure. The tense, bulging fontanel of the infant under one year of age is strongly suggestive of an increased intracranial pressure syndrome and should correlate with other findings consistent with this impression.

For proper assessment of the anterior fontanel, the baby should be relaxed and not crying or straining. The child should be held in the sitting or upright position with the examiner's hand then estimating the degree of elevation and the resistance to gentle pressure. In the normal, quiet infant in the upright position, the anterior fontanel is usually either flat or slightly concave as compared with the surrounding scalp. Perhaps secondary to increased venous pressure, one may observe a bulging fontanel in an infant with congestive heart failure and without other evidence of significant cerebral disease.

The cranial sutures will rapidly become separated with increased intracranial pressure in infants and young children. In infancy, this may be identified by palpation of the skull, whereas in older children, skull roentgenography is necessary to demonstrate it. Suture spread on x-ray may occur in children until at least ten years of age but with considerable variation from case to case. Percussion of the head of young children with abnormal suture spread may cause a "cracked-pot" sound referred to as the Macewen's sign. The ability of the cranial sutures to spread in children may delay or abate some of the symptoms or signs ordinarily associated with the various disorders in question. For example, in infantile hydrocephalus due to aqueductal atresia, marked head enlargement often occurs, whereas papilledema is unusual.

Symptoms and Signs

Recognition of the presence of increased intracranial pressure is usually dependent on the existence of certain symptoms and signs, the finding of characteristic roentgenographic abnormalities, or the demonstration of an abnormally high pressure at the time of lumbar puncture. Ordinarily, the presence of combinations of these findings establishes the presence of increased pressure because any one isolated abnormality may be misleading because of alternative explanations. Thus, headache alone is nonspecific; but headache and papilledema is virtually diagnostic of a syndrome associated with increased intracranial pressure, assuming that the blood pressure is normal. Also, there is great variation of the expression of the various manifestations of increased pressure from patient to patient.

The commonest and most consistent symptoms and signs of increased intracranial pressure include headaches, nausea, vomiting, diplopia, and papilledema. Children in the toddler age group or younger usually express the presence of headache by irritability, fussiness, and anorexia. Older children with intracranial hypertension describe headaches of variable intensity, usually generalized but with a bifrontal predominance. The headache may be persistent but is more often intermittent and frequently is associated with vomiting. When the increased pressure syndrome is due to an intracranial tumor, headaches and vomiting may have a marked tendency to recur in the early morning hours after rising but before breakfast. Vomiting in children with abnormal elevations of intracranial pressure is not different from vomiting due to other causes. The projectile component has been much overemphasized in this regard, because it is considerably less common than generally believed. Projectile vomiting is more consistently observed in infants with hypertrophic pyloric stenosis than in children with increased intracranial pressure.

Personality and behavioral changes are additional common symptomatic expressions of intracranial hypertension. Infants and toddlers become irritable and obstreperous, increasing the difficulties of physical examination. Older children are frequently noted to become indifferent or to show loss of interest. School performance may decline and physical activity diminishes. A previously active youngster may now come home from school and prefer to lie down or play alone within the house rather than be outside with his playmates. Moodiness and ease of tearfulness over trivial matters may become evident.

These personality changes associated with increased pressure pass through stages of subtle indifference to lassitude, and eventually lead to lethargy or drowsiness. Parents often describe progressively increasing complaints of ease of fatigue and tiredness with more and more time being devoted to sleep. As a result of loss of appetite compounded by recurrent attacks of vomiting, significant weight loss supervenes. If persistent long enough and if of a sufficient degree, increased intracranial pressure may lead to significant memory loss and eventually to evidence of progressive dementia. An unusual complication of several conditions associated with severe increase in intracranial pressure is pulmonary edema, probably secondary to an excessive autonomic discharge of central origin (Ducker et al.). In the later stages, vital signs are altered, with slowing of the pulse, elevation of the blood pressure, and irregularity of the respiratory rhythm.

Changes in Vital Signs

The mechanism by which increased intracranial pressure results in slowing the pulse and elevation of blood pressure has been a point of discussion for many years. For a long period of time, the generally accepted concept for the production of these vital sign abnormalities was based on studies by Harvey Cushing. This theory postulated that increased intracranial pressure of sufficient magnitude resulted in medullary anemia with subsequent disturbance of function of the vasomotor centers in the brain stem. It was proposed that anemia of the medullary centers occurs when the intracranial pressure exceeds the systolic blood pressure. Subsequently, various observations were made that seemed inconsistent with this explanation. It was noted that instances of increased intracranial pressure achieving levels as high as systolic blood pressure are unusual in the clinical situation. In addition, it was often observed that with generalized brain swelling, vital sign disturbances infrequently occur, whereas alterations of the pulse and blood pressure might occur in cases of brain tumor associated with considerably less degrees of intracranial hypertension.

Thompson and Malina altered intracranial pressure by various mechanisms and found that a pressure gradient between the posterior fossa and the supratentorial space is necessary for vital sign changes to occur at levels of intracranial pressure below the systolic blood pressure. Their studies suggested that with differences in pressure between the supratentorial and infratentorial compartments, an axial distortion of the brain stem develops. They also concluded that the changes in pulse rate and blood pressure coincide in time with the development of axial distortion of the brain stem. This concept explains many of the inconsistencies apparent in Cushing's postulate of cardiorespiratory failure with increased pressure due to medullary anemia. It might account for the much greater frequency of changes in vital signs seen in patients with cerebral tumors or hemorrhage than in those with conditions such as pseudotumor cerebri.

OCULAR AND FUNDUS ABNORMALITIES

Papilledema

Papilledema is the single most reliable physical sign indicative of increased intracranial pressure. The possibility of pressure elevation is not excluded by the absence of papilledema, however, because some patients show no funduscopic abnormalities, even in the presence of marked increase of the intracranial pressure. Ophthalmoscopic examination should be done with the room partially darkened but with enough illumination available so that the patient can fixate on one object.

If the pupils are small or the patient is uncooperative, it is advisable to dilate the pupils with a mydriatic before the fundus examination is done. Adequate fundus examination is indispensable and its importance far outweighs the disadvantages of temporarily obscuring certain signs by the use of drugs to produce pupillary dilatation. Although induction of pupillary dilatation in lethargic or comatose patients should not be done indiscriminately, it is entirely acceptable when short-acting agents are used and when adequate funduscopy cannot otherwise be accomplished.

The patient's eye to be examined should be rotated slightly medially to facilitate observation of the optic disc. Older children of normal intellect usually sit quietly with eyes directed toward an object, permitting funduscopic examination. Retarded children and those in the younger age group may be more easily examined while lying down. This position stabilizes the child's head and trunk, thus eliminating the usual fidgeting bodily movements characteristic of this group of children. A flashlight directed by the parent and aimed at the ceiling directly above will usually be watched by the child, providing ocular fixation. Funduscopic examination in the infant occasionally can be done without restraint, but assistance may be needed to immobilize the head and arms.

Papilledema is ordinarily an objective finding identified by the examiner and usually does not cause deficits of which the patient is aware. An occasional patient with papilledema describes recurrent, brief periods with momentary disturbance of vision of both eyes. These amblyopic attacks have been referred to as transient obscurations and usually last only a few seconds. Some patients describe a sensation resembling a heavy fog or veil transiently obscuring the visual environment. Others simply describe the sudden appearance of dim vision as though the lights were turned down, with complete recovery seconds later. These episodes are nearly always associated with advanced papilledema but under any circumstances cannot be considered common. The mechanism of such attacks in patients with papilledema remains undetermined.

With the exception of the infrequent occurrence of the transient episodes just described, visual acuity remains unaffected in most people with papilledema. The persistence of the disorder for a long period of time may be followed by secondary atrophic changes in the nerve head, which may be associated with progressive visual loss. The prevention of this late complication of papilledema must always be given due consideration when dealing with patients with increased intracranial pressure, regardless of the cause. The visual field abnormality in patients with choked discs consists of a concentric enlargement of the blind spots, best identified by tangent screen or Goldmann perimetric examination.

As a rule, ophthalmoscopic evidence of edema of the nerve head is present by the time the blind spot is significantly enlarged on formal visual field examination. Thus, it can be used as confirmation of the diagnosis of papilledema but should not be relied upon as diagnostic as an isolated finding. As swelling of the optic disc advances, the edema spreads into the retina toward the macula. This leads to further blind spot enlargement toward the point of fixation, converting an enlarged blind spot into a cecocentral scotoma with slanting margins. The identification of enlarged blind spots is of greatest usefulness in excluding other conditions that may resemble papilledema, such as optic neuritis.

The ophthalmoscopic appearance of the nerve head with papilledema depends on the degree of swelling and the duration of the process (Fig. 1-1). Findings in the adjacent retina also depend somewhat on the nature of the disorder producing increased intracranial pressure. For example, retinal subhyaloid hemorrhages plus papilledema are characteristically seen in conditions in which intracranial pressure becomes elevated precipitously, as with acute subarachnoid hemorrhage, cerebral contusion, or epidural hematoma.

Early ophthalmoscopic evidence of papilledema consists of blurring or indistinctness of the disc margins, which may appear more pronounced on the medial edge than on the lateral margin of the disc. Indistinct disc margins alone need not be abnormal and may be seen in many normal persons. A central erythema or plethora of the nerve head occurs and the diameter of the optic disc increases progressively, as the condition advances. The margin surrounding the optic disc gradually becomes completely obliterated.

The vessels converging on the disc appear to be deflected forward in the vicinity of the junction of the optic disc and the adjacent retina. While the retinal arteries appear to maintain their normal caliber, the retinal veins become progressively distended, altering the normal 3:2 venous to arterial ratio. In addition to distention, the retinal veins become increasingly tortuous, most profoundly so adjacent to the nerve head but extending out a considerable distance on the retina.

The value of the presence or absence of spontaneous retinal venous pulsations as an indicator of the state of intracranial pressure remains in debate. In many normal persons, pulsations can be noted on viewing the veins on the surface of, or just adjacent to, the optic disc. As a general rule, the pulsatile activity of the retinal veins is abolished with early papilledema. Some exceptions must be expected. The sign remains of clinical importance as long as the examiner is aware of the reservations that must be maintained regarding its interpretation. It is important to add that venous pulsations may not be observable in some healthy persons.

With persistence of intracranial hypertension, hemorrhages eventually appear on the disc surface or in the peridiscal region. Retinal hemorrhages in papilledema tend to occur in the nerve fiber layer of the retina, identifiable by the characteristic flame-shaped appearance. With advanced papilledema, punctate white spots may be seen on the disc surface; these are referred to as cytoid bodies which are believed to represent an axonal reaction to injury.

The degree of elevation of the nerve head with papilledema is measured in diopters, corresponding to the numerical designation on the conventional ophthalmoscope. It is generally believed that ophthalmoscopic recognition of papilledema requires that the elevation be at least 2 diopters. Three diopters of elevation corresponds to 1 mm.

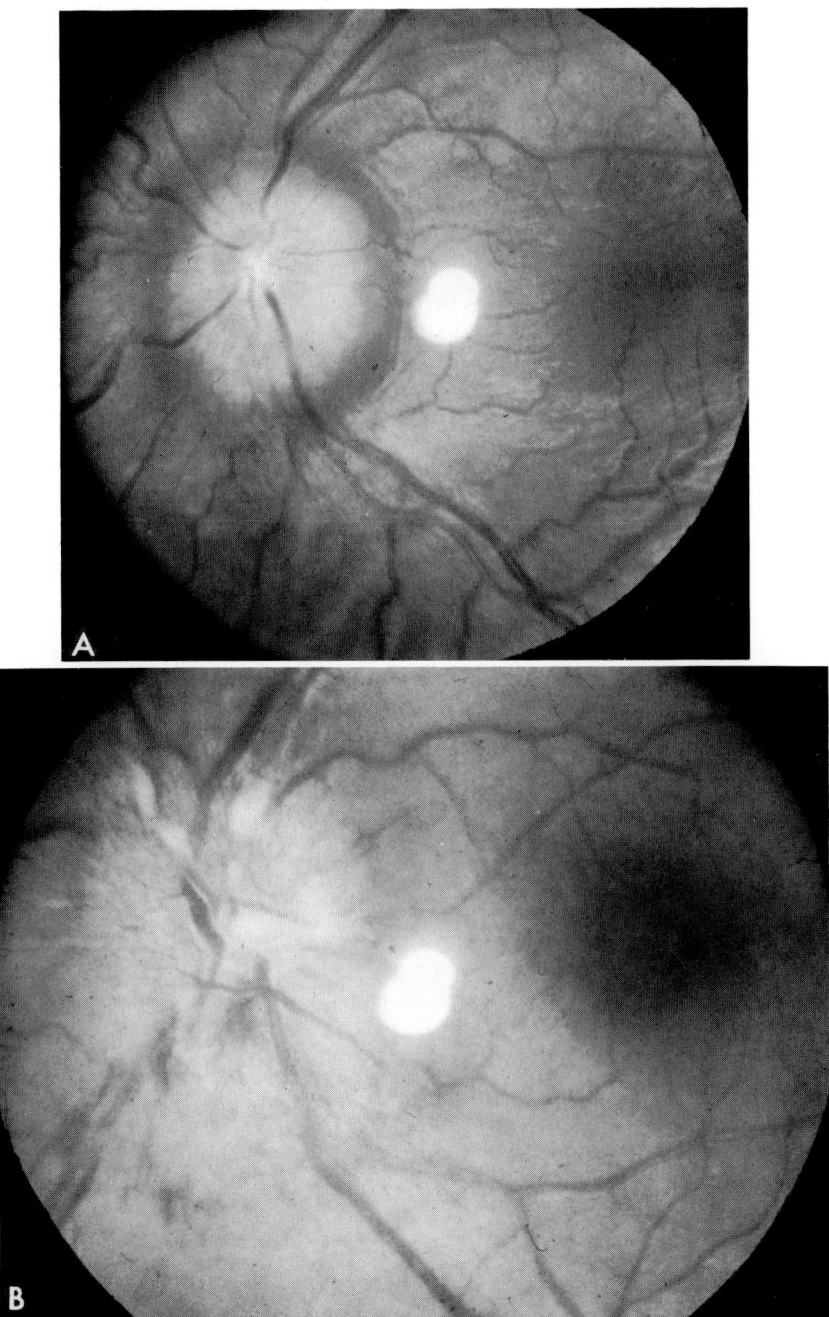

Figure 1-1. Papilledema. *A*, Mild nerve head changes, including elevation of the optic disc margins and venous distention. *B*, Advanced papilledema with obliteration of disc margins and peridiscal hemorrhages.

The ophthalmoscopic abnormalities with papilledema are bilateral in most instances associated with increased intracranial pressure. It is not unusual, however, for the changes to be more advanced on one side than on the other. The degree of elevation may be greater on one side, and hemorrhages may be unilateral despite the bilaterality of nerve head swelling. Variations in the degree of papilledema on the two sides cannot be considered as localizing evidence for the site of intracranial disease.

UNILATERAL PAPILLEDEMA. Unilateral papilledema due to intracranial disease is unusual in childhood. The presence of primary optic atrophy on one side and papilledema on the other is referred to as the Foster Kennedy syndrome. This combination of findings is far more common in adults in whom the most common cause is a meningioma of either the olfactory groove or the tuberculum sellae. Tumors of the orbital surface of the frontal lobe or of the sphenoid ridge may also produce a Foster Kennedy syndrome. The optic atrophy in this syndrome is of the primary type and is produced by direct pressure on the homolateral optic nerve. Increased intracranial pressure due to the mass accounts for papilledema in the opposite eye. Adhesive arachnoiditis is another cause of the Foster Kennedy syndrome, although other ocular findings are far more common.

Unilateral papilledema may also occur in children with unilateral, high grade myopia. Papilledema develops less rapidly on the myopic side and thus a syndrome with increased pressure may result in nerve head swelling in the opposite eye. Intraorbital mass lesions in the absence of increased intracranial pressure may cause unilateral papilledema. Orbital disease with papilledema is usually readily differentiated from intracranial disease by the prominence of other local ocular signs, including exophthalmos.

CHRONIC PAPILLEDEMA. The chronic persistence of papilledema eventually results in degenerative and atrophic changes of the optic nerve head. The end result is secondary optic atrophy with its attendant loss of visual acuity. As atrophic and gliotic changes occur, the disc becomes pale with a gray discoloration. The retinal veins become less congested and the arteries less prominent. The nerve head retains an increased diameter and the margins remain less distinct than normal, as opposed to the findings in primary optic atrophy. With progression of the atrophic changes visual loss advances, possibly resulting in eventual complete blindness.

Visual fields in persons with chronic atrophic papilledema show a progressive concentric constriction of the peripheral fields that parallels the development of decreasing central acuity. With recognition of the importance of long-standing papilledema as a cause of visual loss, appropriate therapy should reduce this complication to a minimum.

Pathogenesis

The pathogenesis of papilledema secondary to increased intracranial pressure remains unclear. Venous obstruction of the central retinal vein behind the orbit has long been considered an important aspect contributing to the development of nerve head edema. However, the marked differences noted on funduscopic examination in central retinal vein obstruction compared with papilledema due to increased pressure suggests that additional factors must also be contributory. A recent reappraisal of the pathogenesis of papilledema (Behrman) suggests that the nerve head edema resulting from increased intracranial pressure may be the result of obstruction of lymph drainage posteriorly from the orbit. Thus, a combination of compromise of venous and lymphatic drainage may account for the abnormalities observed in this condition.

Differential Diagnosis

Certain other conditions may be confused with papilledema because of similarities of appearance on ophthalmoscopic examination. Optic neuritis causes the greatest diagnostic difficulty because the appearance of the nerve head changes may be identical to those of papilledema due to increased pressure. Acute optic neuritis is commonly unilateral, whereas papilledema is generally bilateral. With exception of the absence of other manifestations of increased intracranial pressure with optic neuritis, the visual acuity deficit and visual field abnormality provides the best differentiation of optic neuritis from papilledema.

As already noted, visual acuity generally remains normal in papilledema, and visual fields reveal enlarged blind spots. A marked decrease of visual acuity, often of sudden onset, accompanies optic neuritis. The pupillary response to light is often diminished and may be absent. Patients with optic neuritis often complain of retro-orbital pain, precipitated by horizontal ocular movement. Visual fields in optic neuritis reveal a central or cecocentral scotoma if sufficient acuity is retained for field testing to be accomplished.

Pseudopapilledema is a variation of normal that resembles papilledema resulting from increased intracranial pressure. The disc margins are blurred, apparent elevation of the nerve head may be noted, and retinal veins may be tortuous. The fundus findings may be unilateral or bilateral and may be present in other members of the family. Other somatic anomalies may be present. A combination of pseudopapilledema, macrocephaly, and multiple hemangiomas has been described in several children in a single family (Riley and Smith). The blind spots on visual field examination in pseudopapilledema remain normal and other manifestations of increased pressure should be absent.

Differential diagnosis may be difficult and patients believed to have pseudopapilledema should be reevaluated at periodic intervals to be certain that no additional changes are occurring. It is possible to distinguish early papilledema from pseudopapilledema by fluorescein fundus photography (Miller et al). Following the intravenous injection of 5 ml. of 10 per cent fluorescein sodium, fluorescence can be demonstrated in the region of the optic disc for at least ten minutes in early papilledema. This fluorescence is believed to be the result of extravasation of the dye into the disc tissue because of capillary permeability resulting from the edema. With pseudopapilledema, there is no leakage of fluorescein in the region of the disc and no residual fluorescence ten minutes after the injection. Although the procedure is a valuable technique, limitations of the test include the need for specialized equipment and personnel.

Another anomaly that may resemble papilledema is the presence of drusen, or hyaline bodies, in the optic disc, especially if the drusen are located in the depths of the nerve head, making ophthalmoscopic recognition difficult. When present, drusen are often bilateral and show a yellow coloration rather than the hyperemia more characteristic of papilledema. When superficially placed on the nerve head, they result in the appearance of nodular excrescences of a glistening or glassy nature. Retinal venous distention is not present as in papilledema, and visual fields are usually normal. Extensive involvement of the disc by drusen can cause visual field defects (Rucker). In addition to their presence in normal persons, drusen are observed in some patients with tuberous sclerosis and with other retinal degenerative disorders.

Hypertensive retinopathy may be confused with papilledema secondary to increased intracranial pressure, but certain features allow differentiation. Retinal arterial abnormalities are usually profound in hypertensive retinopathy and consist of narrowing of diameter plus segmental constrictions. As opposed to the hemorrhages with papilledema that are primarily peridiscal in location, retinal hemorrhages with hypertension tend to be diffuse, extending to the periphery of the retina. The characteristic soft exudates in the retina with hypertensive retinopathy serve as another distinguishing feature.

Central retinal vein thrombosis is usually easily distinguished from papilledema because of increased intracranial pressure. Rapid loss of vision occurs with occlusion of the central retinal vein. The disorder is usually unilateral and funduscopic examination reveals marked venous congestion and tortuosity in addition to edema of the optic disc. Retinal hemorrhages assume a radial arrangement and extend far out in the periphery of the fundus as opposed to their peridiscal location with papilledema due to increased intracranial pressure.

False Localizing Signs

The other ocular sign commonly encountered in patients with increased intracranial pressure is abducens nerve paralysis resulting in lateral rectus muscle weakness. This disturbance is directly related to increased pressure within the intracranial space and in this context, not directly from the lesion or disorder causing the increased pressure syndrome. Thus, it has no localizing significance except as a reflection of increased intracranial pressure and is referred to as a false localizing sign.

The disturbance of abducens function is usually unilateral. Mild involvement of the sixth nerve may cause diplopia only on lateral gaze toward the side of the paretic muscle. This may be intermittent or persistent and may not be accompanied by sufficient weakness of ocular movement to be observed by the examiner. As the process advances, diplopia becomes evident to the patient even with the eyes in the primary position. By this time, lag of lateral rectus function on conjugate gaze to the involved side is readily apparent on examination. An internal strabismus may result which, in younger children, may be one of the first objective signs of increased pressure noticed by the parents.

With lateral rectus weakness, the diplopia is horizontal. The difference between the two objects seen by the patient is exaggerated by conjugate horizontal eye movement toward the weak side. If unilateral, double vision is not apt to be present on looking to the side opposite the weak lateral rectus muscle. As a compensatory mechanism to diminish double vision, patients with lateral rectus weakness develop head turning with the face rotated toward the side of the paretic muscle.

The selectivity of involvement of the sixth nerve with increased intracranial pressure is believed to be due to its long intracranial course. After emerging from the ventrolateral surface of the pons, the abducens nerve passes upward to angle over the petrous tip of the temporal bone. After traversing Dorello's canal, the abducens nerve pierces the dura to enter the cavernous sinus en route to the orbit. It is generally believed that the most susceptible site of injury to the abducens nerve in increased pressure is at its point of angulation over the petrous apex. If appropriate medical or surgical therapy can reduce the elevated pressure, the abducens weakness usually gradually regresses. Diplopia may disappear within hours if an obstructive lesion is surgically bypassed or if other methods are successful in reducing intracranial pressure.

Another false localizing sign occasionally encountered with increased intracranial pressure occurs with posterior fossa obstructive lesions resulting in marked distention of the third ventricle. The ballooned anterior third ventricle may compress the optic chiasm, producing a bitemporal hemianopsia. Less often, the pressure exerted by the distended third ventricle results in compression of the chiasm laterally by the adjacent carotid arteries, producing a binasal hemianopsia.

Additional clinical manifestations often included in the category of false localizing signs secondary to increased intracranial pressure are discussed later with tentorial herniations. Although not necessarily related to the site of the primary cerebral hemisphere lesion, these neurologic deficits resulting from internal herniations must be considered to be of significant localizing value, usually indicating the occurrence of midbrain distortion or compression. Thus, it is with considerable doubt that they are appropriately classified as false localizing signs. Included in this category also are oculomotor palsies due to temporal lobe herniation and homonymous field defects due to calcarine infarction. The infarction in the occipital region in this instance is the result of compromise of blood flow of the posterior cerebral artery by the sharp edge of the tentorium.

Paralysis of upward conjugate gaze secondary to temporo-occipital herniation at the tentorium with dorsal midbrain compression may also occur (Johnson and Yates). The abnormality most likely to cause error in diagnostic localization with tentorial herniations is the occurrence of a hemiparesis ipsilateral to the herniation. This may result from lateral displacement of the brain stem away from the hippocampal herniation with pressure on the opposite cerebral peduncle by the edge of the tentorium. As the corticospinal tracts decussate below, at the level of the medulla, the paresis resulting is on the same side as the temporal lobe herniation.

REFERENCES

Behrman, S.: Pathology of papilledema. *Brain*, **89**:1–14, 1966.

Cushing, H.: Concerning a definite regulatory mechanism of the vasomotor centre which controls blood pressure during cerebral compression. *Johns Hopkins Hosp. Bull.*, **12**:290–292, 1901.

Cushing, H.: Some experimental and clinical observations concerning states of increased intracranial tension. *Amer. J. Med. Sci.*, **124**:375–400, 1902.

Ducker, T. B., Simmons, R. L. and Martin, A. M., Jr.: Pulmonary edema as a complication of intracranial disease. *Amer. J. Dis. Child.*, **118**:638–641, 1969.

Johnson, R. T., and Yates, P. O.: Brain stem hemorrhages in expanding supratentorial conditions. *Acta Radiol. Stockholm*, **46**:250–256, 1956.

Miller, S. J. H., Sanders, M. D., and Ffytche, T. J.: Fluorescein fundus photography in the detection of early papilledema and its differentiation from pseudopapilledema. *Lancet*, **2**:651–654, 1965.

Riley, H. D., Jr., and Smith, W. R.: Macrocephaly pseudopapilledema and multiple hamangiomata. *Pediatrics*, **26**:293–300, 1960.

Rucker, C. W.: Defects in visual fields produced by hyaline bodies in the optic discs. *Arch. Ophth.*, **32**:56–59, 1944.

Thompson, R. K., and Malina, S.: Dynamic axial brainstem distortion as a mechanism explaining the cardiorespiratory changes in increased intracranial pressure. *J. Neurosurg.*, **16**:664–675, 1959.

Chapter Two

HEADACHES IN CHILDHOOD

Headache is a common symptom in the pediatric age group. It is a complaint that often occurs in the absence of serious disease but one that usually raises the possibility of a disorder associated with increased intracranial pressure until a detailed history and appropriate examinations are done. Pain in or about the head may be a reflection of a vast number of varied disease states in children, and thus may tax the diagnostic acumen of even the most experienced physician. The very fact that such diversified conditions may cause a headache problem in a child accounts for the need for considerable caution regarding diagnosis in the clinical setting.

Although the complaint may be that of pain in the region of the head, a broad survey of numerous organ systems and physiological processes must be accomplished before one can be reasonably sure of the site of the causative problem. As is often the case with children, seemingly neurologic complaints may represent symptomatic manifestations of disease of other organ systems.

No age group is immune, because even infants surely experience headache but express their discomfort in a different manner than does the older child. Irritability, fretfulness, and poor food intake presumably are manifestations of headache in the preverbal child or toddler. From a broad viewpoint, the age of the child is important in consideration of the diagnostic possibilities. The younger the child, the less likely is headache due to psychogenic disorders, migraine, or visual refractive errors. Disorders with headache in the infant age group are most often those associated with increased intracranial pressure or those of an infectious nature. The causes of headache in the teenage child approximate those in adulthood.

Location of Headache

Location of headache in children is often of little value regarding site of disease because of the peculiarities of innervation of pain-sensitive structures within the head. Intracranial pain-sensitive structures include the major dural venous sinuses and their tributaries, the meningeal arteries, great vessels at the base of the brain, and the dural floor. The dural nerves, derived from the ophthalmic division of the trigeminal nerve, provide a major contribution to the innervation of intracranial structures. Thus, lesions in various areas within the head may result in pain located predominantly in the forehead region. Pain from posterior fossa lesions may be generalized because of increased pressure, or occipital and upper cervical in location because of innervation from the upper cervical nerves. In general, pain from intracranial lesions results from inflammation, displacement, or traction of one or various pain-sensitive structures.

The site of the pain experienced by the patient depends on the source of innervation of the particular intracranial structure involved. Pain from extracranial structures commonly arises from arteries of the external carotid, temporal, or upper cervical muscles, contents of the orbit, membranes of the paranasal sinuses and dental structures. Extracranial vasodilation and muscle contraction represent the most common headache mechanism in the older child as in the adult. The severity of headache experienced is not necessarily related to the seriousness of the underlying disease. Headache with intracranial tumors may be dull and mild in intensity. Pain secondary to extracranial vasodilatation is commonly intense, throbbing, and may be associated with local scalp tenderness.

Historical Aspects

Successful analysis of a headache problem in a child requires time, patience, skillful examination techniques, and knowledge of the possible disease entities associated with this symptom. Hoping for an answer from elaborate laboratory or ancillary studies without pursuing a detailed historical description from the patient or parents usually results in failure and occasionally in diagnostic disaster. The appropriate diagnostic studies and procedures can be decided upon only after the historical data are acquired and the physical and neurologic examinations accomplished.

A properly taken history concerning a child with headaches should provide the physician with considerable insight into the fundamental nature of the problem. The skillful physician usually finds that the physical examination of such a child is simply confirmatory of his anticipations developed from the history. The unexpected discovery of physical signs that totally change the probable diagnosis is unusual in this instance. The most reliable information concerning many points in the history is ordinarily obtained from the child's parents. Certain aspects of the headache problem, however, may be more clearly described by the child, if he is in the older age group. The parents may be able to describe the appearance of the child during a headache episode, but only the patient can usually relate a detailed description of the pain. Thus, the examiner should question both parents and patient to obtain the maximum amount of information concerning the headache.

The total duration of the disorder and the frequency of occurrence of headaches often tend to categorize the problem as far as reasonable considerations. For example, the child with headaches of two or three years' duration, recurring at monthly intervals, can usually be safely handled as an out-patient. However, the child with gradually worsening headaches of three days' duration is apt to require more urgent studies and must be dealt with more cautiously.

In addition to the total duration of the illness and the frequency of headache recurrence, one must obtain a detailed description of the location of the pain, the duration of each headache episode and the intensity of the pain. It is necessary to ascertain if there is a throbbing component to the pain, if it is associated with nausea or vomiting, and what the child does during the headaches. One can usually assume that the pain is farily severe if the child voluntarily ceases to play and lies down during the episode.

Factors that precipitate or relieve the headache may be important in analysis of the problem and should be elicited in the history. Headaches precipitated by coughing or sudden change of position of the head may occur with intraventricular obstructive lesions. Headaches repeatedly occurring in one particular class at school often suggests a stressful situation involving either the subject matter or the teacher conducting the class. Relief of headaches may come from salicylate therapy, from lying quietly, or only after sleep in certain situations.

Time of day of onset may provide clues that aid solution of a headache problem in childhood. Throbbing headache with associated vomiting that wakens the child during sleep may be a migrainous episode but is rarely the case with psychogenic headaches. Late morning and late afternoon headaches in the school-age child may suggest a visual refractive error or ocular muscle imbalance problem requiring ophthalmologic investigation. This is especially apt to be the case if the headache is consistently brought on by visual effort, such as reading, and if symptoms include a burning or uncomfortable sensation in the eyes.

Recurrent, brief headaches occurring in early morning shortly after arising and with vomiting are a common presenting manifestation of a posterior fossa tumor in children. Headaches present on arising and lasting several hours, but occurring at infrequent intervals, may suggest a nocturnal grand mal seizure unobserved by the parents. Other suggestive evidence of this type of problem might include a wet bed coinciding with the headache episode, blood on the child's pillow, or a past history of seizures or a convulsive disorder. Also, recurrent headaches each of sudden onset, perhaps associated with mental confusion or disorientation, and followed by deep sleep at an inappropriate time of day, may represent a seizural manifestation verified by electroencephalography and response to anticonvulsant therapy.

One must inquire into the occurrence of visual abnormalities during the headache episode because of the relationship of such findings to migraine. Scotomas, flickering lights, or field defects that are transient and precede the onset of headache are suggestive of a migrainous syndrome. Also, it is important to ask about the presence of diplopia, blurred vision, or decreasing visual acuity unassociated with headache because of the frequency of such manifestations with space-consuming intracranial lesions in childhood.

History of head trauma must be elicited and if present, details of the events should be recorded. It is important to ascertain how the injury occurred, the presence or absence of loss of consciousness, whether a skull fracture was identified, and the child's emotional response to the traumatic episode. The relation between the child's headache problem and litigation developing from the accident must also be considered. A causal relationship might be entertained if the parents provide a detailed description of the child's symptoms but the child is unable to describe any aspect of his headache problem.

One should inquire about other family members with headaches. If present, a brief description of the characteristics of the headache problem in related persons may be helpful. Childhood migraine is frequently associated with a family history of migraine, especially on the mother's side of the family. Certain aspects in the family history may be of help in the identification of a psychogenic headache disorder in a child. One occasionally finds that the child's headache problem is, by description, nearly a carbon copy of the mother's headache disorder, which she has long recognized to be tension-induced. Psychogenic symptoms in children are often patterned after complaints they have heard in their home environment and have thus learned by experience. If the father has a peptic ulcer or colitis, the child with emotional problems may complain of recurrent abdominal pain. The anxious teenager may develop an intermittent headache problem if one parent has long been susceptible to periodic headaches.

Chronic, recurrent headaches in older children often result from stress situations or disturbed interpersonal relationships within the family. The history should include information about the child's personality makeup and other aspects suggestive of emotional problems. Perfectionistic traits, feelings of inferiority, evidence of sibling rivalry, and signs of anxiety should all be searched for in discussion with the family. Low spirits, depression, frequent crying episodes, or withdrawn and aloof behavior provides further suggestive evidence of an underlying psychologic problem.

It is important to ascertain whether the child and family have recently moved from one community to another. School changes during the academic year in addition to the need to develop new friends and personal relationships may be poorly tolerated by certain children, with headaches resulting.

One must also investigate historically the child's place and relationship within the family setting. Certain children with long-standing feelings of inadequacy may develop a severe headache problem at the time the mother acquires an outside job that temporarily removes her from the home each day. In some instances, with the mother working, the added burden of home responsibilities placed on the oldest child may be stressful enough to cause headaches. Likewise, absence of one parent from the home because of divorce, serious illness, or death may be a source of childhood anxiety or frustration resulting in headaches.

An attempt should be made to assess the parents' relationship with each other, because family discord at this level may be extremely distressful to the child, instilling anxiety and insecurity. Older siblings departing from the home because of marriage, college, or military service may also be upsetting to the younger child remaining behind, particularly if the age difference is not marked and if the siblings are of the same sex. When headaches occur under these circumstances, the child often has considerable insight into the cause of the problem but may resist admitting it.

Additional information to be obtained in the history of a child with headaches pertains to other areas of neurologic dysfunction. One should ask about memory loss, incoordination of gait, limb weakness and sensory abnormalities. Changes of volume of fluid intake or of urine output are of diagnostic importance, if present. The combination of headaches of recent onset and diabetes insipidus provides presumptive evidence of an infiltrative lesion or mass in the anterior region of the hypothalamus. Family history of renal disease, diabetes mellitus, hypertension, or seizures should also be elicited.

Physical Examination

When dealing with a child with headaches, certain observational aspects of the physical examination are profitably begun while the history is being taken. The observant physician may detect evidence of hostility, anxiety, insecurity or depression from the child's demeanor or behavior during the interview. With experience, one often finds that facial expressions reflect many hidden aspects of the total problem. One comes to recognize an appropriate degree of concern about the illness expressed by the patient when it is of an organic nature. If the patient is complaining of headache existent at the time the history is being taken, his appearance and behavior should be consistent with the intensity of the pain he describes. The person who describes intense headache present at the moment but who appears comfortable and acts jovial and superficial presents an obvious incongruity.

Keen observation during the interview also may reveal important aspects about child and parent relationships which may prove important concerning ultimate diagnosis. Points of disagreement in the history may be associated with tell-tale glances indicative of intense hostility between family members or child and parents. Evidence of a domineering mother or overly strict father may also be apparent by careful observation as the history is collected. Frequent yawning by the patient may be noticed during the interview. Although not necessarily of concern, this might be a suggestion of a disorder associated with increased intracranial pressure. Considerable information about the younger child with headaches may be obtained by observation of his playful activity. Evidence of ataxia may be more evident at this time than during the formal examination because of the negative attitude of toddlers concerning examination.

All aspects of the general physical examination are important, because headaches may represent the symptomatic manifestation of many different diseases in childhood. The child's weight and height must be assessed as compared with normal average for his age. The significance of variations from normal is evaluated partly on the basis of physical stature of other family members. Chronic headaches and significant growth failure may occur in children with anterior third ventricle tumors, with hypothyroidism, or with long-standing renal disease. The same combination of abnormalities might occur in children with Turner's syndrome with coarctation of the aorta.

Inspection of the skin of a child with headaches may reveal lesions important for analysis of the problem. Acne and red striae may suggest Cushing's disease, with headaches resulting from hypertension. Headaches, primary optic atrophy, and cutaneous café-au-lait spots direct one's attention to a possible optic nerve glioma associated with neurofibromatosis. Urticaria pigmentosa with systemic mastocytosis may be associated with intermittent histamine release, producing throbbing headache, flushing, diarrhea, and respiratory distress.

The head should be carefully palpated during the examination of children with headache problems. Unilateral, localized occipital or cervical pain may be readily clarified by the identification of tender lymphadenopathy in the area. A highly localized tender area found on palpation may suggest an eosinophilic granuloma of the skull. A pulsating leptomeningeal cyst, developing after skull fracture and producing headaches, may be felt and outlined by careful palpation of the head.

The blood pressure should be determined and femoral pulses palpated. If femoral pulses cannot be felt, blood pressure in both arms and legs should be recorded. Tenderness over the sinuses or mastoid processes or evidence of chronic otitis should be sought. Considerable emphasis should be devoted to the ocular examination in children with headaches because of the wide variety of disorders that have ophthalmologic manifestations. The ocular fundus must be adequately visualized to exclude the possible existence of papilledema or optic atrophy. If difficulty is encountered because of poor cooperation by the child or because of miotic pupils, one should not consider the examination complete until pupillary dilatation is produced with mydriatics and an adequate fundus examination accomplished.

Truncal or limb ataxia must be excluded on examination, plus other evidence of neurologic dysfunction. If one suspects an increased intracranial pressure syndrome in a child with chronic headaches, neck stiffness should be looked for by gentle antiflexion of the head with the child in the supine position. Posterior fossa tumors or cerebellar abscesses in childhood are occasionally associated with neck rigidity.

Diagnostic Studies

The laboratory and ancillary diagnostic studies to be performed when evaluating a child with headache depend on the tentative diagnosis developed from the history and physical examination. If one is satisfied that the problem is one of psychogenic or tension headache, a blood count, urinalysis, and skull x-rays may be all that are needed. Psychometric and psychologic testing may provide further insight into the psychodynamics of the situation and aid the therapeutic approach. Electroencephalography is indicated if a cerebral hemisphere mass lesion or subdural hematoma is considered in differential diagnosis. Differentiation of migraine and seizures in childhood may be difficult clinically, because the symptoms may be similar in the two disorders. Electroencephalographic abnormalities comprising a paroxysmal dysrhythmia are more consistent with a convulsive state, whereas a normal electroencephalogram or one with 14 and 6 positive spikes per second would be suggestive of a migrainous disorder.

The child with headaches who is found to have localizing neurologic signs or signs of increased intracranial pressure usually requires hospitalization for a more extensive diagnostic evaluation. An acute illness of short duration with headaches, fever, and neck rigidity requires lumbar puncture to confirm or exclude bacterial meningitis or an encephalitic disorder. Cerebrospinal fluid examination is of great help in the analysis of several conditions associated with headaches in childhood. However, when high-grade papilledema is present or when the postulated diagnosis is one of epidural hematoma, posterior fossa tumor, or cerebellar abscess, it is usually advisable to defer lumbar puncture. The potential hazard of temporal lobe or cerebellar tonsillar herniation under these circumstances outweighs the probable benefit obtained from the procedure. Air contrast studies or carotid angiography is usually required for diagnostic purposes in children with intracranial mass lesions. The procedure of choice depends on the probable location and type of lesion suspected from previous studies.

Other examinations often utilized in evaluation of children with headaches include sinus or mastoid x-rays, visual field and visual acuity determination, or appropriate consultation with an otolaryngologist or ophthalmologist. One occasionally finds that, after a reasonable diagnostic evaluation, the explanation for a child's headache disorder remains unidentified. The passage of time and periodic re-examinations frequently help clarify the problem, as the natural course of the illness becomes evident.

MIGRAINE

Credit is given to Galen who introduced the term migraine centuries ago. Modern concepts of migraine as a vascular disorder involving both intracranial and extracranial arterial structures are largely constructed on concepts proposed by Wolff. The disorder is now recognized as one with periodic episodes of sudden alteration in the caliber of blood vessels of the head but of unknown etiology. An initial, sudden vasocontriction of intracranial vessels comprises the preheadache phase and results in various neurologic deficits depending on the site of the transient ischemia. Optic nerve involvement results in unilateral visual loss. Vasospasm reducing blood flow to other parts of the visual apparatus may produce scintillating scotoma, homonymous field defects, micropsia or macropsia, or other visual hallucinations. The vasoconstrictive phase may be associated with unilateral limb weakness or numbness, or aphasia if the left cerebral hemisphere is affected.

The initial vasoconstrictive phase is soon followed by the painful, or vasodilatation, phase of the syndrome. Vascular dilatation of branches of the external carotid artery causes stimulation of nerve endings within the vessel wall, with the characteristic throbbing headache resulting. With persistence of the vasodilator component, edema of the involved vessel wall occurs and at times, edema of the surrounding soft tissues. Wolff postulated that the severity of the pain is related to the existence of a substance in the edematous tissue that results in a lowering of the pain threshold. The local accumulation of a polypeptide called neurokinin in the edematous soft tissues adds support to this view (Chapman et al.). The substance is said to cause a sterile inflammatory response contributing to the pain. With prolongation of the vasodiltation process, cervical and occipital muscle contraction adds a tension component to the headache syndrome.

Although there is considerable understanding of pain mechanisms in migraine, there remains little insight into the fundamental cause of the alterations in vessel caliber. Serotonin (5-hydroxytryptamine) has been suggested as possibly related to the basic pathophysiology in migraine, but its role remains unestablished (Dalessio). Interest in this substance in migraine developed with the finding of therapeutic benefits from the antiserotonin agent, methysergide.

Symptoms and Signs

Migraine in childhood varies in several respects from the classic syndrome well known in adults. As opposed to the predominance of females in adult migraine patients, migraine in children is more common in the male (Burke and Peters). The prodromal phase appears to be either less common or less commonly described. The characteristic visual features so often noted in adults with this syndrome are less frequently elicited from youngsters. The gastrointestinal manifestations may be more profound in the younger age group. Some children with migraine are placed in the ill-defined category of "cyclic vomiting" until the headache phase becomes better established and permits proper identification of the process. Recurrent migrainous attacks may be more frequent but with less intense pain in the child as compared to the adult.

For a comparable number of patients with this disorder, ophthalmoplegic migraine and hemiplegic migraine appear to be more common in younger patients. Rarely, migraine in children may present as an acute confusional state with impairment of sensorium (Gascon and Barlow). Diagnosis of migraine may not be evident in such cases until recovery from the acute episode occurs and the associated headache is described.

The onset of a migrainous episode may be at any time of day. Occasionally, the child is wakened from sleep with headache marking the beginning of the attack. Vomiting may occur soon after the appearance of headache or may be delayed for several hours. Vomiting may recur many times during the spell, preventing effective use of oral medication. At times, it is difficult to know whether the vomiting is the result of the basic disorder or results from medication given for pain relief. The duration of a migrainous attack varies from an hour or so up to two or three days in rare instances.

As noted earlier, the initial vasoconstrictive phase is associated with varying symptoms, depending on the site of ischemic involvement. Constriction of branches of the internal carotid system results in transient visual deficits or hemisphere signs. Much less commonly, the vasoconstrictive phase involves the basilar artery system, causing brain stem signs of brief duration (Bickerstaff). These signs may be accompanied by visual disturbances due to occipital cortical ischemia. Sudden, bilateral visual loss followed by various combinations of signs, including vertigo, dysarthria, ataxia, or masseter weakness may occur with basilar artery vasoconstriction. Perioral numbness or dysesthesia of the tongue may also be described. After a brief period, recovery occurs to be followed by throbbing headache usually occipital in location. Regardless of the site of the vasoconstrictive phase in migraine, recovery from neurologic signs resulting therefrom is usually complete. In rare instances, persistence of vasoconstriction may result in focal ischemia resulting in lasting deficits. This has been referred to as complicated migraine (Conner).

Severe throbbing headache and vomiting characterize the vasodilatation phase of the migrainous episode. Initially, the pain is usually unilateral and most often frontal or temporal in location. A complaint of photophobia and local scalp tenderness during the headache phase is not unusual in childhood. The patient usually prefers to lie quietly in a darkened room without noise during the episode. One may find that some relief can be brought about by gentle compression of the common carotid or the superficial temporal artery early in the course of the headache. As the headache abates, some children develop a temporary increase in fluid intake and urine output. A common pattern in migraine is the persistence of headache until sleep ensues. Upon wakening, a feeling of general fatigue persists for a few hours, but the pain is abolished. A peculiar feeling of exhilaration or undue well being may precede a migrainous spell in some persons. More often, a sensation of lassitude or malaise persists a day or so following the end of the episode.

Migraine is usually an episodic disorder but recurrent attacks usually do not follow a specific time pattern. In girls, a relationship between occurrence of attacks and menses may be noted. The disorder in children usually shows a strong familial tendency, a feature that serves as a diagnostic aid. One series revealed a positive family history for migraine in 87 per cent of children with this disorder (Holguin and Fenichel). Although the pathogenesis of the vascular changes remains unclear, there seems little doubt that hereditary factors are important in the migrainous syndrome. Wolff has suggested that the tendency to develop migraine is inherited as a recessive trait.

Stressful or emotionally charged situations may appear to precipitate attacks of migraine in children as in adults. In other instances, migrainous episodes occur in let-down periods, as during weekend days. No definite personality traits can be identified in all cases of migraine. Personality patterns occasionally observed in migrainous children include perfectionism and seriousness. Other children with this disorder are often said to be sensitive, ambitious, or have a driving desire to please. Other somatic traits that have been related to migrainous tendencies include allergies, motion sickness, or epilepsy.

To date, no data provide conclusive evidence of a specific relationship between these disorders and migraine. Some have noted an increased frequency of migraine in patients with familial periodic paralysis. Patients with Melkersson's syndrome also appear to be predisposed to attacks of migraine (Stevens). This disorder is characterized by recurrent facial paralysis, facial edema, and lingua plicata with eventual development of persistent edema of the lips and face. The onset is sudden or gradual and usually in the childhood years. The pathogenesis of Melkersson's syndrome remains unclear, but the relationship to migraine suggests the possibility of some form of vasomotor disturbance of intermittent and recurrent type.

A variant of the migrainous syndrome that may cause difficulty regarding diagnosis is referred to as abdominal migraine. It is seen more commonly in children than adults and may not be recognized as migraine until the child becomes older and develops the more characteristic headache component. Abdominal migraine consists of periodic attacks of abdominal pain with vomiting and with little or no associated headache. The onset and termination of the episode is usually sudden; the duration may be hours or days. If present, a family history of migraine is of help.

HEMIPLEGIC MIGRAINE. In some cases, the visual aura of migraine is associated with or followed by hemiparesis. This pattern may be seen in several members of a family in which case it is referred to as familial hemiplegic migraine (Rosenbaum). The onset of the neurologic abnormality is usually abrupt. Unilateral weakness and sensory loss occurs in stroke-like fashion and is often fully developed before the vasodilatation or headache phase becomes manifest. Varying degrees of mental confusion or disorientation are common. When the process affects the left cerebral hemisphere, dysphasia may be profound, providing further evidence of localizing cerebral involvement.

In one patient the side of the body affected may vary with different attacks. Unilateral throbbing headache ordinarily follows the onset of hemiparesis within minutes or up to an hour. The hemiparesis may be short-lived or may persist for several days before recovery occurs. It is generally believed that the focal neurologic signs in hemiplegic migraine result from transient vasoconstriction with ischemia of one cerebral hemisphere. Complete recovery from any one attack is the rule. Cerebral arterial thrombosis, ruptured arteriovenous malformation, and septic embolization are usual diagnostic considerations due to the sudden onset of the focal signs.

OPHTHALMOPLEGIC MIGRAINE. Ophthalmoplegic migraine is an unusual type of the migrainous syndrome. The disorder consists of a combination of vascular headache of the migraine type and unilateral ophthalmoplegia, which is most often transient. Many cases begin in children and some even in infancy (van Pelt and Andermann) (Fig. 2-1). It appears likely that this variety of migraine more commonly begins in childhood than later in life. In most, the periodic headache pattern characteristic of migraine has been established before the first episode that is associated with extraocular muscle paresis occurs. Other children have the initial

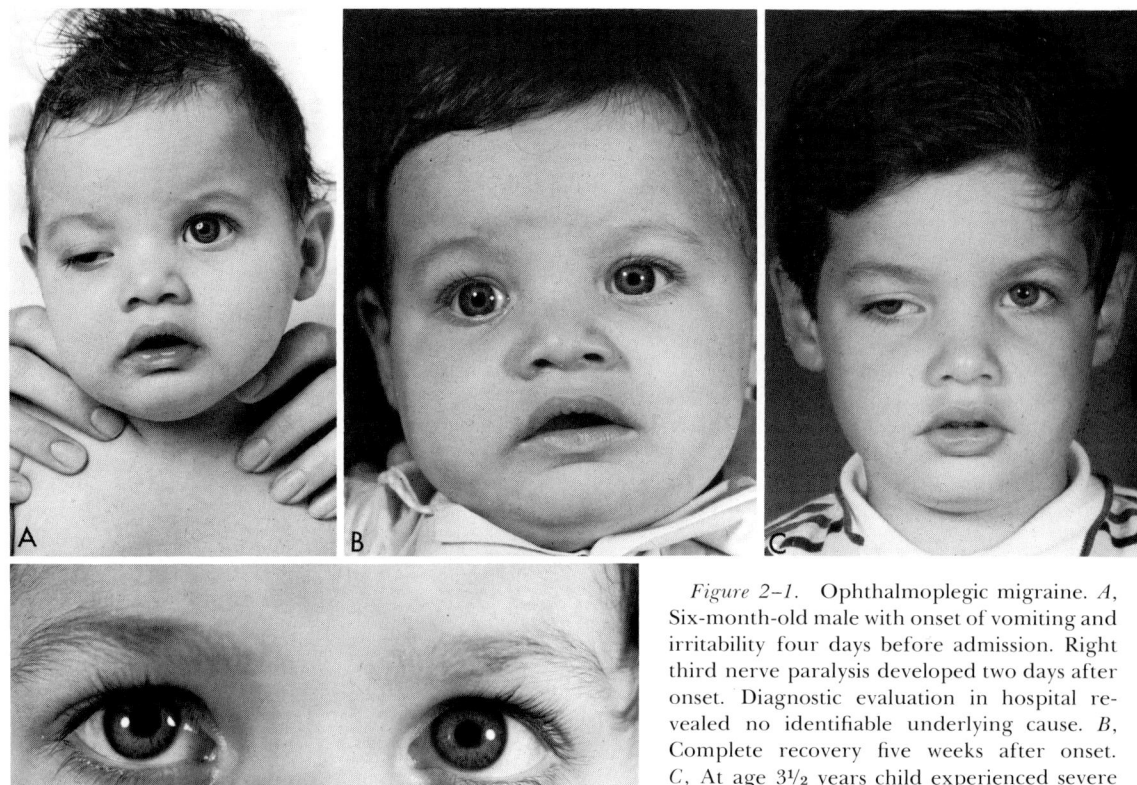

Figure 2–1. Ophthalmoplegic migraine. *A*, Six-month-old male with onset of vomiting and irritability four days before admission. Right third nerve paralysis developed two days after onset. Diagnostic evaluation in hospital revealed no identifiable underlying cause. *B*, Complete recovery five weeks after onset. *C*, At age 3½ years child experienced severe right frontal headache with vomiting. Four days later, he again developed a partial right third nerve palsy. *D*, Four weeks after onset of the second episode, spontaneous recovery had occurred except for slight pupillary dilatation on the right.

bout with migraine complicated by opthalmoplegia.

The unilateral headache is usually present one to four days before evidence of ocular muscle weakness is noted. The ophthalmoplegia occurs on the same side as the headache and is internal and external. Unilateral ptosis, pupillary dilatation, and weakness of muscles innervated by the third nerve are the usual findings. The oculomotor nerve is most commonly implicated, although at times the third, fourth, and sixth nerves may be involved in various combinations. The duration of the ophthalmoplegia varies, but usually ocular function is gradually regained in one to four weeks. On rare occasions, permanent ocular muscle weakness may remain after an attack. Persisting deficits in ocular motility are more likely to occur in persons with repeated episodes of ophthalmoplegic migraine over several years' duration.

The mechanism of ocular nerve dysfunction in the ophthalmoplegic migraine syndrome remains unestablished. Cerebral edema with uncal herniation and third nerve compression has been suggested but has received little support. Compression of the ocular nerves by swollen, edematous arteries within the cavernous sinus or by vessel edema interfering with the vasa nervorum has also been postulated (Walsh and O'Doherty). This mechanism has been suggested by the identification of internal carotid artery constriction in its intracavernous portion by carotid angiography. Others have promoted the concept of oculomotor nerve compression in its peripheral course as it passes between the superior cerebellar and posterior cerebral arteries. Vasodilatation and edema of the vessel wall might cause a compressive third nerve neuropathy and might also account for the high frequency of selective third nerve involvement in this disorder. Narrowing of the lumen of the upper portion of the basilar artery on vertebral angiography would seem consistent with this explanation (Friedman et al.). It is conceivable that the location of ocular nerve impingement may vary in different persons depending on the area of maximum change of caliber of intracranial vessels during the vasodilatation phase.

The combination of severe headache, vomiting, and ocular muscle paralysis in ophthalmoplegic migraine may produce considerable diagnostic confusion. Intracranial aneurysm may produce similar signs but is a rare cause of neurologic dysfunction in childhood. Complete exclusion, however, may require angiography. Myasthenia gravis in childhood may result in sudden onset of ocular muscle weakness but is a painless disorder and thus is easily excluded.

The diagnosis of ophthalmoplegic migraine in infancy cannot usually be established until the natural course with periodic recurrences and symptom-free intervals excludes other causes. Infants with this disorder would manifest headaches with irritability, vomiting, and perhaps low-grade fever. These symptoms followed by a unilateral ophthalmoplegia would more likely be initially interpreted as due to sepsis or dehydration with intracranial vascular thrombosis.

Midbrain tumor or cryptic vascular malformation of the brain stem with subarachnoid hemorrhage might be another consideration until excluded by appropriate studies and the natural course of the illness. Carotid-cavernous fistula would produce similar signs. Pulsating exophthalmos, a bruit over the orbit, and a history of head trauma would be anticipated with this syndrome.

A syndrome similar to ophthalmoplegic migraine and referred to as painful ophthalmoplegia has been reported (Hunt et al.). The orbital pain is usually steady rather than throbbing. Cranial nerve involvement is not usually restricted to the oculomotor nerve but includes dysfunction of all the ocular nerves and the fifth nerve in various combinations. Attacks tend to recur at intervals as in migraine. As opposed to migraine, both pain and cranial nerve deficits often persist for weeks with each recurrence. The syndrome is believed to be due to a low-grade inflammatory process in the cavernous sinus. Corticosteroid therapy has been recommended during the acute phase of the illness with some describing beneficial results.

CLUSTER HEADACHES. A type of recurrent syndrome believed to be a migraine variant is referred to as cluster or histamine headache. Other designations for the same entity have included sphenopalatine neuralgia, vidian neuralgia, and autonomic faciocephalalgia. The disorder occurs most commonly in young adults and only rarely in childhood. The recurrent headache episodes tend to occur in clusters with free intervals of varying duration between the attacks. The onset is usually abrupt and often begins in the nocturnal hours. During a cluster, headaches may recur each night for a week or so, with each attack lasting one to two hours. The pain is exquisite, unilateral, throbbing, and located in the orbital region and temple. Conjunctival injection with tearing occurs on the involved side. Nasal stuffiness or rhinorrhea is usually present during the episode. A transient Horner's syndrome may accompany the headache.

The ocular and headache pain in this disorder appears to result from vasodilatation of the extracranial branches of the external carotid artery. The pathogenesis of the vascular dilatation, however, remains unestablished. The syndrome resembles migraine, but the headache episode is briefer and the prodromal manifestations secondary to intracranial vasoconstriction are usually absent in cluster headaches. As opposed to patients with migraine, who prefer to lie quietly during the painful phase, persons with cluster headaches often move about or pace the floor during the episode.

Histamine desensitization has been advocated therapeutically for this disorder, although benefits remain unproved. Because of the lengthy duration of a desensitization series, the end of the treatment may coincide with a spontaneous remission of the disorder, making interpretation of the therapeutic regimen difficult. Ergotamine therapy in one form or another has been most consistently effective as compared with other therapeutic approaches (Friedman and Mikropoulos). As in migraine, the medication should be taken as soon after the onset of symptoms as possible.

Other Considerations

Electroencephalographic abnormalities have been described in some children with migraine. Tracings are often normal or show only minor slow changes, thus providing diagnostic assistance in cases in which epilepsy is being considered. The most common abnormal electroencephalographic pattern identified with migraine has been 14 and 6 per second positive spikes, now considered by many to be a nonspecific type of disturbance. In one series, this type of electroencephalographic abnormality was found in 46 per cent of children with migraine as compared to 18 per cent of normal controls (Whitehouse et al.).

The natural course of the migrainous syndrom starting in childhood is variable but generally is regarded as favorable. Some children continue to have periodic vascular headaches as adults; but in others, the tendency diminishes or even disappears. Bille followed a number of migrainous children for several years and found that 51 per cent eventually became free of attacks. In another series with a follow-up evaluation of approximately ten years, 79.4 per cent were either well or improved from the migrainous syndrome (Hinrichs and Keith). Although one cannot safely predict the eventual outcome with any one child experiencing migrainous episodes, a generally optimistic outlook may be expressed to the parents.

Treatment

One of the ergotamine tartrate preparations is the drug of choice in treatment of a migraine episode. In addition to drug therapy, however, other aspects of management are necessary if the therapeutic regimen is to be effective. The vascular mechanism of the headache should be explained to the patient and parents to enable them to comprehend the relation between the symptoms and the effect of the medication. This can be conveniently done by quickly sketching the changes in blood vessel size, starting with the normal state and proceeding through the two subsequent stages. Visualizing the drawing of a dilated, throbbing vessel and hearing about pounding headache is easily comprehended by parents. Often they regard it as so logical that it tends to give the family considerable confidence in the physician as well as his diagnosis.

Efforts should be made to provide an explanation of how stressful or environmental factors may precipitate attacks. If certain personality traits that might predispose the child to this disorder are identified, this should also be pointed out to the family. In the case of the perfectionistic or overly ambitious child with migraine, parents may be able to reestablish sense of values and help the child develop realistic goals commensurate with his ability.

The vasoconstrictor effects of ergot preparation are resorted to once the attack has occurred (Table 2-1). Regardless of which preparation or route of administration is used, the ergotamine agents are most beneficial if given during the vasoconstrictor phase or during the very early part of the headache phase. Once the vessel wall has become edematous, the likelihood of relief from ergotrates is remote. Thus, the sooner after onset

Table 2–1. Ergotamine Preparations

Preparation Composition	Amount per Unit
Cafergot (tablet)	
Ergotamine tartrate	1 mg.
Caffeine	100 mg.
Cafergot (suppository)	
Ergotamine tartrate	2 mg.
Caffeine	100 mg.
Cafergot P-B (tablet)	
Ergotamine tartrate	1 mg.
Caffeine	100 mg.
Bellafoline	0.125 mg.
Pentobarbital	30 mg.
Cafergot P-B (suppository)	
Ergotamine tartrate	2 mg.
Caffeine	100 mg.
Bellafoline	0.25 mg.
Pentobarbital	60 mg.
D.H.E. 45 (ampule)	
Dihydroergotamine mesylate	1.0 mg./ml.
Ergomar (sublingual tablet)	
Ergotamine tartrate	2 mg.
Gynergen (tablet)	
Ergotamine tartrate	1 mg.
Gynergen (ampule)	
Ergotamine tartrate	0.5 mg./ml.
Medihaler-Ergotamine (aerosol)	
Ergotamine tartrate	9.0 mg./ml.
Wigraine (tablet, suppository)	
Ergotamine tartrate	1 mg.
Caffeine	100 mg.
Belladonna alkaloids	0.1 mg.
Phenacetin	130 mg.

of the migrainous attack the medication is taken, the more likely it is to be effective.

The agent that will be most effective with any one child with migraine must be determined on a trial basis. Cafergot tablets may be tried initially by the oral route. The oral dose for the younger child is one tablet and for the older child, two tablets. If headache persists 30 minutes after the initial dose, the medication should be repeated. Some children appear to respond better and object less to Ergomar sublingual tablets. This preparation has the advantage of rapidity of absorption and is less apt to be lost by vomiting. In children who have frequent episodes of vomiting from the beginning of the attack, the suppository route is more effective. The young child is given one-half suppository and the older child a full suppository. This also may be repeated in 30 minutes if headache persists. There is little advantage to the use of parenteral ergotamine tartrate in most cases of migraine. In rare instances, this route may be used in intractable patients who respond poorly to other preparations.

Ergotamine preparations should not be used in patients with hypertension, peripheral vascular disease, or sepsis. Side effects are not common if the drugs are used in reasonable quantities. Nausea and vomiting may occur; however, it is often difficult to determine whether gastrointestinal symptoms are due to the drug or the disorder for which it is used. Tingling of the extremities, substernal oppression, and muscle cramps may also occur. Patients should be warned about unnecessary use of ergotrates and advised that such preparations are not analgesics for routine use for headaches of any type. Improper or excessive use of this group of drugs may be hazardous.

With many children with migraine, one finds that if sleep can be induced, the headache will be terminated on waking. As part of the treatment regimen, the child should be encouraged to lie down and attempt to sleep after the ergotrate has been taken. Mild sedatives, including chloral hydrate or short-acting barbiturates, may be helpful in those unable to attain natural sleep. Narcotics should be avoided in patients with migraine because of the chronicity of the disorder.

An occasional child has migrainous attacks that are severe in intensity and intractable to conventional therapy. Vomiting is often profound in this group. Hospital admission may be necessary to abort the episode, and rehydration must be emphasized as an important step in terminating the attack. Sedation and codeine usually suffice in this unusual group of children with severe migraine. Belladonna or atropine may be of value for the intestinal complaints but must be used in children with considerable caution.

Methysergide (Sansert) has been used prophylactically to attempt to prevent recurrences in patients in whom attacks tend to recur at frequent intervals. This antiserotonin agent has been shown to be effective in a number of patients with migraine. Disturbing side effects of the drug include nausea, vomiting, arterial insufficiency, thrombophlebitis, and retroperitoneal fibrosis (Fenichel and Battiata, Graham et al.). The medication is usually given in a dosage of 2 mg. two or three times per day. When it is used, continuous administration should not exceed six months followed by a drug-free interval of several weeks before the agent is reinstituted.

PSYCHOGENIC AND TENSION HEADACHES

Headaches in children, as in adults, may result from stressful environmental situations or anxiety-invoking circumstances. The diagnosis of headaches of psychogenic origin should not be made simply because of the absence of other explanations for the headache problem. First, the description of symptoms should be consistent with, or even suggestive of, psychogenic or tension headaches. Next, one should identify personality deficits, emotional problems, or environmental conflicts that could account for this type of somatic disturbance. Finally, the physical examination, plus additional studies, should help to exclude organic causes of headaches. If such reasonably rigid criteria are adhered to, the possibility of diagnostic error is reduced to a minimum.

Headaches in children of this type are variously described. Some have characteristic muscle contraction, or tension, headache located bitemporally and in the occipital regions. More often in children the pain is poorly and vaguely described, leaving the examiner in question as to the actual characteristics of the headache. Some describe pain located at the vertex of the head. In others, the pain is said to be like a constricting band around the head. The headache may be brief and last only minutes or may be prolonged, persisting throughout the day. Psychogenic headaches are usually steady and persistent, although some may indicate the presence of a throbbing component.

As indicated in the introductory comments, when dealing with a child with a headache disorder, one should search for potential stress situations as the history is obtained. After the historical data is obtained in the conventional way, further information may be obtained by questioning the child in the absence of the parents. Hostile feelings toward one parent or guilt feelings over sexual or other types of activities may remain hidden by the child in the presence of the parents.

The child with significant psychogenic problems often has considerable insight into the fundamental nature of the problem that is bothering him. Although he may not admit a relationship between his headaches and his problems, he is apt to describe at length the source of anxiety or dissatisfaction if the examiner once broaches the appropriate conflict area during the discussion. Thus, one seeks to uncover disturbed interpersonal relationships between child and parents.

One looks for possible sources of anxiety, including fear of school failure, marital discord between parents, or other factors that may remove one parent from the home. Undue responsibility placed on the shoulders of the child, either real or potential, may result in somatic complaints. Older siblings departing from home for college, marriage or military service can cause feelings of insecurity in the remaining child, with headaches resulting. Dissatisfaction with personal appearance may be very distressing to the maturing girl who may regard beauty as synonymous with success with the opposite sex.

Overweight youngsters and those needing to wear dental braces or glasses are common examples of instances in which headaches develop on a basis of feelings of inferiority. Name-calling, so common in the childhood years, serves as a constant reminder to the one less endowed with physical attractiveness. Some respond to this by the development of compensation mechanisms and achieve scholastic superiority. Others react more passively and convert frustration to bodily complaints, including headaches.

Symptomatic manifestations that may accompany psychogenic headaches in childhood include low spirits, crying spells, impulsive outbursts, and depression. Parents may become hostile or guarded if asked directly about such symptoms. They may sense the physician's consideration of a possible emotional problem in the child and at once become negative to his judgment and diagnostic approach. This danger may be circumvented by cautious selection of words as the questions are asked. If asked whether the headache problem has caused the child to be low spirited or unhappy, the parents are less apt to be defensive. If the answer is affirmative, one then asks the parents what they have seen that indicates to them that the child is low spirited, or depressed. This way, the family may be guided to describe the manifestations of the child's emotional turmoil without themselves becoming hostile to the examiner's line of inquiry.

While questioning the child alone, one attempts to uncover emotionally-charged situations that may be related to the origin of the headache problem. Hints to possible problem areas may have been obtained from comments by the parents. Once emotionally painful subjects have been identified, the details of the problem should be pursued to ascertain its significance to the child. The appearance of tears or the occurrence of overt weeping by the child at this point is evidence to the physician of the importance of the particular problem in question.

The management of a child with a headache disorder believed to be psychogenic depends on the circumstances. If the onset of headache is recent and the complaints severe, it is often advisable to admit the child to the hospital. This allows rapid accomplishment of the appropriate diagnostic studies to permit more certainty regarding diagnosis. It also provides the attending physician the opportunity to observe the child's behavior and response to both presence and absence of parents. Under these circumstances, the overindulgent, overprotective mother becomes readily identified and may help point to the psychodynamic explanation of the problem. The patient's response to diagnostic procedures, such as lumbar puncture, may also give clues to personality disorders leading to headaches. The older child who behaves in a hysterical fashion during the performance of a spinal tap and who complains of multiple discomforts for days afterwards suggests emotional instability and immaturity.

When the headache disorder is chronic and the examination is normal, the diagnostic evaluation frequently can be done on an out-patient basis. When one becomes reasonably satisfied that the child's headache disorder is psychogenic, the initial therapeutic approach should be explained to the parents. One indicates how emotional conflicts and anxiety may be converted into somatic complaints, and at the same time, reassures the family of the absence of serious organic disease. Specific points of emotional conflict identified in the history are discussed with them with the hope that environmental adjustments can be made to enable the child to develop emotional stability and maturity. If expected school achievement or goals have been set unrealistically high, this may be corrected to be more consistent with the child's abilities. With insight and understanding, parents can often make the necessary alterations to alleviate basic conflicts resulting in childhood headaches. When the personality deficits are more serious and the problem seems to be getting more unmanageable, psychiatric consultation may be necessary.

HEADACHES DUE TO INTRACRANIAL LESIONS

Headache is a common symptom of any disorder in childhood that is associated with increased intracranial pressure or meningeal irritation. The type and intensity of headache with these syndromes is quite variable. One must depend on other associated symptoms and signs plus appropriate ancillary studies to reach a localizing and etiologic diagnosis.

Tumors

Headaches in children with intracranial tumors are apt to be bifrontal, diffuse, or a combination of both. Children with posterior fossa neoplasms frequently complain of occipital or sub-occipital discomfort in addition to generalized headaches. As a general rule, neither location nor intensity of pain holds much diagnostic value in this group of disorders. A description that may be considered at least as diagnostically suggestive of a posterior fossa tumor pertains to the periodicity and time relationship of the headache problem.

Children with subtentorial tumors often experience recurrent brief headaches in the early morning shortly after arising. Vomiting may follow soon thereafter, often without a feeling of nausea and with a desire to have breakfast moments later. The child may then feel well the remainder of the day only to repeat the episode on subsequent mornings. Recurrent morning headaches in children with brain tumors may occur without associated vomiting, or morning vomiting spells may be present without headache. Morning headaches or vomiting may persist for several weeks before additional symptoms or signs direct one's attention to the possibility of an intracranial mass lesion. Occasionally, the episodic morning complaints spontaneously disappear for a lengthy period of time, giving the physician a false sense of security. Symptoms subsequently recur and are often associated with ataxia or papilledema, making the diagnosis of posterior fossa tumor readily evident.

With the exception of the foregoing headache pattern being suggestive of intracranial tumor in childhood, suspicion of a brain tumor usually is aroused by the combination of recurring headaches and other signs of neurologic dysfunction. The additional signs may be either localizing or signs of increased intracranial pressure, including papilledema and abducens nerve paralysis. Thus, for example, the combination of vague but periodic headaches with visual loss, optic atrophy, and growth failure suggests a mass lesion that is suprasellar. Headaches, unilateral visual loss with associated optic atrophy, and an enlarged optic foramen on x-ray point to an optic nerve glioma. Headaches, unilateral limb ataxia, nystagmus, and papilledema are indicative of a mass lesion in one cerebellar hemisphere. Other children with focal, expanding lesions do not have specific localizing signs on examination but only those of increased pressure. This is commonly seen with midline intracranial tumors and requires definitive contrast studies for identification.

Headaches from increased intracranial pressure occur in children with diffuse neoplastic invasion of the cranial leptomeninges. This occurs most often in the childhood years as a complication of acute lymphoblastic leukemia and often develops during a period of hematologic remission subsequent to drug therapy. The headache pattern is the same as that of other conditions associated with increased pressure. Except for signs resulting from increased pressure, neurologic examination is usually nonrevealing. Neck stiffness may be present. Headache plus other pressure signs commonly are markedly alleviated by therapeutic measures including intrathecal methotrexate, or radiation.

Cerebral Edema

In children, cerebral edema due to any cause produces headaches as a manifestation of increased intracranial pressure. In common with other conditions with increased pressure, the pain is usually generalized with bifrontal predominance and is apt to be persistent but with daily fluctuation in intensity. Pseudotumor cerebri, or benign intracranial hypertension, is associated with few findings except headache and related manifestations of increased pressure. The disorder may occur spontaneously in youngsters or may be related to steroid therapy for arthritic, asthmatic, or other disorders.

Severe headaches commonly precede or are associated with lethargy, seizures, and limb paresis in children with cerebral edema secondary to lead poisoning. The encephalopathy due to chronic lead ingestion usually occurs in young children between one and three years of age, and thus accurate description of the headache in not anticipated.

Headache is also a prominent complaint in children with water intoxication with its attendant cerebral edema. This condition may occur under a variety of circumstances but is most commonly seen when excessive amounts of salt-free fluids are given intravenously. Tapwater enemas may cause water intoxication, especially in patients with abnormal dilatation of the colon, as with Hirschsprung's disease. Gastric irrigation with large volumes of water may also result in excessive water absorption. Generalized headache rapidly becomes more severe. The child appears drowsy and later becomes lethargic. Unless the condition is recognized and promptly corrected, convulsions may occur. When it is suspected, the diagnosis of cerebral edema due to water intoxication can be confirmed by the identification of marked serum hyponatremia and hypochloremia. Therapy includes appropriate volumes of 3 per cent sodium chloride solution given intravenously; recovery usually is prompt.

Subarachnoid Hemorrhage

Subarachnoid hemorrhage in children results in severe, generalized headaches largely due to direct irritation of pain-sensitive meningeal structures. The onset of headache is apt to be explosive and is frequently associated with vomiting, a feeling of faintness, or even a brief episode of disorientation or loss of consciousness. The acutely ill patient finds that lying with the head immobile affords some relief. Sudden movement or change of position makes the pain worse and may precipitate vomiting or excessive perspiration. Severe, diffuse headache of sudden onset with neck stiffness and other signs of meningeal irritation is suggestive of subarachnoid bleeding. Confirmation should follow by the identification of blood in the spinal fluid.

Epidural Hemorrhage

Epidural hemorrhage results in severe headache in association with other signs of increased intracranial pressure and compression of the involved cerebral hemisphere. The headache is ordinarily diffuse and of little value from the standpoint of localization of the side with the lesion. The side involved is usually apparent from the ipsilateral pupillary dilatation, contralateral hemiparesis, and site of skull fracture, if present. Headache with subdural hematoma is usually more chronic and the location varies considerably. Generalized headache is usual, although some patients describe pain lateralized to the side with the lesion.

Vascular Disorders

Cerebral vascular thrombosis in children often is a painless event but occasionally may be associated with sudden, severe headache. Rarely, the headache may even precede other manifestations of cerebral ischemia, such as hemiparesis, field defects, or dysphasia. In such cases, if the headache is unilateral, differentiation of hemiplegic migraine from cerebral thrombosis or embolism may be extremely difficult. Signs of cerebral ischemia with migraine are expected to be transient; those with infarction are more persistent. Carotid angiography may be of diagnostic help if thrombosis is suspected.

INFECTIOUS DISEASE AND HEADACHES

Headache is a very common complaint of children with meningitis or encephalitis, but it may also occur with systemic infections in which the nervous system is not primarily involved. Virtually any febrile disorder may cause headache because of extracranial vasodilatation. In the early stages of infectious hepatitis or infectious mononucleosis, severe generalized headache and malaise may be the most outstanding manifestations, preceding findings usually considered more characteristic of these illnesses. Headache may accompany the febrile phase of measles as well as the other childhood exanthems. Typhoid fever becomes symptomatic with the appearance of headache, fever, malaise, and anorexia. Scarlet fever may cause severe headache and abdominal pain with vomiting before symptoms referable to the pharyngeal region become evident. Likewise, a brief prodromal period with headache and anorexia is common with rickettsial infections, such as Rocky Mountain spotted fever. Psittacosis, Q fever, yellow fever, and dengue are infectious illnesses that characteristically have severe headache notably present at the onset.

Headache is regularly present in older children with bacterial meningitis. The remarkable irritability of infants and toddlers with meningitis probably results from head pain and cervical discomfort, because the irritability is obviously aggravated by any movement of the head. Headache with meningitis is usually diffuse, severe, and often made worse by change of position or coughing. Headache with viral encephalitis is similar to that with meningitis, but the description is more variable. An occasional child with viral encephalitis experiences severe, unilateral, throbbing headache with vomiting at the onset of the illness, virtually identical to that of migraine. One may not consider an encephalitic disorder under these circumstances until fever or lethargy develops or unless lumbar puncture reveals a lymphocytic pleocytosis.

Bacterial infections of the middle ear may be associated with several complications, the clinical picture of which includes headache. These complications are less common now than in years past, because early and widespread use of antibiotics has markedly reduced the frequency of spread of infection from the middle ear or mastoid processes. However, temporal lobe or cerebellar abscesses may still occur in poorly treated or neglected cases of otitis media.

Infection of the middle ear and mastoid processes may extend forward, producing suppuration of the petrous apex, which causes severe retro-orbital and forehead pain. The combination of apical petrositis, lateral rectus paralysis, and severe pain behind the eye on the the same side is referred to as Gradenigo's syndrome subsequent to its description in 1904. Symptoms may appear days or weeks after mastoiditis or mastoidectomy. Fever and signs of toxicity are usually present, and meningitis may result if the process penetrates the dura.

Middle ear and mastoid infections may also result in obstruction of the lateral venous sinus, causing headaches and other manifestations of increased intracranial pressure. The degree of cerebral edema and the severity of symptoms depend on the size and importance for venous drainage of the involved lateral sinus.

Inflammatory disorders of the paranasal sinuses may cause headaches in children, as in adults. Acute sinusitis is more common in the older child than in infancy. Rudimentary maxillary and ethmoid spaces are present soon after birth; however, the wide patency of the ostea of these spaces with the nasal cavity reduces the tendency to infection at this age. The frontal sinuses develop more slowly and are rarely the seat of significant infection under five years of age.

Acute sinusitis may be associated with generalized headache, but it is usually readily recognized by severe pain in the area of the involved sinus. Maxillary sinusitis may cause pain in the region of the upper teeth. Sphenoid sinus disease occasionally is manifested by occipital pain. Acute ethmoiditis may produce retro-orbital and bitemporal pain or pain and tenderness at the bridge of the nose. The ethmoid sinuses are separated from the orbital contents by a thin sheet of bone, which provides poor protection against spread of infection. Acute ethmoiditis in infants and children may extend to one or both orbits with orbital cellulitis resulting. Frontal sinusitis often results in headache typically most severe on wakening in the morning with some relief occurring one or two hours after arising. Pain is frontal and diffuse with tenderness over the sinus commonly present.

Headache due to sinus infection is usually acute in onset and associated with other signs of an infectious process. X-ray evidence of sinus involvement is helpful, although in children under three years of age, the ethmoid sinuses are often hazy roentgenographically in the absence of infection.

HEADACHES DUE TO DISORDERS OF FACIAL STRUCTURES

Face pain and headache may result from a variety of disturbances of the facial structures. Abnormalities of ocular function, sinus and dental disease, and temporomandibular joint dysfunction may be associated with headache in children.

Pain of ocular origin may occur from structural disorders of the orbital contents, from visual refractive errors, and from extraocular muscle imbalance. Pain usually occurs in children with uveitis, orbital cellulitis, and episcleritis. However, localization of the symptoms to the eye plus other overt local signs causes little diagnostic confusion with other causes of headache. Refractive errors may produce headache resulting from sustained traction of the intraocular muscles. Because headache of this sort is brought on by close visual use, such as reading, it is rarely seen in the preschool age child.

Bitemporal, throbbing headache and a heavy or sandy sensation in the eyes is apt to appear in late morning. If sustained visual effort is ceased over the noon hour, the child may then feel better only to have symptoms recur in the afternoon. Cervical and occipital discomfort may develop, adding a tension component to the syndrome. Hyperopia and astigmatism in children are the types of refractive errors found that may cause "eyestrain" headaches. Myopia is not usually associated with symptoms of this type. Ocular muscle imbalance also may result in headache because of a sustained effort to maintain binocular fusion. Scalp and cervical muscle contraction accounts for the generalization of the discomfort in this disorder.

Headache in children due to refractive errors or ocular muscle imbalance is relatively uncommon. Discomfort with these disorders is usually clearly related to sustained visual effort and symptoms are ordinarily alleviated by proper ophthalmologic treatment. One must be cautious not to over-utilize "eyestrain" as a cause of headache in childhood. If the diagnostic evidence is insufficient, it is wiser to defer a specific etiologic diagnosis as to the cause of the headache disorder so that search for the cause will not be abandoned.

Dental disorders characteristically produce pain localized to the site of involvement. Disease of the upper molars, however, may cause pain more prominent in the region of the maxillary sinus, resulting in diagnostic difficulty. The pain also may be felt in the region just anterior to the ear or even in the temporal region on the same side. Dental pain often is altered by changes of position or aggravated by exposure of the diseased tooth to cold water.

Malocclusion may result in disturbance of function of the temporomandibular joint, or the so-called Costen's syndrome. Pain of temporomandibular joint disease is often referred to the external ear canal on the same side, because the joint is innervated by the auriculotemporal branch of the mandibular division of the fifth nerve. Joint motion as occurs with chewing or talking precipitates the pain in this syndrome. An audible and palpable click on opening the jaw is often present and associated with pain in the region at the temporomandibular joint, in the external ear canal, or in the temporal region. The disorder is more common in adults but may occur in older children. Dental consultation is necessary, because treatment includes methods to improve dental occlusion.

CONVULSIVE STATES AND HEADACHES

Headaches are widely recognized as an occasional prodrome of a major convulsive episode or as a disturbing symptom following grand mal seizures in childhood. Postconvulsive headaches are usually mild to moderate in intensity, generalized in location, and last from a few minutes to several hours. The occurrence of headache following an episode of loss of consciousness in childhood may be a valuable diagnostic sign in certain instances. Syncopal episodes are less likely to be followed by significant headache or sleep. Thus, a poorly described or peculiar episode with sudden loss of consciousness is more likely to be seizural if followed by a persisting headache or by deep sleep.

The occurrence of an unobserved nocturnal seizure may be suspected on the basis of periodic morning headaches in a child known to have a convulsive disorder. Such headaches are occasionally the primary lead suggesting the possible existence of a convulsive state and serving as the indication for electroencephalography.

An interesting train of events may be observed after anticonvulsant medication is started in some children with episodic grand mal seizures. Occasionally, one finds that the drug therapy controls overt seizures, but the child now has periodic, brief headaches, at times followed by sleep. Slight increments in drug dosage or addition of a second anticonvulsant agent may cause cessation of the headaches. It is justified to consider the possibility that interictal headaches may represent a seizural phenomenon in a child with a convulsive disorder. However, one must be cautious regarding this interpretation, because both seizures and headaches may be symptoms of an intracranial mass lesion. In addition, children with seizures are susceptible to any other disorder of childhood that may be manifested by headaches.

Much less common is the occurrence of headaches as the sole manifestation of a convulsive state. This is perhaps analogous to the more widely recognized condition with periodic abdominal pain as an isolated manifestation of a convulsive disorder in childhood. The term epileptic cephalea has been used by some to indicate an epileptic condition manifested by headaches (Halpern and Bental). Nonconvulsive epileptic equivalents is another designation suggested for the same disorder (Livingston and Escala).

This type of headache usually appears abruptly, may be either generalized or focal, and is often brief. Mental confusion, disorientation, or inappropriate behavior often accompanies the headache. Vomiting may occur during the episode. Drowsiness or sleep is a frequent event terminating the episode and serves as a hint to the proper diagnosis. A less common description is continuous or persistent headache as a seizural manifestation. If unassociated with variation of behavior or mentation deficit, this pattern may not be considered convulsive until electroencephalography indicates the probability.

A convulsive disorder manifested by sudden onset of localized headache with vomiting can so closely simulate a migrainous episode that clinical differentiation may be impossible. Even transient visual abnormalities may be described indicating further resemblance to migraine. Disturbances in sensorium and a period of sleep after the episode favor a seizural explanation, but these manifestations may not always be present. Electroencephalography and response to medication may ultimately be the only means of distinguishing one disorder from the other.

Epileptic cephalea is treated in the same fashion as other more overt convulsive disorders in children. Either diphenylhydantoin, in a dose of 4 mg. per kilogram per day or phenobarbital, 3 mg. per kilogram per day, is prescribed. It should be emphasized that this diagnosis should not be overutilized as an explanation for headache disorders in childhood. Isolated headaches representing the only manifestation of a convulsive disorder are a rare phenomenon and account for few headache problems in the pediatric age range. Before establishing this diagnosis, other causes of headaches should be excluded, the clinical history should be consistent, and the electroencephalogram compatible with a paroxysmal cerebral dysrhythmia. Response to anticonvulsant therapy might be added as another desired diagnostic criterion. In certain instances, the electroencephalogram is less than diagnostic, but a therapeutic trial with diphenylhydantoin may be attempted. Diagnosis should be deferred, however, and a beneficial response to therapy only signifies that the headache disorder may be a convulsive manifestation.

HEADACHES DUE TO LOW CEREBROSPINAL FLUID PRESSURE

Headaches may follow lumbar puncture; however, this complication appears less common in children than in young adults. Headache may be noted hours after the procedure but occasionally occurs only after a lag period of two or three days. The pain is usually generalized but with a prominent bifrontal component. The most outstanding characteristic of the postlumbar puncture headache is its occurrence with the patient in the upright position and with almost immediate cessation on lying down. The postural head pain may be associated with nausea, vomiting, vertigo, or lightheadedness. It usually persists for two or three days with gradual resolution. In rare cases, postlumbar puncture headache may persist for weeks or even months (Brown and Jones).

The postlumbar puncture headache syndrome is due to low cerebrospinal fluid pressure with traction on pain-sensitive intracranial structures when the head is held upright. Low pressure following lumbar puncture may result from leakage of fluid through a dural tear resulting from passage of the spinal needle (Ingvar). Dana postulated that the procedure inhibits secretory activity of the choroid plexus, thus decreasing cerebrospinal fluid formation.

Most cases of postlumbar puncture headache in children are successfully managed by restricting the child to the lying position for two or three days. In the more intractable case, one might try intramuscular papaverine given at six-hour intervals, attempting to increase cerebrospinal fluid production by choroid plexus vasodilatation. Carbon dioxide inhalation has also been suggested for the same purpose (Shenkin and Novack).

A state similar to the postlumbar puncture headache syndrome may result from a lumbar nerve sleeve tear following trauma (Nosik). Cerebrospinal fluid hypotensive headaches appear soon after the injury and result from fluid leakage into soft tissues in the low back area.

Spontaneous intracranial hypotension with persisting headaches in the upright position has been reported in childhood (Bell et al.). The disorder was first described by Schaltenbrand in 1938 and referred to as aliquorrhea. The syndrome may be of sudden or gradual onset with orthostatic headache the outstanding complaint. In addition to headache, the upright position may be associated with vomiting or vertigo. Mild neck rigidity is sometimes found on examination. Lying supine may produce relief as rapidly as occurs in the postlumbar puncture headache syndrome. The remarkable correlation of the head pain to body position suggests that traction on dural venous sinuses and tributary veins accounts for the headache.

Careful lumbar puncture is necessary for diagnosis of this uncommon syndrome. Pressure determination with the patient in the lateral recumbent position will be less than 40 mm. of water, if measurable at all. If no pressure can be recorded even though one has felt the needle penetrate the spinal dura, the patient should be slowly moved to the sitting position with the needle in place. The fluid will then rise up in the manometer if the needle is in the subarachnoid space. In patients with spinal fluid hypotension, the top of the fluid column will not reach the level of the foramen magnum as occurs in the normal person. Red blood cells may be found in the spinal fluid in this disorder. A mild increase in cerebrospinal fluid protein is also frequent.

In certain instances, small amounts of air in the cerebral ventricles have been demonstrated on x-ray soon after the diagnostic lumbar puncture. It has been postulated that, if the intraventricular pressure is lower than the atmospheric pressure at the time of the lumbar puncture, air may be aspirated through the needle, thereby equalizing the pressures.

The pathogenesis of spontaneous intracranial hypotension is unclear despite many proposed postulates. Schaltenbrand suggested a decrease or cessation of spinal fluid production resulting from a reversible disturbance in vasomotor function of the choroid plexus. The disorder must be rare at any age and especially so in children. Management is essentially the same as with postlumbar puncture headaches, although persisting symptoms might require the use of intravenous hypotonic saline in attempt to increase cerebrospinal fluid formation.

Symptomatic intracranial hypotension may occur following surgical evacuation of a subdural hematoma and after other neurosurgical procedures. Persistence of postoperative drowsiness or lethargy might suggest this complication, which appears to be related to diminished cerebral blood flow in some cases (Shenkin). An intracranial cerebrospinal fluid hypotensive syndrome with postural headaches may also occur after head trauma (Leriche). While these possibilities should be kept in mind in children with headaches after surgery or trauma, intracranial infection or cerebral edema secondary to hyponatremia, remain more likely explanations under these circumstances.

HEADACHES AND SYSTEMIC DISEASE

In eliciting the history from patients with a wide variety of systemic diseases one not infrequently finds that headache preceded other more specific manifestations usually regarded as more specific for the disorder in question. For example, children with Henoch-Schönlein anaphylactoid purpura may experience generalized, nondescript headache and anorexia for a few days before other abnormalities appear. One may be baffled if the child is examined at this time, because no objective findings will be present. Within hours or days, the appearance of arthritis, soft tissue swelling, melena with abdominal pain, and the characteristic urticarial or purpuric eruption with normal platelet count makes the diagnosis clear.

Hypertension in children may cause recurrent headaches, often throbbing and with a tendency to be most prominent during the morning hours. Physical examination in children with headache complaints should never be considered complete until an accurate blood pressure with the proper sized cuff has been determined. If hypertension is identified, the history must be extended to include information concerning the family history of high blood pressure, presence of nerve deafness in the family, or evidence of preexistent renal disease in the patient. One should also inquire whether the child has ever had a previous episode with a transient peripheral facial paralysis. Facial palsy may be a manifestation of hypertension in childhood (Lloyd et al.), and if present in the history, its date of occurrence may help establish an approximate duration of the elevated blood pressure.

Hypertension in children is never considered to be essential in type until an exhaustive search has been made to identify the underlying cause. Renal disease ranks as the leading cause followed by a variety of conditions, including coarctation of the aorta, Cushing's syndrome, pheochromocytoma, and hyperaldosteronism. Severe headaches, stupor, and convulsions are common manifestations of hypertensive encephalopathy in children with acute glomerulonephritis.

Several types of intoxication may produce headache; perhaps best known is that due to carbon monoxide exposure. Headache, nausea, and vertigo are early manifestations of carbon monoxide inhalation followed by stupor, coma, and convulsions if the duration of exposure and concentration of the gas is sufficiently great. Children sleeping in poorly ventilated rooms with defective gas heaters may waken with headache and nausea each morning with symptoms relieved by going outside into the fresh air.

Rheumatoid arthritis in childhood may be associated with headaches resulting from a variety of circumstances. Bitemporal vasodilatation headaches may accompany temperature spikes. Involvement of the upper cervical spine with apophysial joint erosion, atlantoaxial subluxation, or subluxation of other cervical vertebrae may produce severe occipital and upper cervical pain. Iridocyclitis may cause local occular pain or tension, bitemporal headache.

Headaches may occur in patients with hyperparathyroidism or other conditions with chronic hypercalcemia. Hypothyroidism has been associated with chronic headaches, although this appears to be more common in adults than children. Hypoglycemia also may result in headache problems in youngsters.

REFERENCES

Bell, W. E., Joynt, R. J., and Sahs, A. L.: Low spinal fluid pressure syndromes. *Neurology*, **10**:512–521, 1960.

Bickerstaff, E. R.: Basilar artery migraine. *Lancet*, **1**:15–17, 1961.

Bille, B.: Migraine in school children. *Acta Paediat.*, Suppl. 136, pp. 1–151, 1962.

Brown, B. A., and Jones, O. W., Jr.: Prolonged headache following spinal puncture. *J. Neurosurg.*, **19**:349–350, 1962.

Burke, E. C., and Peters, G. A.: Migraine in childhood. *Amer. J. Dis. Child.*, **92**:330–336, 1956.

Chapman, L. F., Ramos, A. O., Goodell, H., Silverman, G., and Woolf, H. G.: A humoral agent implicated in vascular headaches of the migraine type. *Arch. Neurol.*, **3**:223–229, 1960.

Conner, R. C. R.: Complicated migraine. *Lancet*, **2**:1072–1075, 1962.

Dalessio, D. J.: On migraine headache: Serotonin and serotonin antagonism. *J.A.M.A.*, **181**:318–321, 1962.

Dana, C. L.: Puncture headache. *J.A.M.A.*, **68**:1017, 1917.

Fenichel, G. M., and Battiata, S.: Thrombophlebitis secondary to methysergide maleate therapy. *J. Pediat.*, **68**:632–634, 1966.

Friedman, A., Harter, D. H., and Merritt, H. H.: Ophthalmoplegic migraine. *Arch. Neurol.*, **7**:320–327, 1962.

Friedman, A. P., and Mikropoulos, H. E.: Cluster headaches. *Neurology*, **8**:653–663, 1958.

Gascon, G., and Barlow, C.: Juvenile migraine, presenting as an acute confusional state. *Pediatrics*, **45**:628–635, 1970.

Gradenigo, G.: Über circumscripe leptomeningitis mit spinalen symptomen und über paralysis des N. abducens ototischen ursprungs. *Arch. f. Ohrenh.*, **51**:255–270, 1904.

Graham, J. R., Suby, H. I., LeCompte, P. R., and Sadowsky, N. L.: Fibrotic disorders associated with methysergide therapy for headache. *New Eng. J. Med.*, **274**:359–368, 1966.

Halpern, L., and Bental, E.: Epileptic cephalea. *Neurology*, **8**:615–620, 1958.

Hinrichs, W. L., and Keith, H. M.: Migraine in childhood. A follow-up report. *Mayo Clin. Proc.*, **40**:593–596, 1965.

Holguin, J., and Fenichel, G.: Migraine. *J. Pediat.*, **70**:290–297, 1967.

Hunt, W. E., Meagher, J. N., LeFever, H. E., and Zeman, W.: Painful ophthalmoplegia. *Neurology*, **11**:56–62, 1961.

Ingvar, S.: On the danger of leakage of the cerebrospinal fluid after lumbar puncture. *Acta Med. Scandinav.*, **58**:67–101, 1923.

Leriche, R.: De l'hypotension du liquide céphalorachidien dans certaines fractures de la base du crane et de son traitement par l'injection de serum sous la peau. *Lyon chir.*, **17**:638–640, 1920.

Livingston, S., and Escala, P.: Headaches and epilepsy in children. In: *Headaches in Children.* Ed. by Friedman and Harms. Springfield, Ill., Charles C Thomas, 1967.

Lloyd, A. V. C., Jewitt, D. E., and Still, J. D. L.: Facial paralysis in children with hypertension. *Arch. Dis. Childh.*, **41**:292–294, 1966.

Nosik, W. A.: Intracranial hypotension secondary to lumbar nerve sleeve tear, *J.A.M.A.*, **157**:1110–1111, 1955.

Rosenbaum, H. E.: Familial hemiplegic migraine. *Neurology*, **10**:164–170, 1960.

Schaltenbrand, G.: Neuere anschaugen zur pathophysiologie der liguorzirkulation. *Zentralbl. Neurochir.*, **3**:290–300, 1938.

Schaltenbrand, G.: Normal and pathological physiology of the cerebrospinal fluid circulation. *Lancet*, **1**:805–808, 1953.

Shenkin, H.: The cerebral circulation in postoperative intracranial hypotension. *J. Neurosurg.*, **10**:48–51, 1953.

Shenkin, H. A., and Novack, P.: Clinical implications of recent studies on cerebral circulation of man. *Arch. Neurol. & Psychiat.*, **71**:148–159, 1954.

Stevens, H.: Melkersson's syndrome. *Neurology*, **15**:263–266, 1965.

van Pelt, W., and Andermann, F.: On the early onset of ophthalmoplegic migraine. *Amer. J. Dis. Child.*, **107**:628–631, 1964.

Walsh, J. P., and O'Doherty, D. S.: A possible explanation of the mechanism of ophthalmoplegic migraine. *Neurology*, **10**:1079–1084, 1960.

Whitehouse, D., Pappas, J. A. Escala, P. H., and Livingston, S.: Electroencephalographic changes in children with migraine. *New Eng. J. Med.*, **276**:23–27, 1967.

Wolff, H. G.: Headache and other head pain. Ed. 2, New York, Oxford University Press, 1963.

Wolff, H. G., Tunis, M. M., and Goodell, H.: Studies on headache. Evidence of tissue damage and changes in pain sensitivity in subjects with vascular headaches of the migraine type. *Arch. Int. Med.*, **92**:478–484, 1953.

Chapter Three

LUMBAR PUNCTURE WITH INCREASED INTRACRANIAL PRESSURE

The introduction of lumbar puncture into clinical medicine by Quincke in 1891 provided an important diagnostic aid that has proven to be remarkably safe if properly used and cautiously performed. Serious adverse effects of this procedure are largely related to its use with high-grade increase in intracranial pressure or the injudicious application of the Queckenstedt test in circumstances in which it is contraindicated.

Whether or not to perform a lumbar puncture when one suspects a syndrome associated with increased intracranial pressure must be determined by the circumstances surrounding each situation. In certain instances, not only is lumbar puncture contraindicated because of the hazard of tentorial or tonsillar herniation, but also little useful information will be made available by its performance. For example, if one suspects an acute epidural hematoma on the basis of the clinical data, the danger of lumbar puncture far outweighs any possible benefit from the procedure. When this diagnosis has been made clinically, it is extremely doubtful that management of the patient would be altered regardless of the findings, were a lumbar puncture done. Likewise, if the clinical diagnosis is that of a posterior fossa tumor in a child, the information obtained from the lumbar puncture does not ordinarily justify exposing the child to the potential hazard of the procedure.

There are other situations in which lumbar puncture is necessarily performed, despite evidence of increased intracranial pressure. A reasonable possibility of the presence of a central nervous system infection requires the accomplishment of the examination. Tuberculous meningitis and cryptococcal meningoencephalitis cause a multiplicity of abnormal neurologic signs, often including papilledema. If such disorders are seriously considered in the differential diagnosis, one must examine the cerebrospinal fluid regardless of the presence of clinical evidence of increased pressure. Subarachnoid hemorrhage, if suspected from the history and physical findings, must be confirmed or excluded by careful lumbar puncture.

In summary, the decision to do a lumbar puncture in the presence of increased intracranial pressure must be based on several factors. It should not be done when the diagnosis is reasonably definite and when management will not be altered regardless of the findings on lumbar puncture. The procedure is indicated, despite certain potential hazards, when the diagnosis is unclear and when infection or subarachnoid hemorrhage is a likely consideration.

Precautions

Several precautions should be taken during the performance of a lumbar puncture, not only to reduce the danger, but also to allow interpretation of the recorded opening pressure to be meaningful. The less the pain produced by insertion of the needle, the more reliable is the opening pressure. After the needle has penetrated the lumbar subarachnoid space, one should advise the child that the procedure is over and further discomfort will not occur. Immediately after removing the stylet, the manometer is attached to the spinal needle. An effort should be made to avoid loss of more than a few drops of fluid while the manometer is being attached. Because most spinal taps are done with the child lying on one side, it is in this position that the pressure is recorded.

For the pressure to be reliable, the needle tip must be cleanly within the subarachnoid space. This is usually evident by visible spontaneous pulsations at the top of the fluid column in the manometer with the child lying quietly. If the legs are strongly flexed and encrouch on the abdomen, the pressure may be spuriously high. Before the opening pressure is recorded, the legs should be slowly and gently extended at the hips, removing any pressure upon the abdomen. The child's head should be in a neutral position, because any twisting or distortion of the neck may impede venous drainage from the head, falsely elevating the pressure.

Thus, before the opening pressure is determined, one should delay for a short period of time, allowing the child to relax and correcting any postural features that might cause pressure on the neck vessels or abdomen. With a tense or fearful child, simply waiting for three to five minutes after the insertion of the needle and entrance of the subarachnoid space may allow the pressure to drop as much as 100 mm. of water. The infant is not likely to stop crying after the needle is introduced into the subarachnoid space. However, with the needle in place, providing the baby with a rubber nipple to suck or a bottle with a small amount of glucose water may permit an accurate pressure measurement.

Interpretation of the Results

After the opening pressure is recorded, fluid specimens should be obtained for the appropriate studies. When the spinal fluid is bloody, it is important to distinguish whether it was induced by the penetration of the needle or was present before the tap was performed. In the newborn or small infant, the needle may enter the venous plexus on the posterior surface of the vertebral body. Venous blood exudes from the needle hub, indicating the needle tip is not within the lumbar subarachnoid space. In the older child, it is more frequent that one obtains spinal fluid mixed with blood, which may result either from trauma of the procedure or from preexistent subarachnoid bleeding. If fluid is collected sequentially in each of three or four tubes, the fluid will remain equally bloody if due to preexistent bleeding but will usually become progressively clearer if due to needle-induced trauma.

One tube should be centrifuged and the supernatant observed. Xanthochromia of the supernatant fluid adds further evidence of preceding subarachnoid bleeding, whereas crystal clear supernatant fluid indicates that the bleeding is fresh. Microscopic examination of the fluid immediately after it is obtained shows marked crenation of the red cells if they have been present in the fluid for a few hours.

If the opening pressure is abnormally high, the fluid should be obtained slowly, permitting only a gradual drip by retaining the stylet partially within the shaft of the needle. The fluid should not be allowed to spurt out under great pressure, because sudden changes in pressure relationships may be dangerous. An estimate should be made of the quantity of fluid removed and the final or closing pressure recorded before the needle is withdrawn.

The opening pressure is occasionally elevated when the tap is done below the level of a complete spinal block. This is the primary instance in which both opening and closing pressures plus the amount of fluid removed are most valuable for interpretation. While the opening pressure may be high when obtained below the level of a spinal block, removal of even a small amount of fluid results in a marked and precipitous decrease in the pressure. This decrease may be so marked that the closing pressure may be so low that it is unrecordable.

It is clinical suspicion of a spinal block that indicates the advisability of doing a Queckenstedt test at the time of the lumbar puncture. Jugular vein compression results in no rise in the fluid level in the manometer in the presence of a complete spinal block. The obstruction must be virtually complete, however, before no rise will occur with jugular compression. Poppen and Hurxthal demonstrated that if an opening as large as the bore of the lumbar puncture needle at the level of a tumor remains in the spinal canal, a normal rise with jugular compression is expected, assuming the viscosity of the fluid remains constant. A rapid and significant rise and fall is noted in persons without a spinal block if the needle tip is adequately placed in the subarachnoid space.

In clinical practice, there is almost no instance in which the Queckenstedt test is useful with disease above the level of the foramen magnum. In the presence of intracranial disease with increased pressure, jugular vein compression is distinctly hazardous, because the pressure changes induced by this maneuver may precipitate tentorial or tonsillar herniation and death. The main indication for performing a Queckenstedt test is evidence of a spinal block.

The only obvious exception to the lack of value of jugular compression with lumbar puncture in intracranial disease is in the presence of a unilateral transverse sinus thrombosis. This examination is called the Tobey-Ayer test and consists of a normal increase of pressure on jugular compression on the normal side but no increase on compression of the jugular vein on the side with the transverse sinus obstruction. The procedure is not invariably reliable, however, because of the anatomic variations of venous drainage on the two sides of the skull. Because there are better ways to establish this diagnosis and because of the potential danger if the diagnosis is in error, considerable caution is in order regarding application of this test.

The normal cerebrospinal fluid pressure is generally regarded as not exceeding 180 mm. of water with the patient lying in the lateral recumbent position. One assumes that the patient is relaxed and no external pressure is being exerted upon the abdomen or neck vessels. Most accept an opening pressure of 180 to 200 mm. of water as suggestive and over 200 mm. of water as indicative of increased intracranial pressure. When the spinal tap is performed with the patient in the sitting position, these values are no longer valid. In this position, the pressure more commonly increases to a level approximating the level of the foramen magnum; thus the reading on the manometer, if normal, is more dependent on the length of the patient's torso.

The concept of "normal" spinal fluid pressure in regard to the pressure's effect on the ventricular walls appears to be in need of revision in view of recent literature. Studies have shown that the effect of pressure on the ventricular wall is not related to the degree of pressure alone, but also is dependent on the surface area of the ventricles and probably other factors. Adams et al. have pointed out that the force on the walls of a fluid-filled container is equal to the product of pressure and surface area over which the pressure is exerted. Thus, with markedly enlarged ventricles, a recorded spinal fluid pressure one ordinarily would consider normal might be sufficient to produce progressive ventricular enlargement by its damaging effect on the surrounding brain.

REFERENCES

Adams, R. D., Fisher, C. M., Hakim, S., Ojemann, R. G., and Sweet, W. H.: Symptomatic occult, hydrocephalus with "normal" cerebrospinal-fluid pressure. *New Eng. J. Med.*, **273**:117–126, 1965.

Poppen, J. L. and Hurxthal, L. M.: Normal cerebrospinal fluid dynamics in spinal cord tumor suspects. *J.A.M.A.*, **103**:391–393, 1934.

Quincke, H.: Die lumbalpunktion des hydrocephalus. *Berl. Klin. Wschr.*, **28**:929, 965, 1891.

Chapter Four

ROENTGENOGRAPHIC SIGNS OF INCREASED INTRACRANIAL PRESSURE

Roentgenographic evidence of increased intracranial pressure in part depends on the age of the patient and how long the elevated pressure has existed. The degree of increase in pressure is an additional factor that influences the roentgen signs. In some instances, intracranial pressure may be markedly increased with no obvious abnormality evident on skull x-ray. Before it is decided that no such evidence is present, films of technically good quality with proper alignment of the patient's head in the various positions must be obtained. When technically poor x-rays are viewed, the study should be repeated before a final interpretation is made. Simply obtaining x-rays is insufficient if the quality does not permit analysis.

Suture Spread

In the newborn infant, roentgen signs of increased pressure are less reliable than signs evident on observation and palpation of the head. The bony skull sutures are normally unopposed at this time, and differentiation of the normal state from minimal or mild abnormal suture spread on x-ray is extremely difficult. One may see x-ray evidence of bulging of the soft tissues comprising the anterior fontanel in young infants; however, this is better judged clinically than radiographically. In older infants and young children, roentgen evidence of abnormal suture spread is helpful in establishing the diagnosis of increased intracranial pressure.

Although true lateral views of the skull are important for many purposes, films taken with slight oblique rotation of the head may be valuable when one is assessing the possibility of suture spread. True lateral projections cause the two coronal sutures to be overlapped, which can give the false appearance of mild suture separation. With rotation, each coronal suture can be separately visualized, allowing a more accurate interpretation of the degree of apposition or separation. The coronal and sagittal sutures tend to widen first with increasing intracranial pressure, and in more severe cases, the lambdoidal and squamosal sutures also become separated (Fig. 4-1).

In children with the Dandy-Walker syndrome, the reverse may be true, because the lambdoidal sutures are often disproportionately separated as compared with the others. In young infants with advanced hydrocephalus, roentgen demonstration of suture diastasis becomes less obvious as the head progressively enlarges because of associated thinning of the skull generally. Rarefaction of the bones of the skull in this instance results in less striking contrast between bone and cartilage with less clear-cut evidence of suture spread on x-ray.

Skull suture diastasis secondary to in-

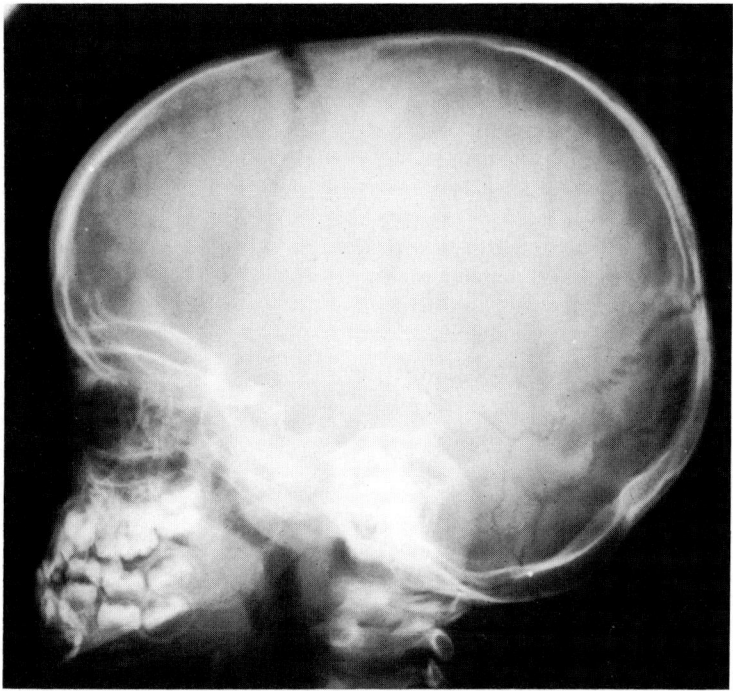

Figure 4-1. Suture spread of acute type due to increased intracranial pressure secondary to multiple cerebral emboli in a 19-month-old child. Coronal sutures are spread more than the lambdoidal sutures, and the sella turcica remains normal.

creased intracranial pressure is not uncommonly seen in children up to 10 years of age. In rare cases, suture spread has been described in persons as old as 16 years (Taveras and Wood). Suture spread beyond this age is most often the result of traumatic diastasis. Children 10 to 15 years of age with delayed skeletal maturation secondary to pituitary insufficiency not uncommonly exhibit suture spread with conditions associated with increased intracranial pressure.

Abnormal suture spread in infants may develop rapidly or may be noted over a few days or a week or so. If one suspects a syndrome with increased pressure in the infant but the initial skull films are normal, repeat films seven to ten days later may show definite suture separation. This may be of particular value in the older infant with closed fontanels who is suspected of harboring a recently acquired subdural hematoma or effusion. Observing such a child in this fashion would be acceptable only if the child is not deteriorating or is not lethargic or stuporous.

Despite the importance of cranial suture spread indicating evidence of increased pressure, it must be emphasized that there are other possible causes of abnormal cranial suture spread on x-ray. Deprived and malnourished children may develop widening of the cranial sutures after correction of the nutritional inadequacies and during catch-up growth (Capitanio and Kirkpatrick, DeLevie and Nogrady). Symptoms and signs of increased intracranial pressure are not observed and the sutures eventually become normally opposed.

In infants with hypophosphatasia, one sees an absence of radiographically demonstrable bone over large segments of the skull. This may be falsely interpreted as evidence of extreme suture separation. The radiolucent areas represent uncalcified osteoid. With subsequent calcification, the syndrome of premature craniosynosis develops. In addition to the skeletal abnormalities, hypophosphatasia is characterized by low levels of serum alkaline phosphatase and the presence of phosphoethanolamine in the urine.

Pycnodysostosis is a generalized bone disease with dysplastic skull abnormalities resulting in a persistently open anterior fontanel and separated sutures (Elmore). These findings persist even into adulthood. Head enlargement, characteristic of this disorder, and apparent suture spread on x-ray might easily lead one to an erroneous diagnosis of hydrocephalus or subdural hematoma. In addition to dysplasia of the skull, other features of pycnodysostosis include short stature, generalized skeletal osteopetrosis with a tendency to recurrent fractures, a double row of teeth, and partial or total aplasia of the terminal phalanges.

Fontanel closure and normal approximation of cranial sutures may also be delayed in cleidocranial dysostosis. Numerous wormian bones arising from accessory ossification centers are usually present in the occipital region in this disorder. The diagnosis is confirmed by chest x-ray revealing bilateral absence or hypoplasia of the clavicles. Cretinism is another disorder with delayed maturation of the skull as well as other bony structures. Retardation of ossification of the membranous portion of the skull delays closure of the fontanels and cranial sutures.

Convolutional Markings

More difficult to interpret and subject to greater variation in childhood are the convolutional or digital markings of the inner table of the skull. Such markings on the skull may be prominent in normal youngsters between four and eight years of age, but they are unusual under 2 years of age (Fig. 4-2). They may also be seen normally in older children but with less frequency than in the age group described. This pattern of convolutional markings on skull x-ray is markedly different from that of craniolacunia, or lückenschädel, seen in the newborn and young infant with meningomyelocoele (Fig. 4-3). Craniolacunia is believed to be an anomaly of skull bone development and probably has no direct relation to the underlying cerebral hemispheres.

Although prominent digital markings on skull x-rays are not infrequently seen in normal children, it is also accepted that they may develop secondary to chronically increased intracranial pressure. Therefore, the digital pattern alone is not usually diagnostic of increased pressure. The finding of marked digital impressions on skull x-ray in a child warrants a search for other clinical and roentgen manifestations of increased pressure. When other evidence of abnormal pressure elevation is found, it can then be assumed that the increased digital markings probably are a reflection of increased pressure.

If the syndrome resulting in increased pressure can be surgically relieved, one often sees a regression or even a disappearance of the digital markings a few months later (Fig. 4-4). Occasionally, the degree of digital mark-

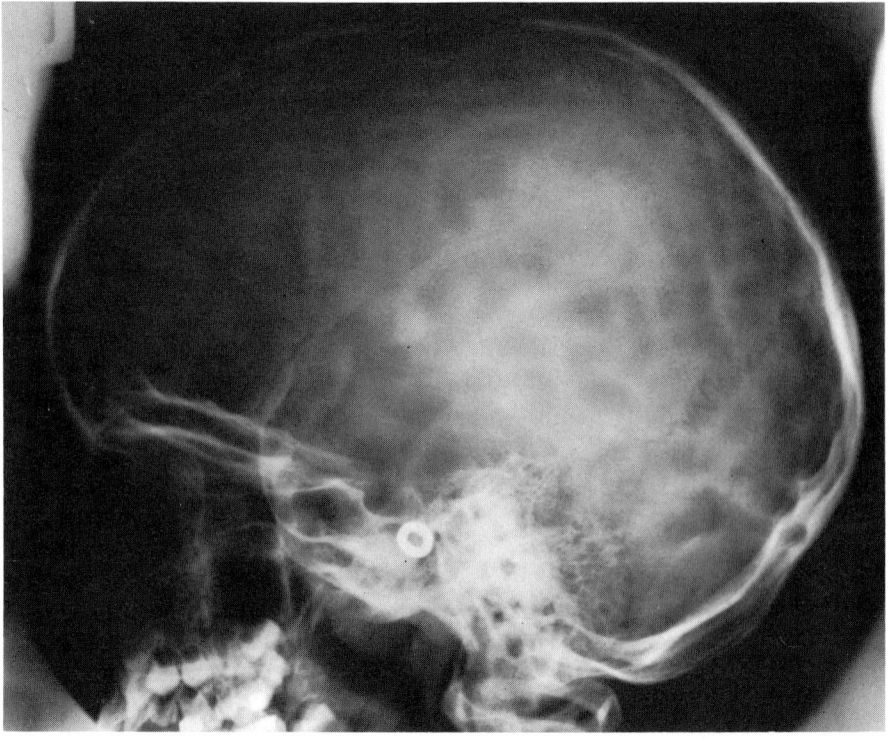

Figure 4-2. Lateral skull x-ray of a normal six-year-old child. Prominent convolutional markings with intact sella turcica and without suture spread is often seen in normal children in this age group.

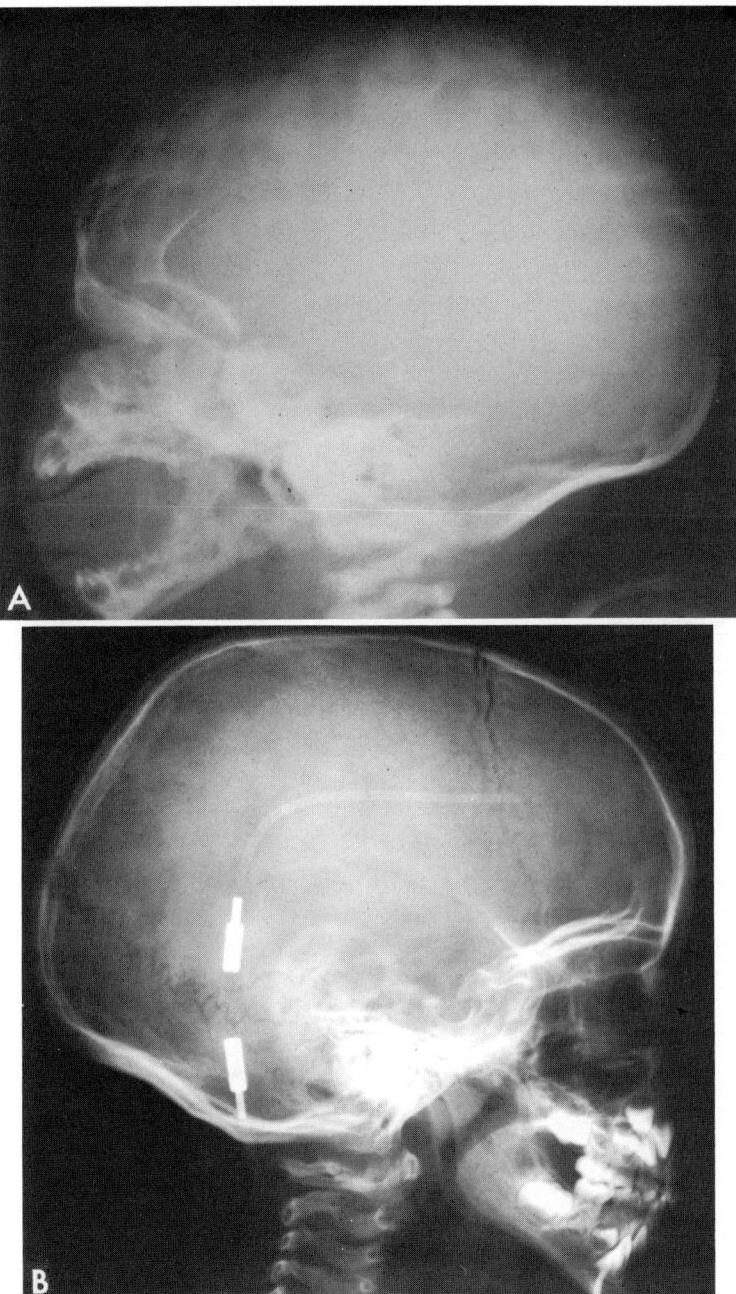

Figure 4–3. Craniolacunia (lückenschädel). *A*, Skull x-ray of a neonate with a meningomyelocoele and hydrocephalus. Honeycombed pattern, or craniolacunia, is probably a defect of membranous bone formation and is to be differentiated from the increased digital markings observed in older children. *B*, Same patient at four years of age. The skull no longer has an abnormal appearance. A ventriculoatrial shunt with valve mechanism is evident.

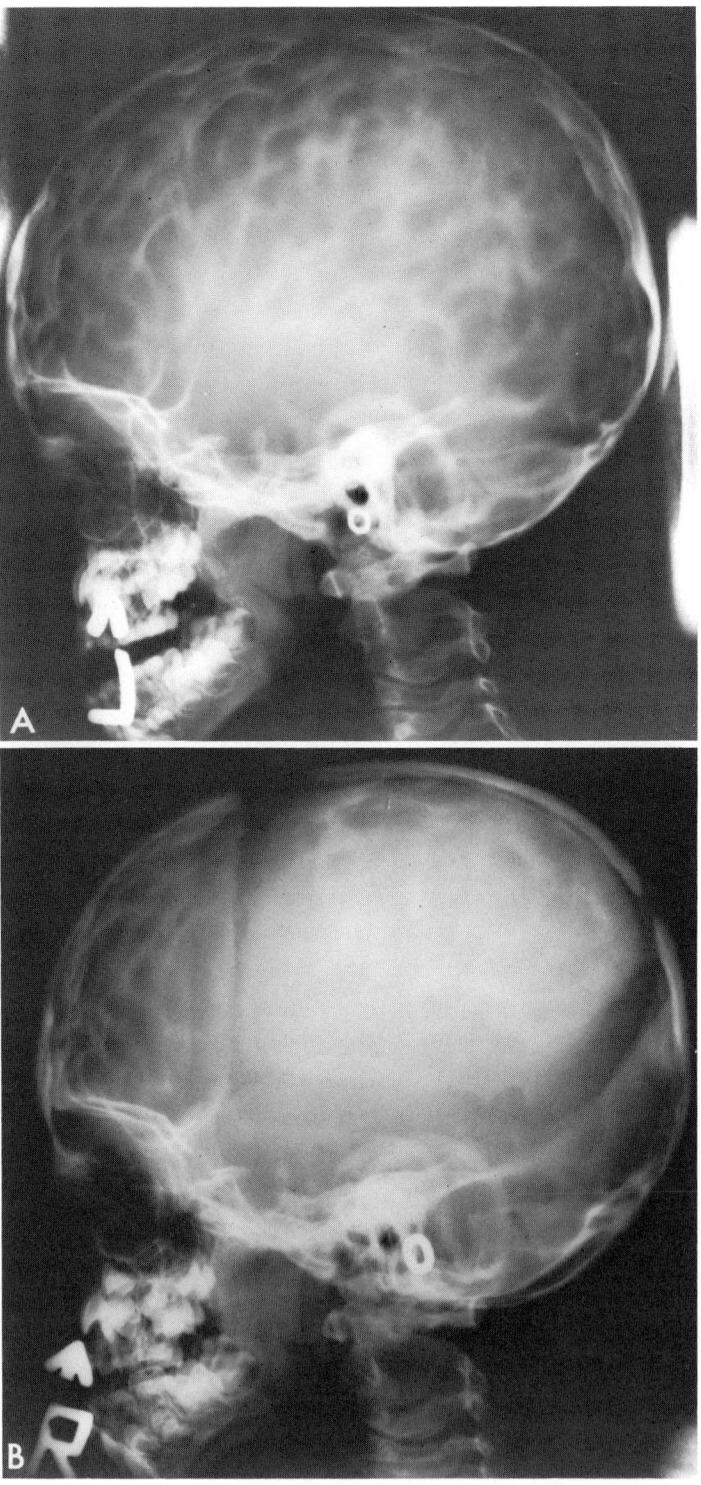

Figure 4–4. Increased convolutional markings secondary to chronic increase in intracranial pressure. *A*, Preoperative skull x-ray of a child with generalized craniosynostosis. The degree of the digital impressions ("beaten silver") and the depression of the floor of the sella turcica indicate long-standing increase in pressure. *B*, Regression of convolutional markings five months after decompression by linear craniectomies.

ings and the thinness of the bones of the skull are so advanced that there is little doubt that these findings are due to long-standing increased pressure. In children, this may be seen with generalized craniosynostosis, aqueductal occlusion, or a posterior fossa tumor. In such cases, other clinical or roentgen abnormalities are usually readily evident.

Alterations of the Sella Turcica

Roentgen changes of the sella turcica including those of the dorsum sella and clinoid processes are valuable indicators of chronic intracranial pressure changes in children, as in adults. Abnormalities that may occur include erosion of the interior of the sella with deepening of the floor into the sphenoid sinus, erosion of the anterior surface of the dorsum sella, and thinning and atrophy of the posterior clinoid processes (Fig. 4-5). Eventually, the posterior clinoid processes may become so attenuated that they are unrecognizable on the lateral skull film. If the process continues unabated, similar atrophic changes will occur in the anterior clinoid processes. In most instances, regressive changes occur in the posterior clinoid processes and dorsum sella before appreciable alterations are noted in the floor of the sella.

Atrophic changes of the anterior clinoid processes in the absence of abnormalities of the posterior clinoid processes or dorsum sella usually suggest local erosion due to a tumor or aneurysm in the immediate vicinity (Taveras and Wood). These destructive changes of the sphenoid bone due to increased intracranial pressure are much more often seen in older children than in infants. The rapid spread of sutures, which occurs in the infant age group, tends to retard atrophic changes in and around the sella.

Pituitary adenomas, rare in childhood, produce changes in the sella that are usually distinguishable from those due to chronic increase in intracranial pressure. The sella harboring a pituitary adenoma usually undergoes a generalized ballooning, with the enlargement in volume being proportionately greater than the destructive effect on the surrounding bony structure. Local le-

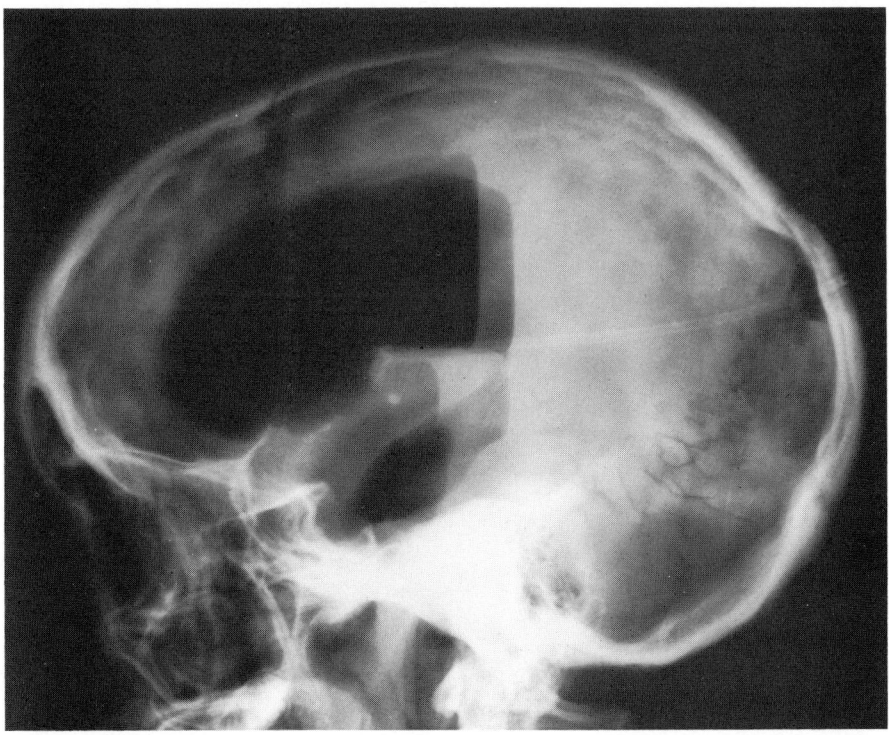

Figure 4-5. Ventriculogram in a 16-year-old girl with intraventricular obstructive hydrocephalus secondary to a cerebellar neoplasm. Alterations in the sella turcica due to chronically increased intracranial pressure include enlargement of the sella, depression of its floor into the sphenoid sinus, and marked attenuation of the posterior clinoid processes. Note the extension of the enlarged anterior third ventricle into the chiasmatic region.

sions above the sella, such as the craniopharyngioma, may result in changes of the sella that are more difficult to distinguish from those secondary to generalized increase in intracranial pressure. Other clinical signs, the presence of calcification within the tumor, or perhaps ventriculography will suffice for localization of the primary site of the disorder.

With long-standing elevation of intracranial pressure due to posterior fossa obstructive lesions, erosion of the clivus may occur, producing an apparent thinning and curvilinear distortion of the clivus on lateral skull x-rays. Chronic increase in pressure may also result in decalcification of the petrous tips of the temporal bones.

REFERENCES

Capitanio, M. A., and Kirkpatrick, J. A.: Widening of the cranial sutures. A roentgen observation during periods of accelerated growth in patients treated for deprivation dwarfism. *Radiology,* **92**:53–59, 1969.

DeLevie, M., and Nogrady, M. B.: Rapid brain growth upon restoration of adequate nutrition causing false radiologic evidence of increased intracranial pressure. *J. Pediat.,* **76**:523–528, 1970.

Elmore, S. M.: Pycnodysostosis. A review. *J. Bone and Joint Surg.,* **49**-A:153–162, 1967.

Taveras, J. M., and Wood, E. H.: *Diagnostic Neuroradiology.* Baltimore, The Williams and Wilkins Company, 1964.

Chapter Five

TRANSTENTORIAL AND CEREBELLAR HERNIATIONS

A constant hazard in the presence of increased intracranial pressure is tentorial or cerebellar tonsillar herniation resulting in midbrain or medullary compression. It is the possibility of such internal herniations with an abrupt change in pressure relationships that warrants caution regarding lumbar puncture in the presence of increased intracranial pressure. Herniations of cerebral or cerebellar tissue may occur in acute, fulminating fashion, leading to necrosis of the herniated tissue and compression of vital structures producing distinctive clinical signs. In other patients, slowly progressive increase in intracranial pressure is associated with chronic herniations that remain asymptomatic but are capable of decompensation at any time.

TRANSTENTORIAL HERNIATIONS

In 1920, Adolf Meyer demonstrated the occurrence of cerebral herniation into the tentorial incisura in patients with increased intracranial pressure. Tentorial herniations have been classified as anterior, posterior, and complete (Azambuja et al.). Such herniations may be either unilateral or bilateral, in part depending on the type and location of the causative cerebral hemisphere lesion. In addition to the location of the herniated tissue, the rapidity of production of the herniation is important in regard to the clinical signs that result.

With anterior herniations, the uncus and hippocampal gyrus descend through the tentorial opening and may be associated with downward displacement of the brain stem. With progressive herniation of tissue of the medial temporal lobe, distortion of structures below the tentorium results in a variety of neurologic deficits. Pressure on the displaced uncus and hippocampus by the tentorial edge results in grooving of the undersurface of these structures. Eventual hemorrhagic necrosis of the herniated structures may occur.

Angulation of the homolateral oculomotor nerve across the petroclinoid ligament or against the posterior cerebral artery may result in varying degrees of third nerve paralysis (Fig. 5-1). The pupil on the involved side often becomes dilated before other deficits of oculomotor function become evident. With large herniations, the posterior cerebral artery may be compressed upon the sharp tentorial edge, producing occipital lobe infarction (Fig. 5-2). This may be either unilateral or bilateral and causes significant visual field defects noted on examination.

Herniations through the tentorial opening produce a variety of long-tract signs depending on the site of compression. The cerebral peduncle may be compressed on the side of the herniation, resulting in a contralateral hemiparesis. In other instances, the opposite cerebral peduncle may be pressed against the

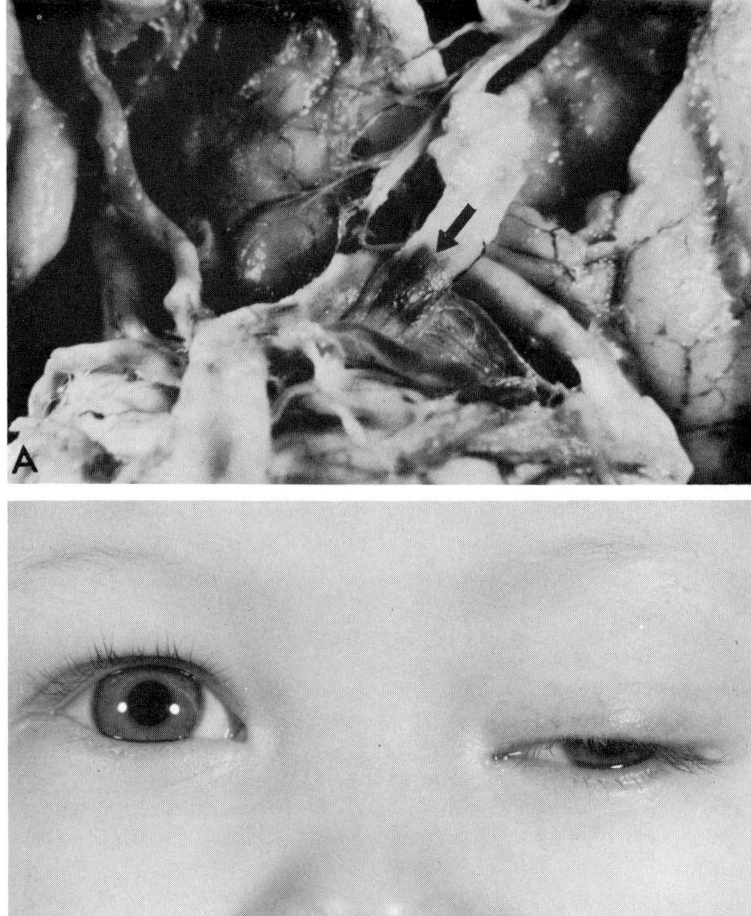

Figure 5–1. *A*, Transtentorial herniation resulting in hemorrhagic changes in the oculomotor nerve (arrow) from compression. Third nerve compression occurs on the side of the uncal herniation and results in homolateral pupillary dilatation with loss of the light response and drooping of the eyelid. This is followed by weakness of the extraocular muscles innervated by the oculomotor nerve. *B*, Child with left oculomotor paralysis secondary to transtentorial herniation. In addition to ptosis and pupillary dilatation (not seen), the left eye is deviated slightly laterally and inferiorly due to retained function of the lateral rectus (abducens nerve) and the superior oblique muscles (trochlear nerve).

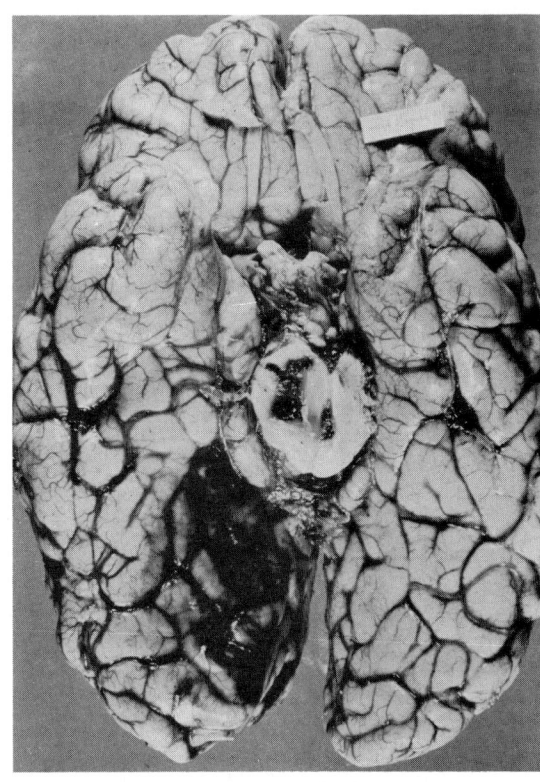

Figure 5–2. Transtentorial temporal lobe herniation secondary to increased intracranial pressure. Medial temporal lobe structures on the right side have herniated beneath the tentorium, compressing the brain stem and displacing it to the opposite side. Note the secondary midbrain hemorrhages and the necrosis of the peduncle on the left side. Compression of the right posterior cerebral artery against the edge of the tentorium has resulted in hemorrhagic infarction of the medial surface of the right occipital lobe.

tentorium, producing a hemiparesis ipsilateral to the side of the herniation (Kernohan and Woltman). The resulting groove in the peduncle opposite to the side with the herniation has been referred to as "Kernohan's notch" (Fig. 5-3). Further compression of the midbrain results in obstruction of the aqueduct. This factor further aggravates increased pressure above the tentorium, producing a vicious cycle with each event tending to complicate and accelerate the total problem. With progressive distortion of the brain

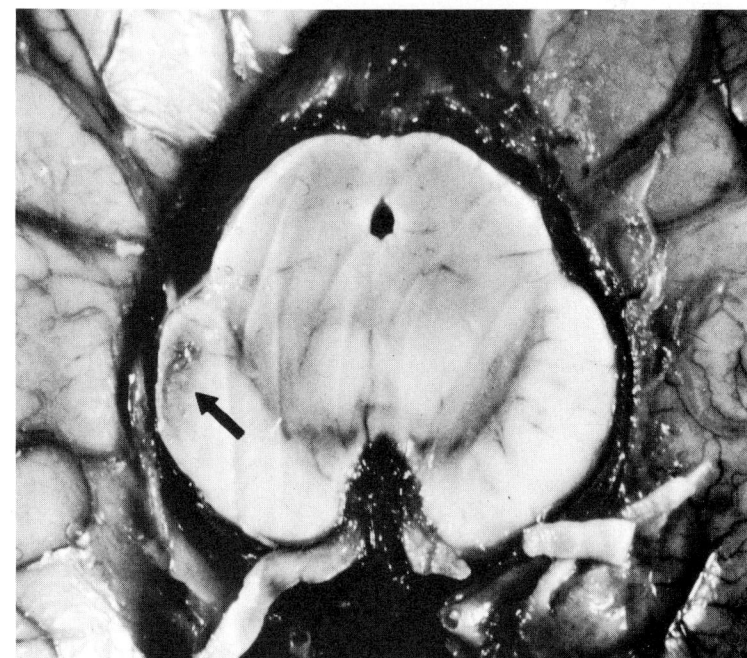

Figure 5–3. Transtentorial herniation on the right side has displaced the midbrain, resulting in compression of the *left* cerebral peduncle against the tentorial edge. Grooving and subsequent necrosis of the peduncle (arrow) opposite to the side of the herniation is referred to as "Kernohan's notch." This may result in a spastic hemiparesis on the *same* side as the tentorial herniation and thus may result in misleading localizing clinical signs.

stem, disturbances of responsiveness become more profound and signs of decerebration emerge. Midbrain hemorrhage and death soon follow if the process cannot be relieved.

Symmetrical movement of both hemispheres toward the tentorial incisura may result in posterior tentorial herniations. The posterior temporo-occipital herniation results in side-to-side compression of the dorsal half of the midbrain, producing a pear-shaped elongation of the upper part of the brain stem. Tectal compression may cause paralysis of upward gaze in addition to bilateral pupillary abnormalities. The downward displacement of the brain stem associated with this and other tentorial herniations may cause angulation of the pituitary stalk across the clivus. Pituitary necrosis and diabetes insipidus may be explainable on this basis (Johnson and Yates).

Many of the clinical signs observed in association with tentorial herniations are due to direct compression of structures by the impacted tissue or due to angulation of nerves or arteries against normal structures in the area. The most life-threatening aspects of these complications of increased intracranial pressure include the various possible distortions of the brain stem in addition to midbrain and pontine tegmental hemorrhages (Fig. 5-4).

Many postulates have been presented to explain the pathogenesis of these secondary brain stem hemorrhages. Scheinker supported the view that midbrain and pontine hemorrhages in this condition are of venous origin. Convincing studies by Johnson and Yates, however, have strongly implicated an arterial source for these devastating lesions. These authors felt that one factor important for the production of midbrain hemorrhages due to increased supratentorial pressure is the resultant caudal displacement of the brain stem. Many of the arterial branches passing from the basilar artery to supply the midbrain tegmentum enter at right angles to the axis of the brain stem. The superior end of the basilar artery is firmly anchored to the tentorial edge by its relation to other portions of the circle of Willis. Thus, downward displacement of the brain stem with relative immobility of the basilar artery causes the penetrating arteries to enter the midbrain and pons obliquely and also to become elongated. The resulting tension on the paramedian and circumferential branches of the basilar artery causes vessel disruption and brain stem hemorrhage.

The second factor Johnson and Yates considered important in the production of such hemorrhages is midbrain distortion in the anteroposterior direction. With bilateral tem-

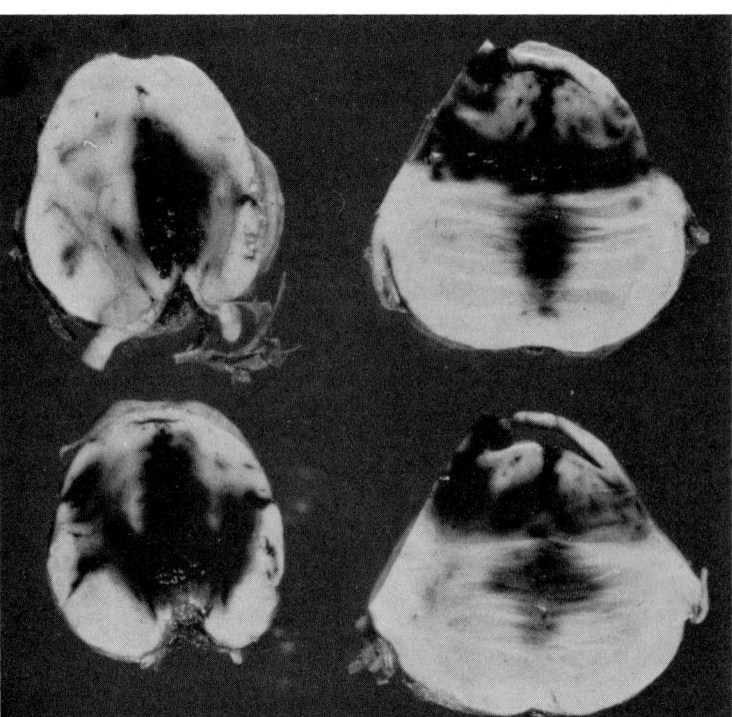

Figure 5–4. Brain stem (Duret) hemorrhages secondary to transtentorial herniation. Hemorrhage tends to be symmetrical and shows a predisposition for pontine tegmental involvement.

poro-occipital herniations, the dorsal part of the midbrain is compressed from both sides. In addition to flattening of its dorsal and lateral surfaces, the midbrain becomes elongated anteroposteriorly. This produces a stretching effect on the vessels penetrating from the basilar artery with eventual disruption and hemorrhage.

The combination of this type of elongation of the midbrain plus downward displacement of the brain stem would be additive with respect to the development of hemorrhagic lesions within the midbrain. The parenchymal hemorrhages that occur in the brain stem secondary to tentorial herniation appear to occur at the terminal branches of the penetrating vessels. The mechanism proposed for these arterial hemorrhages suggests that ischemia in the territory of the involved vessels precedes the occurrence of bleeding.

The presence of a tentorial herniation resulting from increased pressure above may be suspected or identified by carotid angiography. Uncal herniation results in medial displacement of the anterior choroidal artery visualized on the anteroposterior view. On the lateral angiogram, the anterior choroidal artery becomes stretched and straightened, while the posterior communicating artery may be displaced downward. With posterior hippocampal herniations, the anteroposterior carotid angiogram reveals medial displacement of the posterior cerebral artery and the lateral view shows downward displacement of this vessel (Fig. 5-5). Pneumoencephalographic demonstration of tentorial herniation depends upon the presence

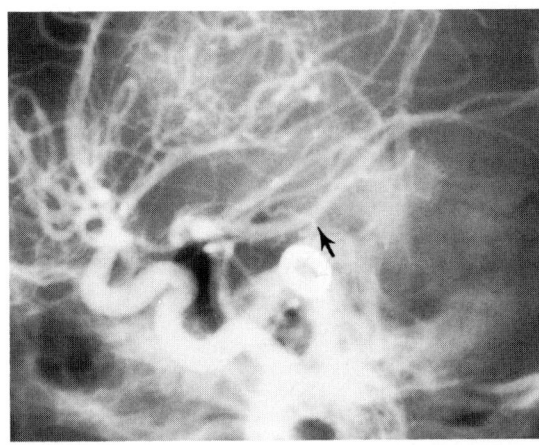

Figure 5–5. Carotid angiogram in a child with a deep-seated cerebral glioma. Downward displacement of the posterior cerebral artery (arrow), as compared to that on the opposite side, indicates transtentorial temporal lobe herniation.

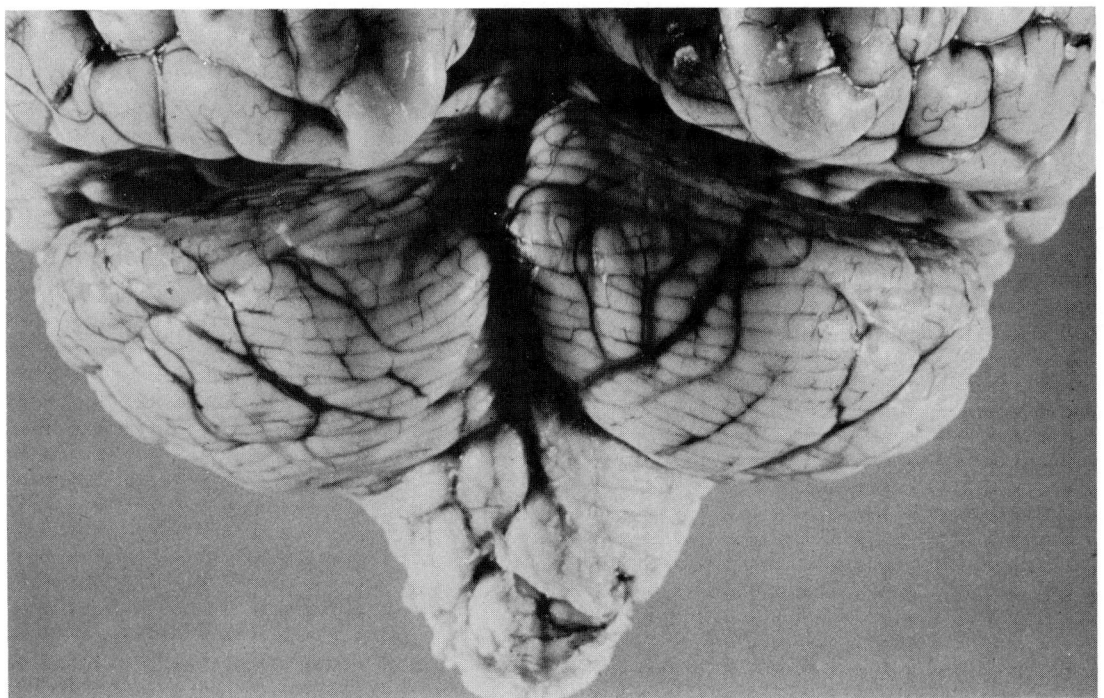

Figure 5–6. Cerebellar tonsillar herniation. View from the posterior aspect of the cerebellum demonstrates the caudal displacement of the cerebellar tonsils secondary to increased pressure from above. The cone of herniated tonsillar tissue impinges upon the dorsal surface of the cervical spinal cord.

of abnormalities of the ambient, quadrigeminal and crural cisterns (Azambuja et al.). This method of roentgen diagnosis is generally less reliable and more subject to variation than the angiographic abnormalities described previously.

CEREBELLAR HERNIATIONS

Cerebellar herniations may be directed upward through the tentorial notch or downward with impaction of the cerebellar tonsils through the foramen magnum. Upward herniation causes compression of the dorsal aspect of the midbrain and the adjacent vessels. The pineal gland may be displaced superiorly and the posterior third ventricle elevated. Obstruction of the flow of cerebrospinal fluid at the level of the aqueduct or the ambient cisterns further aggravates the intracranial pressure abnormalities. Cerebellar tonsillar herniation through the foramen magnum may obstruct the outflow of fluid from the fourth ventricle and compress the medulla (Fig. 5-6). Compression of the posterior inferior cerebellar artery against the edge of the foramen magnum may also occur.

Neck stiffness may be present when there is a cerebellar tonsillar herniation but should be searched for on examination only with caution. Forceful antiflexion of the neck may further injure the involved structures and can precipitate cardiorespiratory failure. This maneuver may enhance compression of the medulla or may further compromise involved vascular structures producing local ischemia.

Herniation of the cerebellar tonsils is demonstrable during pneumoencephalography as a filling defect projecting below the foramen magnum into the upper cervical canal. Tonsillar herniation does not necessarily require termination of the procedure although ventricular filling may not be possible. If air does not proceed into the fourth ventricle, the procedure should be abandoned and ventriculography subsequently performed. Tonsillar herniation may occur under a variety of circumstances but is particularly common with posterior fossa mass lesions.

REFERENCES

Azambuja, N., Lindgren, E., and Sjögren, S. E.: Tentorial herniations. *Acta Radiol. Stockholm.* **46**:215–223, 1956.

Azambuja, N., Lindgren, E., and Sjögren, S. E.: Tentorial herniations. Pneumography. *Acta Radiol. Stockholm.* **46**:224–231, 1956.

Johnson, R. T., and Yates, P. O.: Brain stem hemorrhages in expanding supratentorial conditions. *Acta Radiol. Stockholm.* **46**:250–256, 1956.

Johnson, R. T., and Yates, P. O.: Clinico-pathological aspects of pressure changes at the tentorium. *Acta Radiol. Stockholm.* **46**:242–249, 1956.

Kernohan, J. W., and Woltman, H. W.: Incisura of the crus due to contralateral brain tumor. *Arch. Neurol. and Psychiat.* **21**:274–287, 1929.

Meyer, A.: Herniation of the brain. *Arch. Neurol. and Psychiat.*, **4**:387–400, 1920.

Scheinker, I. M.: Transtentorial herniation of the brain stem. Characteristic clinicopathological syndrome. Pathogenesis of hemorrhages in the brain stem. *Arch. Neurol. and Psychiat.*, **53**:289–293, 1945.

PART II

Causes of Increased Intracranial Pressure in Childhood

Chapter Six

GENERAL COMMENTS

When the presence of increased intracranial pressure has been ascertained from the manifestations already described above, the possible etiologic causes must next be considered. The causes of increased intracranial pressure do not necessarily differ in various pediatric age groups. Certain conditions of this type, however, are more often seen in infancy, whereas others may occur later and only rarely in the infant age group. A few disorders in this category are almost limited to the infant age group.

THE NEWBORN PERIOD AND INFANCY

Marked increased intracranial pressure in the newborn child is usually the result of either congenital hydrocephalus or of a complication of the birth process. Perinatal anoxia may cause brain swelling and diffuse parenchymal cerebral bleeding. Birth anoxia or trauma may produce intraventricular hemorrhage, especially in the low birth weight baby. Tentorial or falx laceration secondary to distortion of the skull during birth is associated with subarachnoid and parenchymal hemorrhage, identified by lumbar puncture. Subtentorial subdural hematoma in the newborn is infrequent but is a life-threatening condition because of brain stem compression and obstruction of the aqueduct and fourth ventricle.

Any of these complications of delivery may be associated with increased intracranial pressure. The status of the infant, however, is usually more closely related to the primary insult to the brain. The elevated pressure reflects the presence of the injury but is generally less important in this age group. Infants with significant subarachnoid hemorrhage at birth without increased pressure may subsequently acquire it, as a result of a communicating hydrocephalus.

In early infancy beyond the newborn period, disorders with increased intracranial pressure can be arbitrarily divided into those with and those without abnormal head enlargement. More chronic conditions are usually associated with an abnormal rate of head enlargement; acute illnesses occur without significant change in the head size. In acute disorders the anterior fontanel is often more impressively bulged. The one obvious exception to this classification is generalized craniosynostosis (Fig. 6-1). This disorder is gradually progressive in early infancy with marked increase in pressure but without head enlargement. Because all cranial sutures are prematurely closed, growth of the brain is impeded by the unyielding skull. Papilledema develops early and skull x-rays reveal evidence of increased pressure plus the absence of patent sutures.

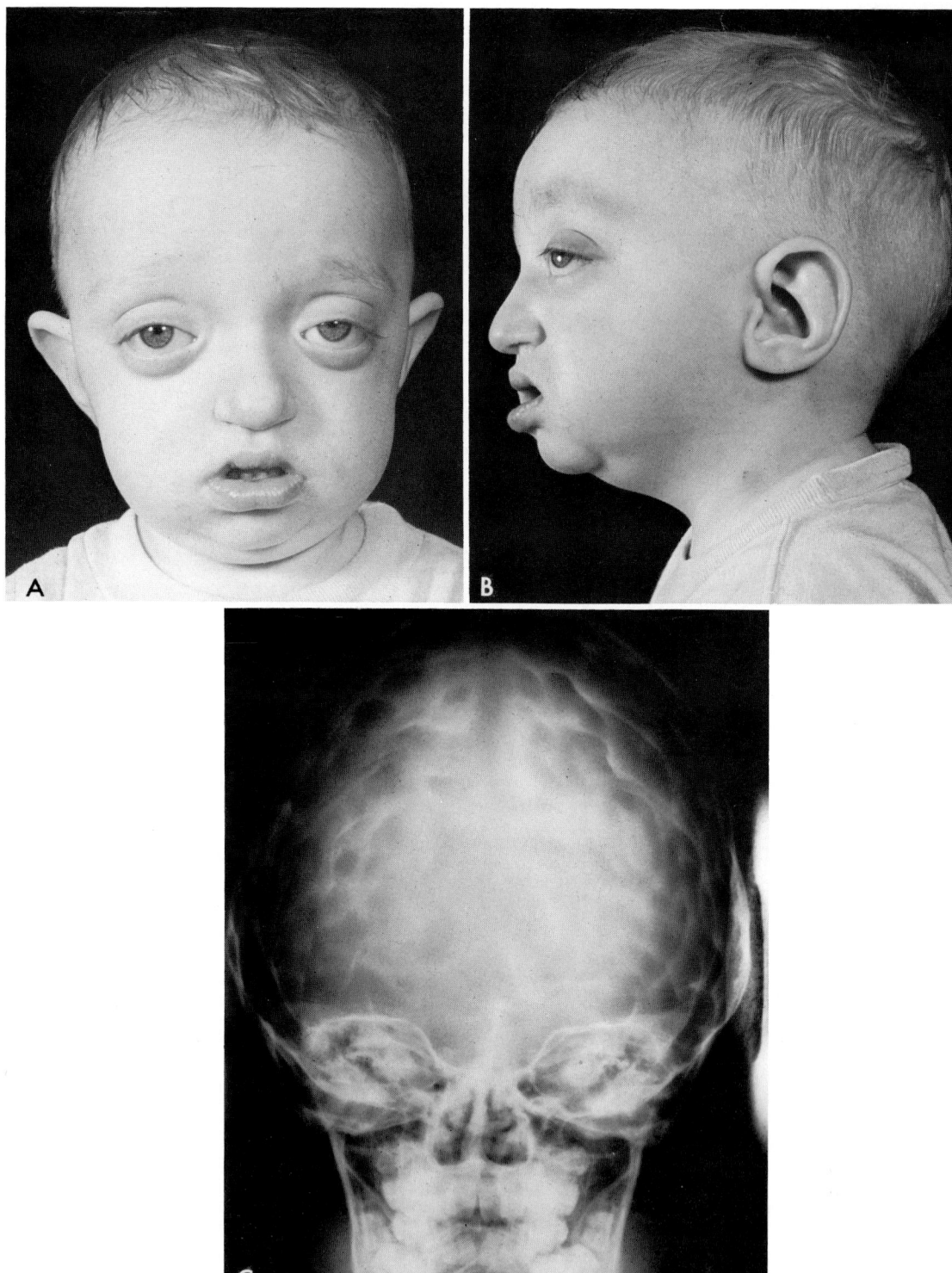

Figure 6–1. Generalized craniosynostosis (Crouzon's syndrome). Chronic increase in intracranial pressure in infancy without abnormal head enlargement. *A* and *B*, Characteristic facial appearance with bilateral proptosis, beaked nose, and mandibular hypoplasia. *C*, Anteroposterior skull view shows thinning of the skull, absence of visible sutures, and digital impressions.

Hydrocephalus

Conditions in early infancy with increased pressure and abnormal head enlargement include noncommunicating hydrocephalus due to congenital anomalies and communicating hydrocephalus secondary to subarachnoid bleeding, infection, or unknown factors. Noncommunicating hydrocephalus secondary to congenital anomalies is most often due to obstruction in the region of the aqueduct of Sylvius. Abnormal head enlargement may be present at birth or may not become apparent for the first few weeks or months of life.

The clinical manifestations are primarily those of increased pressure and include feeding problems, irritability, and eventually increase in muscle tone and hyperreflexia. Seizures are unusual in this group of infants, and papilledema is not expected, despite considerable abnormal head enlargement. The Dandy-Walker syndrome is a type of hydrocephalus in which generalized head enlargement may occur, but the most striking enlargement is in the region from the external ears to the occiput. The rate of head enlargement may be either rapid or slowly progressive.

Neonatal bacterial meningitis is often complicated by the development of hydrocephalus of either the communicating or the noncommunicating type. Evidence of increased intracranial pressure is obvious from the abnormal rate of head growth and the degree of suture spread. The physical abnormalities, however, frequently result from the parenchymal damage of the brain from the infectious illness. Clinical abnormalities, including blindness, optic atrophy, and spasticity are greater in the child with postmeningitic hydrocephalus than in the infant with uncomplicated hydrocephalus due to a congenital anomaly of the aqueduct. Congenital toxoplasmosis with hydrocephalus may be suspected in the infant with hepatosplenomegaly, intracranial calcification, macular chorioretinitis, and xanthochromic ventricular fluid with a high protein content.

Subdural Hematoma

Subdural hematoma in early infancy is often associated with progressive head enlargement with increased intracranial pressure. Most instances result from trauma, either at birth or subsequent to a head injury in the first few months of life. In most instances, the subdural hemorrhages are bilateral. Subdural hematomas are often clinically recognized between two and eight months of age. In addition to the abnormal head size, this disorder is suspected by the high incidence of convulsions, the presence of anemia, and evidence of papilledema or retinal hemorrhages.

Diagnosis is established by the performance of bilateral subdural taps. Whenever subdural hematomas are identified in an infant, chest and long bone x-rays should be obtained to search for other possible evidence of physical abuse. Newborns with osteogenesis imperfecta may have increased pressure and abnormal head enlargement at birth due to subdural hematomas acquired prenatally or during the birth process.

Tumors

Intracranial tumors are less common causes of increased pressure syndromes with head enlargement in infancy than are the disorders previously described. Posterior fossa neoplasms may result in increased pressure because of the bulk of the lesion or obstruction of the fluid pathways causing hydrocephalus. Papilloma of the choroid plexus is a rare tumor but with a predisposition to occur in early infancy. The mechanism of increased pressure in patients with this tumor primarily involves increased cerebrospinal fluid formation from the lesion, with a resultant communicating hydrocephalus.

Hydrocephalus in infancy secondary to primary brain tumor may be indistinguishable clinically from hydrocephalus due to congenital anomalies. Papilledema is more often seen in those with tumor but is not invariably present. Adequate ventriculography is the most precise differential diagnostic technique. Aneurysms of the great vein of Galen may act much like midline neoplasms in infancy. Obstruction of the aqueduct produces hydrocephalus in the absence of other localizing signs. A loud bruit may be heard on auscultation of the head, and high output cardiac failure can precede other signs indicative of intracranial disease. Tumors metastatic to the intracranial contents may occur at any time in infancy and childhood. Infiltrative leptomeningeal lesions occur with metastatic neuroblastoma, producing increased pressure with extreme suture spread. Retinoblastoma may infiltrate the subarachnoid space and ventricular system, causing increased pressure by a variety of mechanisms.

Infections

Disorders of a more acute nature in infancy resulting in increased intracranial pressure produce a tense fontanel and suture spread but with less effect on the head size of the child. If the acute process persists or becomes chronic abnormal head enlargement is expected. Acute infectious diseases, including bacterial meningitis and viral encephalitis, are often associated with increased pressure. Other signs more specifically related to the infectious process are usually much more profound than those secondary to intracranial pressure elevation. Subdural effusion and, rarely, subdural abscess may occur as complications of bacterial meningitis in infancy, markedly accentuating the degree of increased intracranial pressure.

An additional group of disorders in infancy and early childhood associated with marked brain swelling include the encephalopathies related to systemic infections (Lyon et al.). This condition is sometimes referred to as acute toxic encephalopathy and develops as a complication of a more generalized viral or bacterial illness. During or near the end of a systemic infection, the child abruptly develops high fever, stupor or coma, convulsions, or manifestations of increased pressure due to cerebral edema. Spinal fluid examination reveals a high pressure but is otherwise normal. The agent that is toxic or injurious to the brain in these cases remains unclear. Although related to an infectious disorder, this complication does not appear to be the result of invasion of organisms into the brain, as occurs with meningitis or encephalitis. The mortality rate is significant and the morbidity rate is high.

A related condition manifested by an acute encephalopathy associated with fatty degeneration of the abdominal viscera was described by Reye et al. in 1963. Cerebral swelling without overt evidence of central nervous system infection is present in this illness, usually following a mild upper respiratory infection. Hepatomegaly, elevation of the serum glutamic oxaloacetic transaminase level, hypoglycemia, and ketonuria have been noted in variable combinations. Cerebral edema with increased pressure may be fulminating and become life-threatening in this group of toxic encephalopathies.

Bulging of the fontanel with transient and benign increased intracranial pressure may also occur as a rare complication of roseola infantum (Oski). The pathogenesis has not been clarified; however, it does not seem to represent an encephalitic manifestation of roseola.

Trauma

Head trauma in infancy or childhhod may result in increased intracranial pressure by a variety of ways. Cerebral trauma with contusion and edema is one of the more common causes of subarachnoid hemorrhage in children. Acute subdural hematoma is generally associated with other evidence of trauma to the brain and thus with a combination of factors producing increased pressure. Acute epidural hematoma may occur in small infants as well as in older children and need not be associated with a temporal skull fracture as is usually the case in adults. The degree and rate of development of increased intracranial pressure with an epidural hematoma is often profound and may cause rapid deterioration unless properly managed.

Vascular Disorders

Parenchymal cerebral bleeding may result in a precipitous increase in intracranial pressure because of the substance of the mass and the associated edema. In addition to trauma, bleeding into the brain in infancy may occur with arteriovenous malformations (Fig. 6-2) and with various hematologic disorders, including hemophilia, leukemia, and conditions with thrombocytopenia. Intracranial venous thrombosis may also result in severe hemorrhagic infarction with associated cerebral edema. This is most commonly seen in infants with dehydration and metabolic acidosis secondary to diarrhea. If dehydration is of the hypernatremic type, evidence of cerebral swelling may become apparent following fluid and electrolyte therapy. This is especially likely to occur if the repair fluids do not contain adequate salt, thus causing a precipitous decrease in the serum osmolarity. The result is brain edema, often associated with convulsions. Water intoxication with

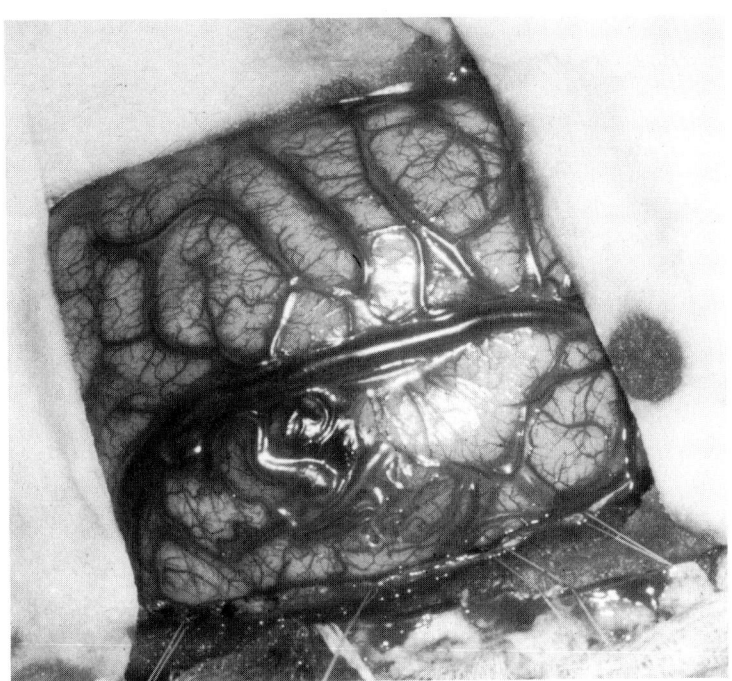

Figure 6–2. Cerebral (right) arteriovenous malformation in a ten-year-old girl. Child was well and without symptoms until sudden onset of severe headache and vomiting. Physical findings included neck stiffness, hyperreflexia on the left side, and left homonymous hemianopsia. Lumbar puncture revealed bloody spinal fluid with a xanthochromic supernatant. Diagnosis confirmed by carotid angiography. Photograph during the craniotomy reveals the superficial vascular anomaly located in the right temporo-occipital region. Increased intracranial pressure resulted from an intracerebral hematoma and cerebral edema adjacent to the mass. The intracerebral clot was aspirated and the vascular anomaly was successfully excised with minimal residual deficits.

serum hypo-osmolarity in infants and children is associated with manifestations of increased pressure due to cerebral edema. Seizures are often present in addition to headaches, lethargy, and papilledema.

Tetracycline

Infants may respond in a peculiar fashion to tetracycline, resulting in a bulging fontanel syndrome (Fields, O'Doherty). The tense fontanel may be noted within hours after initiation of the drug or may not occur for a few days thereafter. It may develop after a single dose of tetracycline and, unless recognized, can be associated with progressive signs, including back-arching, vomiting, and lethargy. Lumbar puncture or withdrawal of the drug is followed by rapid recovery.

The mechanism by which tetracycline causes an increased intracranial pressure syndrome has not been established. Meningitis is often suspected until the lumbar puncture is done, revealing normal findings except for increased pressure and resulting in clinical improvement of the child. Intracranial hypertension secondary to tetracycline therapy has been observed mainly in infants but has been reported in older children (Maroon and Mealy) and even in adults (Koch-Weser and Gilmore).

Vitamin A

Abnormalities of vitamin A intake are a rare but widely recognized cause of increased intracranial pressure (Feldman and Schlezinger). Acute hypervitaminosis A occurs with ingestion of a large quantity of the agent over a short period of time. Symptoms and signs develop within hours and include bulging of the fontanel, vomiting, and irritability. Symptoms tend to abate promptly on cessation of administration of vitamin A.

Chronic vitamin A intoxication is characterized by a more insidious onset with anorexia, dry skin, coarsening and loss of hair, angular fissures at the lips, hepatosplenomegaly, and cortical thickening of long bones. This picture with chronic ingestion is rarely observed in children under one year of age. It is generally believed that the minimum toxic dose for chronic vitamin A poisoning is approximately 75,000 units per day.

In rare instances, a child may show manifestations of chronic vitamin A intoxication with superimposed increased intracranial pressure, more characteristic of the acute variety (Woodard et al.). This may occur with or without cutaneous manifestations and has been observed in adolescent patients receiving large doses of vitamin A for acne vulgaris (Morrice et al., Lascari and Bell). The cause of the increased pressure in this disorder remains speculative. However, the case described by Woodard et al. included a pneumoencephalogram that showed mildly dilated lateral ventricles. Hypovitaminosis A likewise may result in increased intracranial pressure (Cornfeld and Cooke, Wolf). The cases described in infancy have shown regression of the syndrome with adequate vitamin A therapy although several weeks may be required for the tense fontanel to subside.

Little information regarding pathogenesis is available in humans. Animal investigations have shown that maternal vitamin A deficiency during pregnancy results in offspring with increased pressure due to hydrocephalus with ventricular enlargement (Millen and Woollam). Whether the hydrocephalic process is due to increased secretion or decreased absorption of cerebrospinal fluid remains to be clarified.

CHILDHOOD AND ADOLESCENCE

Head trauma with its various complications, nervous system infections, and hemorrhagic disorders continues to be a cause of increased pressure in childhood, as described in infancy. Among infectious conditions, herpes simplex encephalitis has a special tendency to involve primarily one temporal lobe. The localized swelling may reach a degree sufficient to cause ipsilateral hippocampal tentorial herniation.

After 18 months of age, lead encephalopathy, to be described later, becomes a consideration in differential diagnosis as a cause of cerebral swelling. A disorder with similarities to that produced by lead ingestion is hypertensive encephalopathy, also notable for its intracranial hypertension. In children, severe systemic hypertension may result from a variety of causes, such as acute glomerulonephritis, chronic renal disease, pheochromocytoma and coarctation of the aorta. The retinal abnormalities of severe hypertension, including exudates and arterial constriction, aid in the differentiation of this condition from those primarily due to intracranial disease.

In children, cerebral artery occlusion due to thrombosis or embolization causes signs due to local tissue ischemia and occasionally, increased pressure due to cerebral edema. The degree of edema is extremely variable but may be severe with a ventricular shift resulting. Increased intracranial pressure secondary to cerebral edema has also been described in children with diabetic ketoacidosis (Young and Bradley). Clements et al. monitored cerebrospinal fluid continuously in five patients with diabetic acidosis and found that an abnormally high pressure developed in all after therapy had resulted in a significant decrease in serum glucose and osmolarity. Decline in state of awareness corresponded with the development of increased pressure in these patients.

Pseudotumor Cerebri

A syndrome described later in greater detail is referred to as benign intracranial hypertension. This condition is more common in young adults but may occur at any age in childhood. The clinical findings are those of increased intracranial pressure without focal neurologic signs. The disorder must be distinguished from a midline tumor which it may resemble in all respects.

A syndrome identical to benign intracranial hypertension of unknown cause may result from lateral sinus thrombosis as a complication of middle ear or mastoid infection. The degree of brain swelling resulting from lateral sinus thrombosis depends on the anatomic arrangement of the venous drainage at the torcula. If the major portion of the blood in the superior sagittal sinus normally drains through the thrombosed lateral sinus, marked cerebral edema will result. Other conditions frequently discussed with the pseudotumor cerebri syndrome include increased intracranial pressure secondary to hypoparathyroidism (Sugar) or to Addison's disease (Walsh).

Tumors

In early childhood, intracranial tumors become progressively more common as an important cause of increased intracranial pressure. A multiplicity of signs may occur in a child with an intracranial tumor, depending on the location and size of the lesion. Those located in the cerebellum or dorsal to the midbrain are most likely to produce pressure manifestations early in the illness because of the tendency to cause hydrocephalus.

With certain midline tumors, such as colloid cysts of the third ventricle, craniopharyngioma, or ependymoma of the fourth ventricle, the manifestations of increased pressure can be strikingly intermittent and evanescent. The remarkable intermittency of symptoms and signs occasionally seen with intracranial tumors may be the result of slight changes in position of the lesion. In some instances, it may be secondary to alterations occurring in surrounding brain tissue because of transient volume changes occurring with variation of factors such as arterial blood flow, venous drainage, or respiratory changes.

Infiltrative meningeal disease with leukemia, reticulum cell sarcoma, neuroblastoma, or metastatic melanoma causes communicating hydrocephalus with associated increased pressure. Cerebral or cerebellar abscesses become more common after two years of age and are almost always associated with marked increased pressure.

Burns

Minor or extensive cutaneous burns may be associated with brain swelling (Emery and Reid, Warlow and Hinton). Clinical signs can be those mainly of increased pressure or may encompass a variety of deficits, including spastic hemiparesis, visual loss, and convulsions. Although the pathogenesis of brain swelling in the burn patient is unclear, the degree may be sufficient to result in tentorial herniation and death. A burned child who becomes lethargic or drowsy, or who develops headaches or repeated vomiting, should undergo a careful funduscopic examination. Considerable improvement occasionally follows intravenous mannitol therapy if brain swelling has occurred.

Pulmonary Disease

Chronic respiratory insufficiency with respiratory acidosis may result in increased intracranial pressure, or in papilledema in the absence of an elevated pressure. Cameron first described papilledema in patients with respiratory acidosis in 1933. Two broad groups of pulmonary disorders associated with hypercapnia and possible optic nerve changes have been described. The first consists of those with intrinsic lung disease and with subsequent carbon dioxide retention. These include emphysema, cystic fibrosis, and other pulmonary parenchymal disorders. The second group includes disorders with alveolar hypoventilation but without significant pulmonary parenchymal disease. Examples in this category are extreme obesity with hypoventilation in the Pickwickian syndrome (Burwell et al.), severe kyphoscoliosis (Chapman et al.), and poliomyelitis (Whittenberger and Ferris). Muscular dystrophy also may result in sufficient skeletal muscle weakness to cause hypoventilation, hypercapnia, and retinopathy (McCormack and Spalter).

Regardless of the type of pulmonary involvement, the retinal or increased pressure syndromes described with these conditions are believed to be related to carbon dioxide retention. Cerebral and retinal vessels respond to hypercapnia with marked vasodilatation and subsequent increase in blood flow. These factors appear to be of primary importance in the pathogenesis of papilledema secondary to respiratory insufficiency. It is likely, however, that other metabolic factors such as hypoxia, elevated venous pressure, and compensatory polycythemia with increased blood viscosity may contribute to the retinal and cerebral abnormalities.

Rare Causes

Rare causes of increased intracranial pressure in childhood include congenital aqueductal stenosis, which may remain partially compensated until the child becomes several years of age at which time headaches, papilledema, and perhaps ataxia are identified. These findings are usually assumed to be due to a posterior fossa tumor until ventriculography and craniectomy establish the true nature of the problem. Likewise, the Dandy-Walker syndrome may remain surprisingly silent for several years before clinical symptoms appear. Such children usually have abnormally large heads for age, but its significance may be over-looked until other more impressive abnormalities develop.

In these unusual cases, the manifestations of increased intracranial pressure may be precipitated by a mild head injury or generalized infectious illness. Adhesive arachnoiditis of unknown etiology is an additional rare cause of hydrocephalus due to fourth ventricle outlet obstruction. Ventriculography and craniectomy are required to establish the diagnosis.

Increased intracranial pressure with papilledema has been described in adolescent females with iron deficiency anemia (Lubeck). Symptoms and signs subside with therapeutic administration of iron and correction of the anemia. Papilledema and other aspects of increased pressure may occur with or even represent the initial manifestations of subacute sclerosing panencephalitis (Tibbles et al., Glowacki et al.). An intracranial tumor is apt to be suspected in this instance, however, the type of recurrent seizure so characteristic of this disease suggests a more generalized cerebral process. Diagnosis may become evident from the first zone colloidal gold rise and increased gamma globulin in the spinal fluid, the suppression-burst abnormality on electroencephalography, and elevated serum and cerebrospinal fluid measles antibody titers. Increased pressure may be observed as a rare manifestation of certain degeneration brain diseases in childhood, including sudanophilic leukodystrophy.

Papilledema and other evidence of increased pressure rarely accompany certain spinal cord tumors (Browder). Love et al., described two patients with spinal cord tumors in whom papilledema coexisted. One was an intramedullary glioma of the spinal cord; the other was an ependymoma of the filum terminale. Some authors have postulated that increased intracranial pressure with intraspinal lesions is the result of obstruction of the arachnoid villi secondary to an elevated spinal fluid protein content (Gardner et al.). In other instances, subarachnoid hemorrhage occurs from spinal cord or filum terminale tumors with increased intracranial pressure resulting therefrom (Nassar and Correll).

The Guillain-Barré syndrome also is rarely complicated by papilledema, although the mechanism remains in debate. Certain authors have suggested that cerebral edema coexists with the peripheral nerve disease (Joynt). Others have ascribed the increased pressure to hydrocephalus secondary to an arachnoidal block due to the elevated spinal fluid protein.

The Wiskott-Aldrich syndrome has been described with associated increased pressure of unknown cause (Greer). This is an unusual manifestation of a rare disease that is inherited as a sex-linked recessive trait. A more common explanation for increased intracranial pressure in this disease is the result of intracranial hemorrhage secondary to thrombocytopenia. A few children with the Wiskott-Aldrich syndrome have been described with reticuloendothelial malignancies involving the brain and increased pressure therefrom (ten Bensel et al.).

Osteopetrosis is a rare cause of chronic head enlargement and increased pressure in infancy (Fig. 6-3). Clinical suspicion of this illness is based on the combination of head enlargement, hepatosplenomegaly, pancytopenia, and multiple cranial nerve palsies.

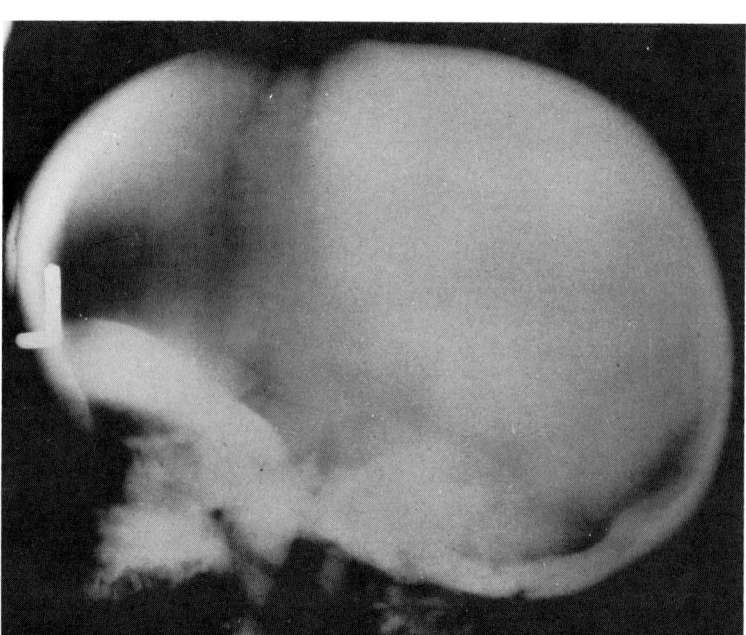

Figure 6–3. Skull x-ray of a 15-month-old child with abnormal head enlargement secondary to osteopetrosis. Note the marked increase in density and thickness of the skull, especially at the base. Bilateral optic atrophy, deafness, and hepatosplenomegaly were found to be present on examination.

Skull and skeletal x-rays establish the diagnosis.

REFERENCES

Browder, J.: Tumors of the spinal cord. *Amer. J. Surg.*, **24**:1–10, 1934.

Burwell, C. S., Robin, E. D., Whaley, R. D. and Bickelman, A. G.: Extreme obesity associated with alevolar hypoventilation–a Pickwickian syndrome. *Amer. J. Med.*, **21**:811–818, 1956.

Cameron, A. J.: Marked papilledema in pulmonary insufficiency. *Brit. J. Ophth.*, **17**:167–169, 1933.

Chapman, E. M., Dill, D. B., and Graybiel, A.: The decrease in functional capacity of the lungs and heart resulting from deformities of the chest. Pulmonocardiac failure. *Medicine*, **18**:167–202, 1939.

Clements, R. S., Jr., Blumenthal, S. A., Morrison, A. D., and Winegrad, A. I.: Increased cerebrospinal-fluid pressure during treatment of diabetic ketosis. *Lancet*, **2**:671–675, 1971.

Cornfeld, D., and Cooke, R. E.: Vitamin A deficiency: case report; unusual manifestations in a 5-1/2 month old baby. *Pediatrics*, **10**:33–38, 1952.

Emery, J. L., and Reid, D. A. C.: Cerebral edema and spastic hemiplegia following minor burns in young children. *Brit. J. Surg.*, **50**:53–56, 1962.

Feldman, M. H., and Schlezinger, N. S.: Benign intracranial hypertension associated with hypervitaminosis A. *Arch. Neurol.*, **22**:1–7, 1970.

Fields, J. P.: Bulging fontanel: a complication of tetracycline therapy in infants. *J. Pediat.*, **58**:74–76, 1961.

Gardner, W. J., Spitler, D. K., and Whitten, C.: Increased intracranial pressure caused by increased protein content of the cerebrospinal fluid. *New Eng. J. Med.*, **250**:932–936, 1954.

Glowacki, J., Guazzi, G. C., and Van Bogaert, L.: Pseudotumoral presentation of certain cases of subacute sclerosing leukoencephalitis. *J. Neurol. Sci.*, **4**:199–225, 1967.

Greer, M.: Benign intracranial hypertension (Pseudotumor cerebri). *Pediat. Clin. N. Amer.*, **14**:819–829, 1967.

Joynt, R. J.: Mechanism of production of papilledema in Guillain-Barré syndrome. *Neurology*, **8**:8–12, 1958.

Koch-Weser, J., and Gilmore, E. B.: Benign intracranial hypertension in an adult after tetracycline therapy. *J.A.M.A.*, **200**:345–347, 1967.

Lascari, A. D., and Bell, W. E.: Pseudotumor cerebri due to hypervitaminosis A. Toxic consequence of self-medication for acne in an adolescent girl. *Clin. Pediat.*, **9**:627–628, 1970.

Love, J. G., Wagener, H. P., and Woltman, H. W.: Tumors of the spinal cord associated with choking of the optic discs. *Arch. Neurol. and Psychiat.*, **66**:171–177, 1951.

Lubeck, M. J.: Papilledema caused by iron-deficiency anemia. *Tr. Amer. Acad. Ophth. Otolaryng.*, **63**:306-310, 1959.

Lyon, G., Dodge, P. R., and Adams, R. D.: The acute encephalopathies of obscure origin in infants and children. *Brain*, **84**:680–708, 1961.

Maroon, J. C., and Mealy, J., Jr.: Benign intracranial hypertension. Sequel to tetracycline therapy in a child. *J.A.M.A.*, **216**:1479–1480, 1971.

McCormack, W. M., and Spalter, H.: Muscular dystrophy, alveolar hypoventilation, and papilledema. *J.A.M.A.*, **197**:957–960, 1966.

Millen, J. W., and Woollam, D. H. M.: Vitamins and the cerebrospinal fluid. In: *Ciba Foundation Symposium: The cerebrospinal fluid.* Ed. by Wolstenholme and O'Conner. Boston, Little, Brown Co. 1958, pp. 168–188.

Morrice, G., Jr., Havener, W. H., and Kapetansky, F.: Vitamin A intoxication as a cause of pseudotumor cerebri. *J.A.M.A.*, **173**:1802–1805, 1960.

Nassar, S. I., and Correll, J. W.: Subarachnoid hemorrhage due to spinal cord tumors. *Neurology*, **18**:87–94, 1968.

O'Doherty, N. J.: Acute benign intracranial hypertension in an infant receiving tetracycline. *Develop. Med. Child. Neurol.*, **7**:677–680, 1965.

Oski, F. A.: Roseola infantum. *Amer. J. Dis Child.*, **101**:376–378, 1961.

Reye, R. D. K., Morgan, G., and Baral, J.: Encephalopathy and fatty degeneration of the viscera. A disease entity in childhood. *Lancet*, **2**:749–752, 1963.

Sugar, O.: Central neurological complications of hypoparathyroidism. *Arch. Neurol. and Psychiat.*, **70**:86–107, 1953.

ten Bensel, R. W., Stadlan, E. M., and Krivit, W.: The development of malignancy in the course of the Aldrich syndrome. *J. Pediat.*, **68**:761–767, 1966.

Tibbles, J. A. R., Donohue, W. L., Kofman, O., and Prichard, J. S.: Subacute inclusion encephalitis: A clinical and pathological review. *Canad. Med. Ass. J.*, **90**:401–408, 1964.

Walsh, F. B.: Papilledema associated with increased intracranial pressure in Addison's disease. *Arch. Ophthal.*, **47**:86, 1952.

Warlow, C. P., and Hinton, P.: Early neurological disturbances following relatively minor burns in children. *Lancet.*, **2**:978–982, 1969.

Whittenberger, J. L., and Ferris, B. G.: Alteration of respiratory function in poliomyelitis. *Amer. J. Phys. Med.*, **31**:226–237, 1952.

Wolf, I. J.: Vitamin A deficiency in an infant. *J.A.M.A.*, **166**:1859–1860, 1958.

Woodard, W. K., Miller, L. J., and Legant, O.: Acute and chronic hypervitaminosis in a 4-month-old infant. *J. Pediat.*, **59**:260–264, 1961.

Young, E., and Bradley, R. F.: Cerebral edema with irreversible coma in severe diabetic ketoacidosis. *New Eng. J. Med.*, **276**:665–669, 1967.

Chapter Seven

CEREBRAL EDEMA

Cerebral edema is a response of brain tissue to a variety of insults and consists of an abnormal accumulation of fluid associated with a volumetric enlargement of the involved brain substance. Reichardt attempted to distinguish brain edema from brain swelling, largely on the basis of the appearance and texture of the brain examined grossly. The terms cerebral edema and swelling are now generally used interchangeably. Cerebral edema may be diffuse, involving both cerebral hemispheres, or it may be relatively focal, as occurs in the area of a neoplasm or abscess (Fig. 7-1). A metastatic tumor in the cerebrum may be associated with marked and widespread edema that becomes more life-threatening than the primary lesion.

With diffuse cerebral edema, flattening of the cortical gyri and narrowing of the sulci are seen on gross observation of the surface of the brain. If swelling is symmetrical in the two hemispheres, the lateral ventricles retain midline position but may be reduced in size. Unilateral cerebral edema results in shift and distortion of the ventricular system and, at times, with asymmetrical internal herniations previously described. Edema may occur in the cerebral cortex or white matter or both. As a rule, the process tends to be much more pronounced in the cerebral white matter (Feigin and Popoff). With lesions deep in the centrum semiovale, extensive swelling may occur in the area but spare the subcortical arcuate fibers.

The location of edema fluid in brain tissue had been controversial for many years. Light microscopic examinations produced conflicting postulates in this regard. The development of electron microscopy also initially resulted in concepts that tended to vary in different laboratories. In recent years, however, electron microscopic studies have clarified many of the problems of the pathology of cerebral edema. Certain early electron microscopic examinations suggested that the edema fluid accumulation was intracellular

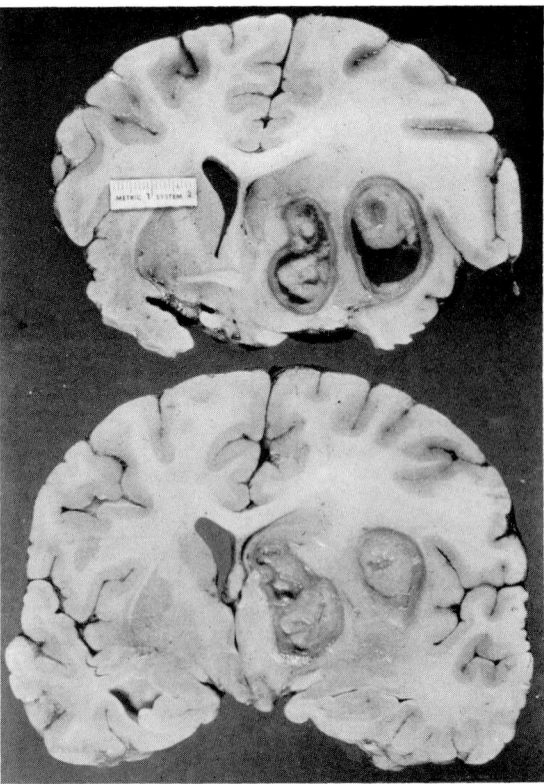

Figure 7-1. Marked edema of the cerebral white matter secondary to multiple abscesses. Swelling is largely unilateral and results in flattening of the surface gyri and narrowing of the sulci.

and virtually confined to glial cells (Gerschenfeld et al, Luse and Harris). The involved cells in these initial investigations were interpreted by some as being oligodendroglial (Luse and Harris). Despite the predominance of white matter involvement in cerebral edema, these initial studies focused attention on the histologic changes in the cortical gray matter.

Continued observations with the use of the electron microscope revealed a difference in the extracellular compartments of white and gray matter in normal brain tissue. Lee and Bakay demonstrated that the intercellular space in normal white matter may obtain a distance of 800 angstroms, while that in the normal cerebral cortex more constantly measures 150 to 200 angstroms. Because of this difference in the space between cell membranes in gray and white matter, it is not surprising that the abnormal accumulation of fluid in cerebral edema is different in gray as compared to white matter.

In cortical tissue, edema fluid is generally confined to astrocytes and astrocytic processes. Extension of fluid to the extracellular spaces occurs when marked distention of the cell results in rupture of the cell membrane with subsequent extravasation into the extracellular space. In white matter, edema fluid is characteristically found in both the extracellular space and the astrocytic processes (Klatzo).

From a pathogenetic standpoint, cerebral edema has been categorized into two types (Klatzo). The first, or vasogenic, type is related to injury to cerebral vessel walls with alteration in permeability leading to an escape of water and plasma components into the parenchyma. The second variety of cerebral edema is called the cytotoxic type in which the fundamental pathogenic mechanism is a direct effect on parenchymal cellular elements. Vascular permeability in this type remains essentially unaltered and the fluid collection is predominantly intracellular. The immediate source of fluid that accumulates in cell processes in the cytotoxic type of cerebral edema is believed to be from the extracellular compartment.

While recognizing the clinical limitations of such a classification, Klatzo has suggested that the therapeutic approach might be more rationally devised if cases could be divided in this manner. Thus, in the vasogenic type of cerebral edema, hypertonic solutions might be of little benefit or could conceivably be harmful. With increased vascular permeability, it is postulated that hypertonic substances would have ready access to the edematous tissue, increasing its osmolarity and producing a further shift of fluid into its substance.

Corticosteroids might be more appropriate in the vasogenic type of cerebral edema because of proposed effect on vascular integrity. Because vascular permeability is not significantly altered in the cytotoxic variety, hypertonic substances administered intravenously would seem more rational. Although this kind of classification of pathogenic types of cerebral edema is useful, its limiting factor is that most insults that produce cerebral edema in the clinical setting cause injury to both vasculature and parenchyma.

Treatment

Management of cerebral edema is a vitally important aspect of treatment in a great number of neurologic conditions. In cerebral trauma, the ability to control brain swelling may determine life or death of the patient. This factor may play a determining role during and after neurosurgical procedures in which edema may be fulminating because of manipulation or traction on brain tissue. Likewise, proper management of brain swelling may decide the outcome in meningitis, encephalitis, intoxication, neoplasm, cerebral hemorrhage, and infarction. In some instances, correction of cerebral edema is dependent primarily on recognition and correction of the cause. Hyponatremia with brain swelling due to the administration of excessive quantities of salt-free intravenous fluids responds promptly to hypertonic saline.

The most commonly used therapuetic approaches for cerebral edema at present include hypertonic urea, mannitol, corticosteroids, and surgical subtemporal decompression. Shenkin and Bouzarth have advised caution with the use of osmotic agents when there is a possibility of active intracranial bleeding. An increase in the cerebral blood flow that accompanies use of these preparations may enhance bleeding, either spontaneously or during an operative procedure. Conversely, the increased cerebral blood flow resulting from the osmotic agents provides an added beneficial effect when used to reduce cerebral edema secondary to cerebral ischemic disease.

Subtemporal decompression is currently less popular than in the past and is generally regarded to be a last resort if other more effective and less hazardous measures fail. In certain instances, however, subtemporal decompression may prevent death in intractable cases or may prevent visual loss from secondary optic atrophy with chronic papilledema. A more extensive surgical decompressive procedure has been proposed by Kerr for progressive cerebral edema following severe head trauma. The purpose of more extensive or bilateral decompressions is to avoid herniation and necrosis of cerebral tissue at the margin of the craniectomy and to prevent shift of the brain stem, which may occur with the conventional subtemporal procedure.

Urea. Urea was first proposed as an agent to reduce increased intracranial pressure in 1927 by Fremont-Smith and Forbes. Its use did not become clinically popular, however, until emphasized by Javid and Settlage in 1956. Hypertonic urea given intravenously draws fluid from the brain into the vascular compartment because of the resulting osmotic gradient existent before urea gains entrance into brain tissue.

Using C-14-labeled urea, Reed and Woodbury have shown that following administration of urea, eight hours are required for osmotic equilibrium to occur between blood and brain substance. The reduction of fluid in the brain is greatest between 30 and 60 minutes after urea is given. The effect is associated with, but not dependent upon, a marked diuresis. When urea is used in stuporous or lethargic patients, an indwelling urethral catheter may be necessary to prevent distention of the bladder. When urea becomes equilibrated with the intracellular space, the osmotic gradient is no longer present and may even be reversed. In this case, fluid may again enter cell processes and a rebound effect may result.

Intravenous urea is currently used in a 30 per cent solution in 10 per cent invert sugar. The agent is administered in a dosage of 1 gram per kilogram of body weight over a period of 60 minutes. Repeated use of hypertonic urea over a short period of time can become hazardous because of serum hyperosmolarity. Escape of hypertonic urea into the subcutaneous tissue at the site of the needle produces tissue necrosis.

Mannitol. Intravenous mannitol has advantages over urea as an agent to reduce cerebral edema. Mannitol is confined chiefly to the extracellular vascular space and is excreted rapidly. Because it has less tendency to enter cells, the rebound effect is not as pronounced as with urea (Wise and Chater). Intravenous mannitol is used in a 20 per cent solution in distilled water in a dose of 2 grams per kilogram of body weight. It is given over a period of 20 minutes with the maximum reduction of brain edema occurring in two to four hours.

A transient increase in the total blood volume is expected when this dosage is administered. Thus, use of mannitol may create difficulties in a child with impending or frank cardiac failure. Furthermore, adequate renal function must be present for excretion of hypertonic substances such as mannitol and urea. Administration of these agents to a child in renal failure would markedly overload the vascular system, possibly leading to cardiac failure and pulmonary edema.

Corticosteroids. In recent years, corticosteroids have been used extensively for reduction of cerebral edema. Drowsiness in a patient with cerebral edema surrounding either a metastatic or primary neoplasm may be diminished remarkably with the use of corticosteroids, allowing sufficient time for diagnostic studies before specific therapy can be accomplished. Even children with posterior fossa obstructive lesions may show symptomatic improvement with steroid therapy, although the mechanism remains unexplained.

Galicich et al. first suggested steroid therapy for the reduction of cerebral edema in 1961, but the mechanism by which it is accomplished has remained unclear. With cerebral edema produced by psyllium seed implantation, Long et al. demonstrated by electron microscopic examination that large dose dexamethasone therapy reduces the fluid content of swollen astrocytic processes and extracellular spaces. It was also shown that the effect of steroids is greater if initiated 48 hours before the edema is induced in the cerebral white matter. Once swelling has developed, the effect of administration of steroids, although definite, is less marked. Thus, if the development of cerebral edema is anticipated, as with certain neurosurgical procedures, corticosteroid therapy may be more advantageously utilized if begun before the operation and continued for several days postoperatively. The suggestion that steroids act by enhancing the integrity of vessel walls may partially explain the prevention of the formation of cerebral edema but would not seem to account for its reduction, once formed.

Dexamethasone has been the agent most widely used in treatment of cerebral edema. This glucocorticoid is extremely potent—0.75 mg. of dexamethasone is equal to approximately 30 mg. of cortisone acetate. It may be given in a dose of 0.25 to 0.50 mg. per kilogram of body weight per day either intramuscularly or intravenously. The drug is given at six-hour intervals with improvement usually beginning 8 to 24 hours after initiation of therapy.

In instances in which rapid reduction of brain swelling is deemed necessary, intravenous mannitol may be given initially along with the more slowly acting steroid preparations. In addition to dexamethasone, methylprednisolone sodium succinate has also been effective in large doses for the control of cerebral edema. This preparation is given in a dosage of 1 mg. per kilogram of body weight per day in four divided doses.

Glycerol. Glycerol (1,2,3-propanetriol) has been used by oral or nasogastric tube administration to reduce cerebral edema with favorable results (Cantore et al., Buckell and Walsh). Advantages include its prompt edema-reducing action, its relative freedom of toxicity, the lack of evidence of a rebound effect after intracranial pressure has been reduced, and the ability to give the agent two or four times per day for several weeks.

Glycerol may be given in an immediate dose of 2 grams per kilogram of body weight by tube in the comatose patient with severe brain swelling, or in a dose of 0.5 gram per kilogram orally every six or eight hours in an alert patient less seriously ill. Its use three or four times per day on an out-patient basis may provide a valuable method of management of the patient with pseudotumor cerebri in whom maintenance treatment is required. When glycerol is used in this fashion, the nauseating qualities may be diminished by the addition of fruit juice or prior administration of an antiemetic agent.

REFERENCES

Buckell, M., and Walsh, L.: Effect of glycerol by mouth on raised intracranial pressure in man. *Lancet,* **2**:1151–1152, 1964.

Cantore, G., Guidetti, B., and Virno, M.: Oral glycerol for the reduction of intracranial pressure. *J. Neurosurg.,* **21**:278–283, 1964.

Feigin, I., and Popoff, N.: Neuropathological observations on cerebral edema. *Arch. Neurol.,* **6**:151–160, 1962.

Fremont-Smith, F., and Forbes, H. S.: Intraocular and intracranial pressure: experimental study. *Arch. Neurol. and Psychiat.,* **18**:550–564, 1927.

Galicich, J. H., French, L. A., and Melby, J. C.: Use of dexamethasone in treatment of cerebral edema associated with brain tumors. *J. Lancet,* **81**:46–53, 1961.

Gerschenfeld, H. M., Wald, F., Zadunaisky, J. A., and DeRobertis, E. D P.: Function of astroglia in the water-ion metabolism of the central nervous system. An electron microscopic study. *Neurology,* **9**:412–425, 1959.

Javid, M., and Settlage, P.: Effect of urea on cerebrospinal fluid pressure in human subjects: preliminary report. *J.A.M.A.,* **160**:943–949, 1956.

Kerr, F. W. L.: Radical decompression and dural grafting in severe cerebral edema. *Mayo Clin. Proc.,* **43**:852–864, 1968.

Klatzo, I.: Neuropathological aspects of brain edema. *J. Neuropath. and Exper. Neurol.,* **26**:1–14, 1967.

Lee, J. C., and Bakay, L.: Ultrastructural changes in the edematous central nervous system. *Arch. Neurol.,* **13**:48–57, 1965.

Long, D. M., Hartman, J. F., and French, L. A.: The response of experimental cerebral edema to glucosteroid administration. *J. Neurosurg.,* **24**:843–854, 1966.

Luse, S. A., and Harris, B.: Electron microscopy of the brain in experimental edema. *J. Neurosurg.,* **17**:439–446, 1960.

Reed, D. J., and Woodbury, D M.: Effect of hypertonic urea on cerebrospinal fluid pressure and blood volume. *J. Physiol.,* **164**:252–264, 1962.

Reichardt, M.: Zur entstehung des hirndrucks bei hirngeschwulsten und anderen hirnkrankheiten und über eine bei diesen zu beobachtende besondere art der hirnschwellung. *Deutsche Ztschr. Nervenh.,* **28**:306–355, 1905.

Shenkin, H. A., and Bouzarth, W. F.: Clinical methods of reducing intracranial pressure. *New Eng. J. Med.,* **282**:1465–1471, 1970.

Wise, B. L., and Chater, N.: The value of hypertonic mannitol solution in decreasing brain mass and lowering cerebrospinal-fluid pressure. *J. Neurosurg.,* **19**:1038–1043, 1962.

Chapter Eight

HYDROCEPHALUS

Hydrocephalus refers to a group of conditions associated with ventricular enlargement which, in the majority of cases, is secondary to obstruction of the normal egress and flow of cerebrospinal fluid from its points of origin to its sites of absorption. In this context, hydrocephalus implies the presence of an increased quantity of cerebrospinal fluid under increased pressure, the latter being present either intermittently or persistently, and either currently or at some time in the past.

Ventricular enlargement due to primary atrophic or hypoplastic cerebral conditions is not related to pressure relationships in most cases and thus should not be included in the hydrocephalus category. The term "hydrocephalus ex vacuo" is mentioned only to be condemned because of its misleading implications. In these disorders, the primary site of disease is the substance of the brain with enlargement of the ventricles occurring passively and secondarily. However, atrophic conditions of the brain may be associated with absorptive abnormalities, allowing both mechanisms to become operational.

Abnormal enlargement of the head is often present when hydrocephalus begins prenatally, in the newborn period, or in early childhood, but does not occur when the onset is in later childhood or the adult years. This observation was made as early as 1761 by Morgagni and accounts for many of the differences in symptoms and signs seen in hydrocephalic patients of different age groups.

Dorothy Russell has credited Vesalius (1514 to 1564) with the first clear description of hydrocephalus, although the condition had been recognized centuries before. Robert Whytt, in 1768, was able to distinguish internal and external forms, descriptive terms no longer widely used because of lack of clarity. Continued study over the years has clarified many of the problems related to the pathogenesis and physiologic principles associated with hydrocephalus, although a great deal remains to be learned, especially in regard to treatment.

Our current level of knowledge indicates that in most instances, hydrocephalus in humans results from obstruction at some point along the cerebrospinal fluid pathways. For this reason, the time-honored reference to intraventricular obstruction as "obstruc-

Table 8-1. Classification and Types of Hydrocephalus

Noncommunicating (intraventricular obstructive)
1. Maldevelopments of the aqueduct
   stenosis
   forking ("atresia")
   septum
   gliosis
2. Obstruction due to mass lesions (neoplasm, cyst, hematoma, aneurysm of the vein of Galen)
3. Obstruction secondary to exudate, hemorrhage, or parasites
4. Obstruction of the fourth ventricle outlet foramina (Dandy-Walker, arachnoiditis)

Communicating (extraventricular obstructive)
1. Postinfectious, posthemorrhagic, or developmental adhesions of basilar cisterns or surface subarachnoid space
2. Arachnoid villi obstruction by erythrocytes
3. Communicating hydrocephalus with the Arnold-Chiari malformation
4. Developmental failure of arachnoid villi (presumptive)
5. Hypovitaminosis A (experimental animals)

Communicating hydrocephalus due to excessive cerebrospinal fluid formation (choroid plexus papilloma)

tive" hydrocephalus needs qualification or revision. Since virtually all hydrocephalus is obstructive, designations such as intraventricular obstructive (or noncommunicating) and extraventricular obstructive (or communicating) convey greater meaning and avoid the confusion engendered by terms otherwise commonly used.

Intraventricular obstructive, or noncommunicating, hydrocephalus is most likely to occur because of abnormalities in areas where pathways are narrow, including the aqueduct of Sylvius, the fourth ventricle, or the foramina of Monro. Developmental anomalies, especially of the aqueduct, neoplasms, cystic lesions, aneurysms, and ependymal changes secondary to infection or hemorrhage are the commonest causes of blocks within the ventricular system leading to hydrocephalus.

Extraventricular obstructive hydrocephalus is synonymous with communicating hydrocephalus, an acceptable term that implies free communication of the ventricular system with the cervical subarachnoid space and the region of the basilar cisterns. It indicates that the obstruction is at some point distal to the outlet foramina of the fourth ventricle, usually at the level of the basilar cisterns, or within the arachnoid over the surface of the brain, or at the presumed absorptive site, the arachnoid villi.

The only recognized exception to the rule that hydrocephalus results from obstruction either within or external to the ventricular system occurs with the rare choroid plexus papilloma. Ventricular enlargement in infants with this tumor is attributed to cerebrospinal fluid secretion from the lesion in excess of the system's absorptive capabilities (Matson and Crofton). Although communicating hydrocephalus in patients with choroid plexus papillomas may result from excessive fluid formation in many or even most cases, hemorrhage from the lesion also may cause a basilar or arachnoid villi block, thus adding another causative factor (Laurence et al).

CEREBROSPINAL FLUID PHYSIOLOGY AND ANATOMY

The mechanisms related to cerebrospinal fluid formation and absorption, the factors that influence its direction of flow, and anatomic correlates of these physiological principles have been subjects of intensive investigation for many years. Yet, many of the details of the function of this system remain unknown. One might summarize our current level of knowledge by stating that most authorities agree that cerebrospinal fluid is secreted at least in part, by the choroid plexuses, and that the arachnoid villi are probably important sites of absorption of some of the cerebrospinal fluid into the venous system.

In 1825, Magendie discovered the midline, posterior fossa outlet foramen now known by his name and demonstrated that communication normally exists between the ventricles and the surface subarachnoid spaces. This was confirmed by Luschka in 1855 who added the existence of two lateral foramina through which fluid departed from the fourth ventricle. The classic work of the Swedish investigators Key and Retzius appeared in 1875 and provided a detailed description of the anatomy of the cerebrospinal fluid pathways.

Research published by Lewis Weed in 1917 revealed that in the pig embryo corresponding to the six week human embryo, the fluid-containing ventricular system is still closed posteriorly and is normally distended. At approximately this time in embryonic development, the choroid plexus appears, and by the eighth week, pressure on the fluid filtering through the membranes of the fourth ventricle or rhombic roof produces a complete dissection of the potential subarachnoid spaces and thus, absorptive surfaces. Eventual dissolution of the membranes in the posterior fossa results in a patent system with communication of the fourth ventricle with the cervical and cerebral subarachnoid spaces.

Lack of resorption of the semipermeable membranes of the rhombic roof in embryonic life has been proposed as an explanation for numerous conditions, including congenital hydrocephalus, hydromyelia, and syringomyelia (Gardner). This theory is based on the premise that the central canal of the spinal cord shares progressive distention with the ventricular system if the outlet foramina do not become patent. Dissection of the contained fluid from the central canal into the surrounding spinal cord, resulting in a syrinx and rupture of the neural tube, is presumed to be the pathogenesis of a myelocoele. Gardner suggests that support for this postulate is the high incidence of hydromyelia with either the Dandy-Walker syndrome or myelocoele and also the frequent relationship of any of these disorders with congenital hydrocephalus.

Weed postulated that if permeability of the rhombic membranes does not develop at this critical period in embryonic life, fluid is retained in the ventricular system and the surface subarachnoid spaces are not opened and rendered functional. Thus, even if the outlet foramina in the posterior fossa subsequently become patent, the absorptive surfaces have not formed and communicating hydrocephalus is present. The validity of this postulate remains questionable although in certain situations, especially the Dandy-Walker syndrome, surgical opening of the outlet foramen obstruction may convert noncommunicating hydrocephalus to one of communicating type.

Studies by Milhorat and colleagues (1971) have cast considerable doubt upon previously developed concepts regarding formation of the subarachnoid space in patients with congenital hydrocephalus. These authors have shown that, at least in some cases, occlusion of the aqueduct is associated with a cisternal block demonstrated by isotope cisternography but that reexpansion of the subarachnoid space may follow ventricular drainage. It was therefore proposed that the subarachnoid space is potentially open but mechanically compressed in infants with congenital intraventricular obstructive hydrocephalus. Histologic examination of the brain and meninges of 52 patients with congenital hydrocephalus revealed the subarachnoid space to be present in all even though pathological changes were often evident.

Cerebrospinal Fluid Formation

The site of cerebrospinal fluid formation has intrigued many investigators for years and remains incompletely established. In 1914, Cushing observed the formation of drops of clear fluid on the surface of the choroid plexus in the lateral ventricles during surgical exposure. Dandy (1919) found that surgical occlusion of one foramen of Monro causes distention of the lateral ventricle on the same side if the choroid plexus remains intact. Schaltenbrand and Putman added further evidence of the role of the choroid plexus in fluid formation by the intravenous injection of fluorscein, which yielded greenish fluid on the plexus surface. The interpretation of these observations generally was that cerebrospinal fluid was formed by an active secretory process of the choroid plexus.

All investigators did not agree with these conclusions, however, and evidence was put forth to oppose the earlier findings. For example, Hassen demonstrated iron pigment granules in the epithelium of the choroid plexus following intraventricular hemorrhage and postulated that plexus function is concerned with removal of certain waste products from the cerebrospinal fluid. The consensus of opinion remains that the choroid plexus is responsbile for part but not all of the cerebrospinal fluid formed within the ventricles. More recent experiments (Bowsher) utilizing radioactive isotope entrance into the cerebrospinal fluid have indicated that different components of the cerebrospinal fluid enter at different rates and by various mechanisms. Certain substances, such as protein and electrolytes, are actively secreted by the choroid plexus while other substances pass by diffusion from plasma into cerebrospinal fluid across membranes, including ependyma. These studies propose that water enters and leaves at many sites and with great rapidity.

Milhorat performed choroid plexectomy on hydrocephalic monkeys and found the composition of the cerebrospinal fluid to be normal after the procedure. Furthermore, only a slight decrease in cerebrospinal fluid production followed the operation, suggesting that the choroid plexus is not the sole or even major source of cerebrospinal fluid. Additional experiments by Milhorat et al. on hydrocephalic children have indicated an absorptive as well as a secretory role of the choroid plexus. Albumin injected into the ventricle was removed considerably slower in patients after choroid plexectomy, possibly a manifestation of the dual function of these structures. The rate of cerebrospinal fluid formation in children has been estimated at approximately 0.35 ml. per minute (500 ml. per day), thus suggesting that the cerebrospinal fluid is renewed about five times per day (Cutler). The rate of formation in hydrocephalic children is only slightly less, approximately 0.30 ml. per minute (Lorenzo et al.).

Cerebrospinal Fluid Absorption

The sites and mechanisms of absorption of cerebrospinal fluid have been even more elusive, and subject to many and varied interpretations. Dandy and Blackfan, in 1913, studied absorption using phenolsulfonphthalein dye and formed the opinion that absorption occurs through veins of the subarachnoid space. Dandy (1921) later estimated that approximately 75 to 80 per cent of the cerebrospinal fluid is absorbed from the cranial subarachnoid spaces. Cooper has placed greater emphasis on the absorptive capabilities of the spinal subarachnoid pathways than have other investigators. In 1914, Weed developed the concept that absorption occurs through the arachnoid villi into the venous system intracranially, and to a lesser degree into lymphatic vessels in the spinal region.

In 1960, Bowsher summarized the data available to that time which stated that absorption occurs in many regions, including across the ependyma within the ventricles, via arachnoid villi into venous channels, and through spinal perineural spaces into lymphatic vessels. An eloquent study of the arachnoid villus by Welch and Friedman has revealed this valvular structure to be a labyrinth of small tubes that communicate with the subarachnoid space and the venous channels of the dura. The tubes open when pressure of the cerebrospinal fluid is greater than that of the venous blood. The reverse pressure relationship causes effacement of the villus in a valvular fashion, thereby preventing reflux of blood into the subarachnoid space under conditions of low spinal fluid pressure.

ETIOLOGIC AND PATHOLOGICAL CONSIDERATIONS

In a significant number of hydrocephalic infants and children lesions are identified that account for the condition even though the cause is unknown. For example, neoplasms within the posterior fossa or of the choroid plexus, arachnoid cysts, or aneurysms of the vein of Galen produce hydrocephalus by obvious mechanisms, although the etiology of the primary abnormality is not explainable. A posterior fossa subdural hematoma in the newborn results in fourth ventricle obstruction by compression and originates from hemorrhage secondary to head trauma. Likewise, acquired hydrocephalus usually of the communicating type, frequently is etiologically related to a preceding subarachnoid hemorrhage (Fig. 8-1) or meningeal infec-

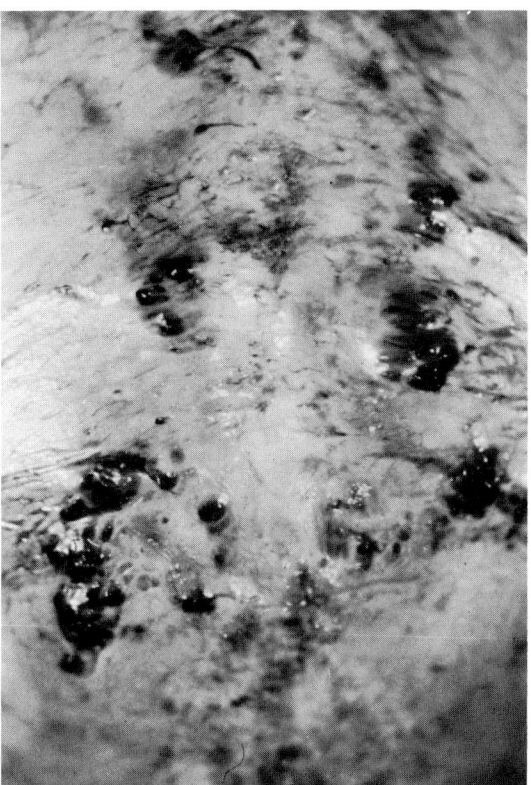

Figure 8-1. Blood in arachnoid villi on internal surface of the skull in a child following subarachnoid hemorrhage. Mechanical obstruction to cerebrospinal fluid absorption at this level may result in temporary or permanent communicating hydrocephalus.

tion. Intracranial bleeding may accompany birth trauma or be delayed for several days after perinatal hypoxia (Lourie and Berne). In either instance, block at the level of the basilar cisterns can lead to communicating hydrocephalus.

By far the most common type of congenital hydrocephalus is that associated with other major anomalies, including meningomyelocoele and encephalocoele (Fig. 8-2). Among 558 infants with hydrocephalus reviewed by Lorber and Bassi, 478 had spina bifida cystica. Of the remainder, 67 with congenital hydrocephalus had no obvious cause and 41 were infants with *acquired* hydrocephalus secondary to hemorrhage or meningitis early in infancy.

Hydrocephalus associated with meningomyelocoele is usually due to aqueductal obstruction, although some are of the communicating type with disturbance of subarachnoid flow secondary to the Arnold-Chiari malformation. Lorber (1961) found that 80 per cent of newborn infants with

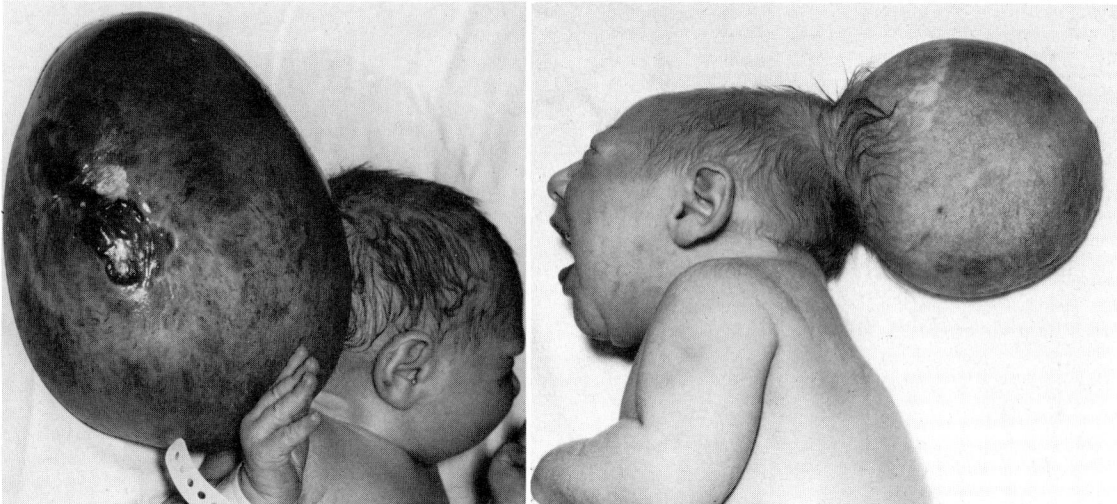

Figure 8–2. Two infants in the newborn period with hydrocephalus and large encephalocoeles. Malformed, gliotic brain tissue containing enlarged ventricles is usually present in lesions of this size.

meningomyelocoeles had associated hydrocephalus. Infants with lumbar myelocoeles with paraplegia had a 96 per cent incidence of hydrocephalus. Hydrocephalus was usually demonstrable in the newborn period, and surgical repair of the meningomyelocoele did not appear to influence the development or progression of hydrocephalus. In many babies in this series, Lorber demonstrated the presence of hydrocephalus even though the head circumference was normal.

Excluding the foregoing categories of hydrocephalus secondary to an obvious compressive lesion, the etiology of many cases of congenital hydrocephalus and those appearing in early infancy remains unidentified. Infections, including toxoplasmosis, cytomegalovirus disease, and syphilis, account for congenital hydrocephalus in a relatively small proportion of cases. Another small percentage of infants with hydrocephalus due to aqueductal stenosis inherit the disease as a sex-linked recessive trait (Bickers and Adams, Edwards et al., Edwards, Needleman and Root, Warren et al.). Except for the clustering of males within a family and the occasional maldevelopment of thumbs (Edwards, Warren et al.), this form of hydrocephalus is not distinguishable from many other types in the neonate. Genetic factors in congenital hydrocephalus otherwise remain speculative.

Among siblings of patients with primary congenital hydrocephalus without spinal defects, the incidence of anencephaly and spina bifida cystica has been estimated to be five times greater than expected in the general population (Lorber and De). The empirical risk of a major congenital malformation in subsequent offspring following birth of a child with congenital hydrocephalus is approximately 1 in 25 (Lorber and De).

Aqueductal Lesions

The most common site of intraventricular obstruction in infants with congenital hydrocephalus is within the aqueduct. The underlying pathology may be one of several types, which in most instances are separable only by histologic examination. Forking (atresia) of the aqueduct consists of a nonpatent system in which the aqueduct at various levels consists of multiple channels lined by ependyma that may or may not communicate with one another and are separated by fairly normal neural tissue (Fig. 8-3). This lesion may occur as an isolated abnormality causing hydrocephalus or may be associated with other nervous system anomalies, especially meningomyelocoele and the Arnold-Chiari malformation.

Stenosis of the aqueduct was described by Russell as an aqueduct that is histologically normal but abnormally small in caliber. There is no excessive subependymal glia or other evidence of an inflammatory reaction. Little is known of the origin of this lesion. It may represent a form of hydrocephalus that is slowly progressive or may even remain silent until later in childhood (Fig. 8-4). Aqueductal stenosis has been assumed to be

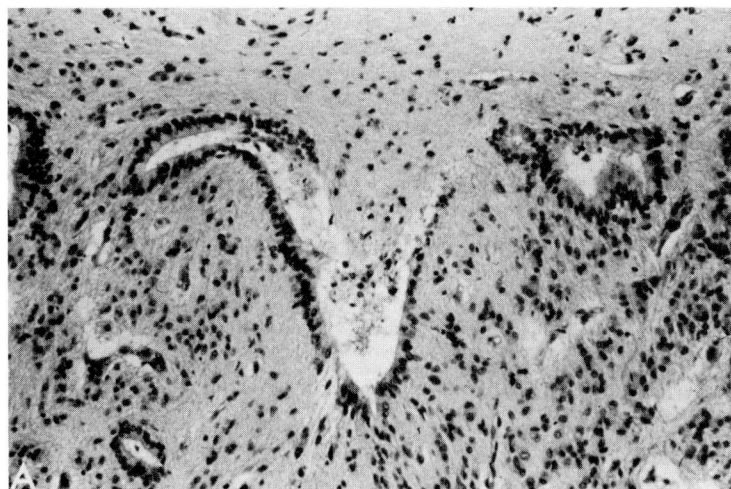
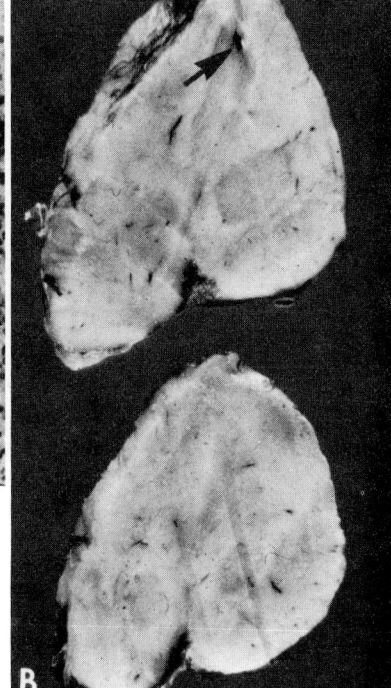

Figure 8–3. Congenital aqueductal occlusion. *A*, The aqueductal configuration is grossly disorganized with multiple, poorly formed channels. A mass of gliosis protrudes into the lumen of the central channel. *B*, Sections through the mesencephalon at different levels illustrate the patent but stenotic aqueduct above (arrow) but no identifiable aqueduct below.

an unusual cause of hydrocephalus (Russell, Laurence).

The origin of gliosis of the aqueduct also has defied explanation and it may result in hydrocephalus in older children and even adults. The aqueduct is narrowed or occluded by overgrowth of subependymal glia while the ependymal lining may be replaced by gliosis. No definite relation to preceding infection has been established in such cases. Laurence (1959) mentioned four patients with gliosis of the aqueduct associated with neurofibromatosis. Drachman and Richardson described one child in whom gliosis and forking of the aqueduct were found at different levels.

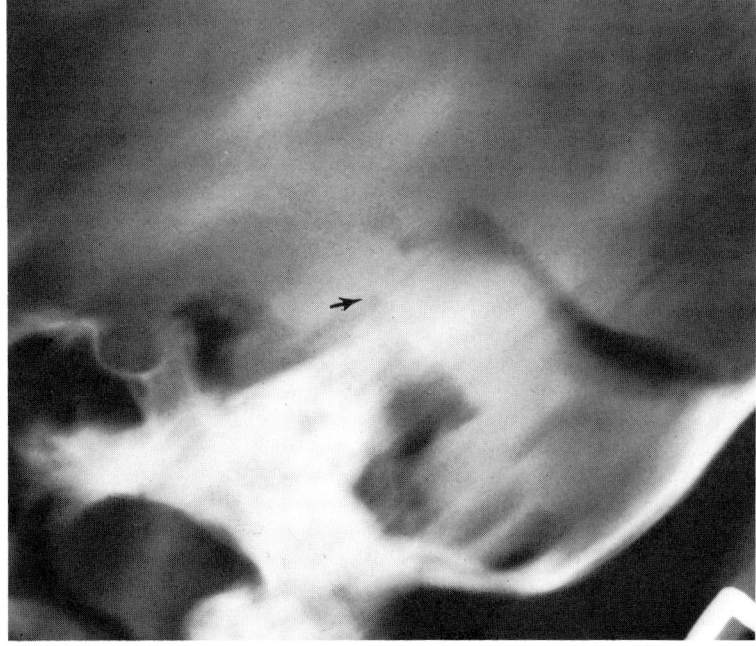

Figure 8–4. Aqueductal stenosis or membrane. Twelve-year-old girl was well until three months before admission when she developed recurrent headaches and vomiting. Bilateral papilledema was present and head circumference was normal for her age. Pneumoencephalogram demonstrates a normal fourth ventricle but obstruction at the junction of the fourth ventricle and the aqueduct (arrow). A subsequent ventriculogram showed dilated ventricles with obstruction of the distal aqueduct, at approximately the same level noted on the pneumoencephalogram. Symptoms were completely relieved following a ventriculoatrial shunt.

Another rare obstructive lesion of the aqueduct is a neuroglial septum. Russell reviewed the previously described cases with septum formation and suggested several possible etiologic theories.

Of considerable interest in regard to the aqueductal lesions already described is the recent discovery of experimental viral infections as a cause of structural abnormalities of the aqueduct. Intracerebral injection of polyoma virus in rodents has produced hydrocephalus but with a marked inflammatory reaction unlike the aqueductal lesions presumed to be maldevelopments (Li and Jahnes, Holtz et al.).

Experimental hydrocephalus has been produced in suckling hamsters by the inoculation with reovirus type I (Margolis and Kilham). Hydrocephalus due to aqueductal stenosis without inflammatory changes was induced in hamsters by intracerebral injection of mumps virus (Johnson and Johnson). Fluorescent antibody staining indicated that virus growth was limited to the ependymal cells in these animals.

Timmons and Johnson subsequently described a child with mumps encephalitis followed by recovery but with manifestations of hydrocephalus developing almost two years later. Narrowing of the aqueduct was demonstrated by air encephalography and was presumed to be a sequela of the previous viral illness. Findings such as these suggest the possibility of intrauterine viral infections as a cause of some cases of congenital hydrocephalus with aqueductal occlusion.

White Matter Alterations

Regardless of the site of obstruction, progressive hydrocephalus is associated with progressive attenuation of the cerebral white matter. Alterations of the white matter long precede cerebral cortical changes, probably explaining the relative preservation of intellect despite even enormous dilatation of the lateral ventricles. The relative sparing of the cerebral cortex and deep nuclear gray matter in contrast to the rapid loss of white matter has been attributed to the plentiful blood supply to the more metabolically active gray matter (Bowsher).

The concept that ventricular enlargement and thinning of white matter is simply due to back pressure of blocked cerebrospinal fluid circulation was challenged by Bering. He concluded that ventricular enlargement is caused by an undampened arterial pulse wave originating from the choroid plexus. Wilson and Bertan supported this view with experiments in which they ligated the anterior choroidal artery, the major arterial supply to the choroid plexus. This reduced the amplitude of the ventricular cerebrospinal fluid pulse in the ventricle on the side that had been operated on, while the mean pressures remained the same within the two ventricles. Reduction in size of the ventricle on the side with the diminished pulsatile activity suggested the causative effects of choroid plexus pulsation to these investigators also.

Changes of the cerebral white matter that occur as the ventricles enlarge have aroused great interest because if hydrocephalus can be corrected, considerable reconstruction of the thinned cerebral mantle can occur. Fishman and Greer created hydrocephalus in dogs by the intracisternal injection of kaolin and studied the effects on the cerebral cortex and white matter. Water and electrolyte composition of the hydrocephalic cerebral cortex was not altered but the white matter had increased water, sodium, and chloride content despite its reduction in volume. There was a significant loss of lipid and protein from the white matter.

Milhorat et al. (1970) produced acute hydrocephalus in monkeys by using an inflatable balloon in the fourth ventricle and demonstrated that marked ventricular enlargement occurred within six hours after obstruction was produced. The frontal horns dilated intially and by 24 hours the aqueduct also was enlarged. The rate of ventricular distention was precipitous during the first six hours, but thereafter the rate abruptly decreased. Ependymal disruption and tears were found at the angles of the frontal horns, which permitted migration of ventricular fluid to penetrate the periventricular tissues. These investigators surmised that the cessation of rapid ventricular enlargement after six hours depended upon the compromised integrity of the ventricular surface.

Further evidence of the disturbed ependymal barrier in hydrocephalic subjects is the rapid migration into brain tissue of radioisotope injected directly into the ventricle (Milhorat and Hammock). Escape of cerebrospinal fluid into adjacent brain tissue partially compensates the system with fluid being absorbed after its penetration through the ependymal tears. Thus, the increased water content in hydrocephalic white matter observed by Fishman and Greer may have represented flow of ventricular fluid into the brain substance.

CLINICAL ASPECTS OF HYDROCEPHALUS

Symptoms and signs observed in patients with hydrocephalus vary with the age of the child, the acuteness of onset, and the rapidity of progression. Complete ventricular obstruction with abrupt onset may result in a precipitous deterioration of the state of awareness and responsiveness plus other signs of increased pressure. Recognition of acute ventricular dilatation as the cause of the patient's worsening condition may be obscured by the primary illness that caused it, such as meningitis, subarachnoid hemorrhage, or hemorrhage into a posterior fossa tumor (Milhorat, 1970).

Children with acquired disorders that cause progressive hydrocephalus of a more insidious nature exhibit the usual symptoms of headaches, nausea, vomiting, and diplopia if lateral rectus paresis occurs. In a previously normal older child with hydrocephalus of recent onset, posterior fossa tumor is the most common explanation, but aqueductal stenosis may rarely present in the same fashion. The latter diagnosis is a difficult one requiring detailed air studies, usually from both above and below.

Very slowly progressive hydrocephalus in children and adults may remain occult from the standpoint of increased pressure manifestations and is discussed under the title of normal pressure hydrocephalus. In such patients, clinical progression may be evidenced by deteriorating mental capabilities, disturbances of coordination, and primary optic atrophy with its attendant loss of vision.

In the newborn period and in early infancy, there is a wide variation of clinical manifestations, depending in part on the rapidity of progression of the illness. Occasionally, the head of the hydrocephalic infant is so large at term that normal birth is impossible unless the head is decompressed by insertion of a needle into the ventricle. Most authorities believe that birth by cesarean section is not justified because of dystocia due to fetal head enlargement.

As a generalization, infants with intraventricular obstructive hydrocephalus show more rapid progression of head enlargement and other clinical signs than do those with communicating hydrocephalus. In some instances, the baby may show no abnormalities of behavior, feeds well, and progresses adequately regarding motor skills with the only clue of a medical problem being the abnormality rapid rate of growth of the head. More often, the infant with congenital hydrocephalus is irritable, feeds poorly, has recurrent vomiting, and shows inadequate weight gain. Seizures in infants with hydrocephalus are not common and papilledema is infrequent, even in those with marked head enlargement. If the condition proceeds unarrested, optic atrophy may eventually develop.

Developmental motor skills are occasionally delayed but some hydrocephalic infants progress in a remarkably normal fashion during the first year. Mild hydrocephalus does not account for profound developmental delay by 6 to 12 months of age unless the retardation is due to the disorder that caused the hydrocephalus. As hydrocephalus progresses, the disproportion between the size of the head and the facial structures becomes more apparent. Distention of scalp veins and enlargement and bulging of the anterior fontanel reflect elevated intracranial pressure.

Increased muscle tone and hyperreflexia in the lower limbs has been attributed to stretching of fibers arising in the parasagittal area, which must project around the angle of the lateral ventricle to enter the internal capsule enroute to supply the legs (Yakovlev). These fibers would be affected earlier with progressive ventricular enlargement than would the descending fibers to the upper limbs, which arise more laterally on the motor strip.

Late signs in hydrocephalic infants include distortion of the orbital structures causing the "setting sun" sign (Fig. 8-5) and the "cerebral cry" characterized by its brevity and high-pitched, shrill quality. A variety of ocular signs can occur in the infant with congenital hydrocephalus, although lack of cooperation and irritability make analysis difficult. Internal strabismus is occasionally observed and limited vertical gaze may be present. Horizontal nystagmus also may be evident. Smith et al. described cortical blindness in older children with congenital hydrocephalus, all of whom had had multiple shunt procedures, perhaps with occipital lobe injury.

Rare or unusual manifestations of hydrocephalus include a variety of endocrine disturbances and metabolic abnormalities. It is surprising that clinical evidence of hypothala-

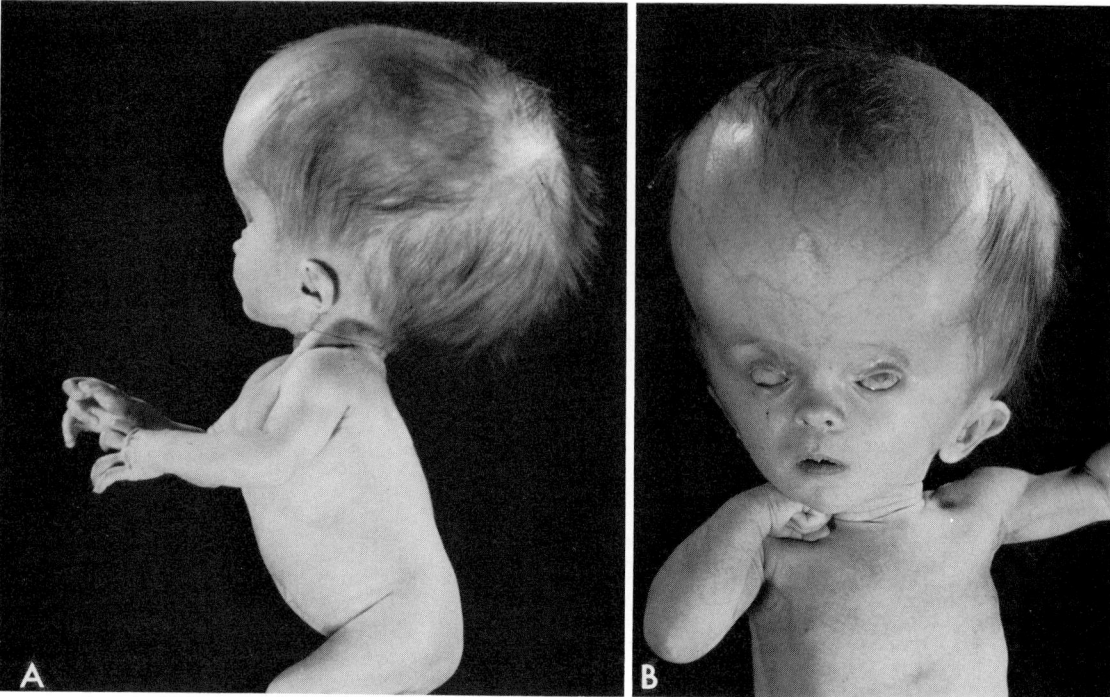

Figure 8–5. Advanced hydrocephalus present at birth and secondary to atresia of the aqueduct. *A*, Lateral view reveals striking disproportion between size of the head and that of the body. *B*, The skin of the scalp is thinned and stretched, and superficial veins are prominent. Note the profound depression of the orbital contents referred to as the "setting sun" sign.

mic dysfunction is not observed more often in advanced infantile hydrocephalus. Third ventricle distention would be expected to disrupt certain hypothalamic pathways or nuclear groups. Precocious puberty (Dorff and Shapiro), diabetes insipidus (Guillame and Roge), and hypopituitarism (Pollock) have only rarely been described as consequences of chronic hydrocephalus but probably have been infrequently sought . Hogan and Woolsey described a child with polydipsia but with normal urine concentrating ability in whom chronic hydrocephalus was due to obstruction of the aqueduct. Conversely, absence of the thirst mechanism has been reported with occult hydrocephalus (Hays et al.). Disturbances of thermoregulation with advanced hydrocephalus are additional manifestations of hypothalamic dysfunction.

Another rare manifestation of hydrocephalus due to aqueductal stenosis described by Nellhaus is a rhythmic to-and-fro bobbing of the head referred to as the "bobble-head doll syndrome." This peculiar movement disorder has also been observed in children with hydrocephalus secondary to a cyst within the third ventricle (Benton et al.).

An equally strange disorder that has been described in children with hydrocephalus with meningomyelocoele is severe stridor with laryngeal palsy (Kirsch et al., Morley, Fitzsimmons, Adeloye et al.). Stridor has usually occurred several weeks or months after birth in these patients, and in some it seemed to correspond to the development of increased pressure secondary to hydrocephalus. In certain cases, marked improvement followed the reduction of intracranial pressure by shunt procedures (Adeloye et al., Kirsch et al.), although this has not occurred in others. Kirsch and colleagues performed suboccipital craniectomies on two patients with stridor with rapid improvement following the decompression.

The cause of respiratory obstruction in these cases has not been clarified and several postulates have been proposed. Caudal displacement of the medulla with traction on the vagus nerve has been suggested as well as "coning" of the medulla with pressure at the foramen magnum. Morley described two patients with severe stridor in which localized medullary hemorrhages were found at autopsy.

DIFFERENTIAL DIAGNOSIS

Differential diagnostic considerations are especially important in the newborn and young infant because the possible spectrum of causes of abnormal head enlargement tends to be more complex in this age group. The older child with acquired hydrocephalus usually either has an obvious explanatory cause, such as preceding meningeal infection or hemorrhage, or is expected to have developed an obstructive lesion within or adjacent to the ventricular system.

The prematurely born infant is often erroneously considered to be hydrocephalic because of the normal rapid rate of head growth frequently observed in the first two weeks and the usual disproportion between head and body size. The mean head circumference of the 1500- to 2000-gram infant at birth is 30 cm. (Ylppö). Occasionally, within ten days after birth, growth plus correction of molding acquired during the labor process result in head enlargement of 1.5 to 2 cm. Overinterpretation of the significance of these findings in premature babies can be tempered by watchful observation and attention to the anterior fontanel.

Mass Lesions

Two important principles to be remembered are that all infants with abnormally large heads do not have hydrocephalus and that all infants with hydrocephalus need not have congenital anomalies as the cause. The later in infancy the abnormal head enlargement develops, the more likely is the second premise.

Intraventricular and posterior fossa tumors may bear close resemblance to the more common infantile hydrocephalus, and often can be distinguished only by adequate contrast studies. This is also true of arachnoid cysts which may be located in various intracranial positions causing head enlargement because of the space they occupy or because of ventricular obstruction (Kruyff, Anderson and Landing). An aneurysm of the vein of Galen may obstruct the aqueduct in the newborn or young infant, resulting in hydrocephalus resembling that due to more common causes (Fig. 8-6). A loud cranial bruit or high-output cardiac failure is characteristic of this lesion, which is demonstrable by angiography.

Infants with subdural hematomas may masquerade as hydrocephalus with few signs evident except for irritability, vomiting, and abnormal enlargement of the head. A history of convulsions or the presence of anemia may be a clue to the presence of subdural collections of blood but positive identification depends upon transfontanel subdural taps. A posterior fossa subdural hematoma in the newborn results in abrupt head enlargement because of fourth ventricle obstruction (Carter and Pittman). This lesion is usually fatal unless surgical evacuation can be performed, and air ventriculography is required for its detection. Communicating hydrocephalus frequently develops in patients who survive and requires a shunt procedure.

Megalencephaly

Megalencephaly has been variously described and defined, but descriptively refers to a brain of abnormally excessive weight (Laurence, 1964). Brains of excessive weight may occur as a congenital malformation otherwise unrecognized as a syndrome, as a component of identifiable conditions such as achondroplasia or cerebral gigantism, or with certain degenerative diseases, including Tay-Sachs disease, Canavan's spongy degeneration, or Alexander's disease. Because head size is related to brain size, children with megalencephaly are often considered to have hydrocephalus until air studies are done.

Excessive brain weight does not necessarily correlate with functional or intellectual abnormalities. Lord Byron's brain weighed 1807 grams and that of Bismarck weighed 1790 grams (Laurence, 1964). Children with megalencephaly, however, often have severe developmental and intellectual retardation in addition to seizures and other neurologic signs. The lateral ventricles are normal or only slightly dilated while other anomalies may include absence of the corpus callosum, excessive gliosis, subcortical heterotopias and disturbances of the gyral pattern. Syringomyelia has been noted in certain cases (Benda, Dyggve and Tygstrup). On rare occasion, the cerebral enlargement may be unilateral (Laurence, 1964).

Megalencephaly may occur as a familial trait (Riley and Smith) and may not be associated with other defects in such persons. Unless recognized by the familial aggregation, megalencephaly as previously described

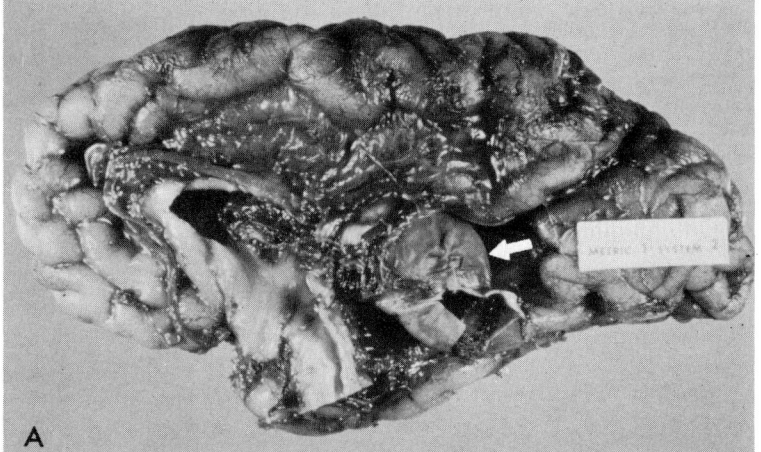

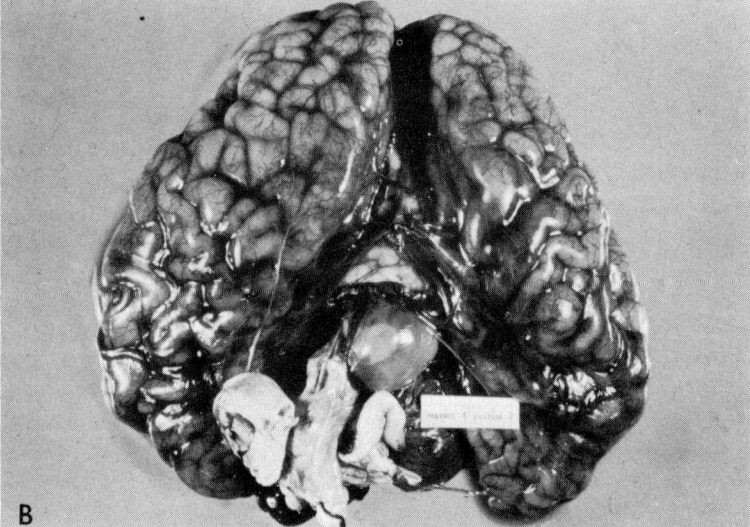

Figure 8-6. Aneurysm of the vein of Galen. *A*, Aneurysm (arrow) is located in the midline, posterior to the brain stem, resulting in hydrocephalus by compression of the aqueduct. Numerous dilated vessels are evident on the medial surface of the cerebral hemisphere anterior and superior to the lesion. *B*, View of the aneurysm from its posterior surface by spreading the occipital lobes laterally.

can usually be differentiated from hydrocephalus only by air encephalography. Isotope encephalography may also be useful in this regard.

Achondroplasia

The head usually appears disproportionally large in comparison to the trunk in achondroplastic children (Fig. 8-7). The reason is speculative and in some cases may be due to a combination of factors. Dennis et al. studied the brains of five children with achondroplasia and attributed head enlargement to megalencephaly. Cohen et al. reviewed 15 such children, 13 of whom had head circumferences exceeding the ninety-seventh percentile for age. Eight of these children had air encephalograms, all revealing ventricular dilatation. Two patients in this series required ventriculoatrial shunts because of evidence of progressive hydrocephalus.

Skull x-rays in achondroplasia reveal a large calvarium and a constricted skull base. The frontal region is prominent and sutures are generally not separated to an abnormal degree. Retardation of cartilagenous growth at the base of the cranium results in an increased vertical diameter and the characteristic brachycephalic configuration of the achondroplastic skull.

Although the head is larger than normal in circumference, the curve of head growth in infancy parallels that of the normal child unless hydrocephalus is present. Despite the large head size, the anterior fontanel is soft, intellect is usually normal, and signs of increased intracranial pressure are generally

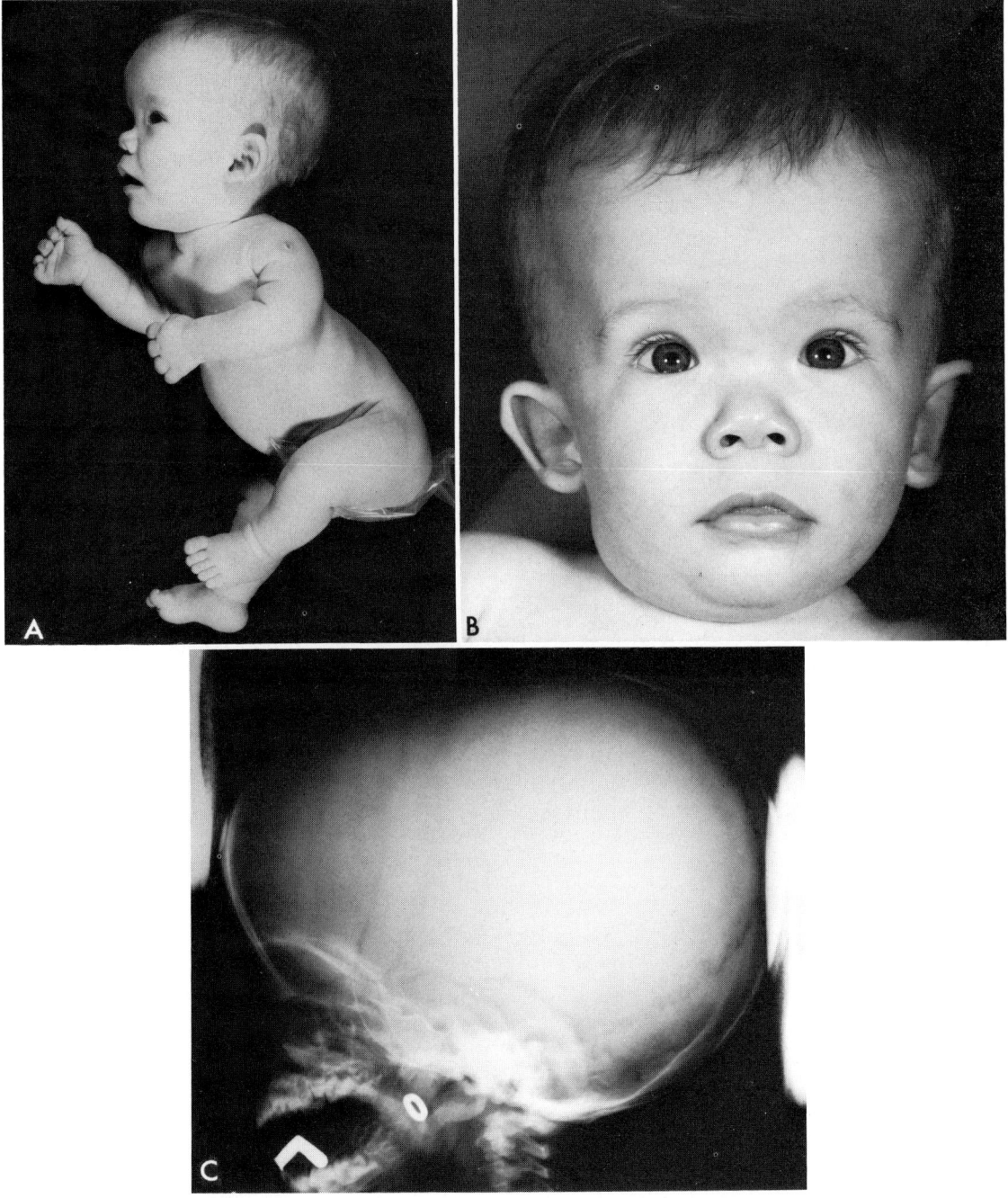

Figure 8–7. Achondroplasia with megalencephaly. Nine-month-old child with head circumference of 49 cm. Anterior fontanel was soft and developmental skills normal for age. *A*, Extremities are short in comparison to the trunk and the head is disproportionately large with a dolicocephalic shape. The fingers are short and stubby and the hand is broad. *B*, The forehead is prominent and the bridge of the nose is flattened. *C*, Lateral skull x-rays show large calvarium but without suture spread or digital impressions. The sella is elongated but the base of the skull is shortened.

absent. In the small percentage of patients who develop progressive hydrocephalus, obstruction to cerebrospinal fluid flow at the level of the constricted foramen magnum is the most plausible explanation.

Skeletal Disorders

An additional form of dwarfism associated with large head size in comparison to the remainder of the body is referred to as the Russell dwarf (Szalay, Holden, Fuleihan et al, Russell). Infants with this syndrome are born with a low birth weight but of term gestation. The upper limbs are disproportionately short and other minor anomalies are usually present.

The abnormally large appearance of the head is due in part to the poorly developed facial structures, which remain abnormally small. The head circumference is approximately normal for the usual term infant. The anterior fontanel remains open longer than normal but is soft and without other manifestations of increased pressure. Intellect has been normal in most reported cases.

Other skeletal disorders in which head size is abnormally large include Hurler's disease, familial osteoectasia (Bakwin et al.), cleidocranial dysostosis (Forland, Keats), osteopetrosis (Johnson et al.), and pycnodysostosis (Elmore, Maroteaux and Lamy). These conditions are usually recognized by the identification of characteristic physical signs and confirmed by appropriate radiologic examinations.

Cerebral Gigantism

Infants and young children with the syndrome referred to as cerebral gigantism may also be erroneously assumed to have hydrocephalus because of the large size and rapid growth rate of the head. This syndrome was described in 1964 by Sotos et al. who suggested derangement of hypothalamic function as the cause of excessive growth. While cerebral dysfunction is present in children with this disorder, no consistent abnormality of growth hormone or other hypothalamic factors has been identified (Bejar et al., Hook et al.).

The birth weight of these patients is usually greater than average and somatic growth is excessively rapid in the first few years of life (Ott and Robinson). Skeletal maturation likewise, is accelerated. Facial characteristics include hypertelorism, depressed nasal bridge, a downward slant to the eyes, high arched palate, and prominence of the mandible (Fig. 8-8). The hands and feet are frequently enlarged. The head is dolicocephalic and, even at birth, is larger than average in circumference.

Cases in which pneumoencephalography has been done have shown mildly dilated lateral ventricles, and occasionally, a disproportionately large third ventricle (Milunsky et al). The evidence available to date suggests that these findings reflect an abnormally large brain with generous sized ventricles and not communicating hydrocephalus. Mental dullness is characteristic of these children, who also may exhibit hyperactivity, poor coordination, and seizures. The facial configuration and the excessive growth rate are the most important diagnostic features.

Degenerative Diseases

Abnormal enlargement of the head may occur in certain degenerative brain diseases in infancy, usually because of expansion of the brain rather than hydrocephalus. Excessive head size has been commonly observed in Canavan's disease, or spongy degeneration, although it is not invariable. In the original case reported by Canavan in 1931, the brain weight at autopsy was 1890 grams.

Alexander's disease (Alexander), a type of leukodystrophy with eosinophilic deposits in astrocytic cytoplasm (Schochet et al.), is also frequently associated with abnormal head enlargement. While the brain may be excessive in weight at postmortem examination (Sherwin and Berthrong), the ventricles also may be enlarged. Whether an extraventricular obstructive factor is related to ventricular distention in these cases remains unestablished. Children with Tay-Sachs disease may develop megalencephaly if they survive into the second year of life. Volk has attributed the increased bulk of the brain in the later stages of this disease to profound astrogliosis that accompanies neuronal degeneration.

Meningeal Infiltration

On rare occasion, neuroblastoma may spread to the dural surfaces, producing symptoms of increased pressure and head

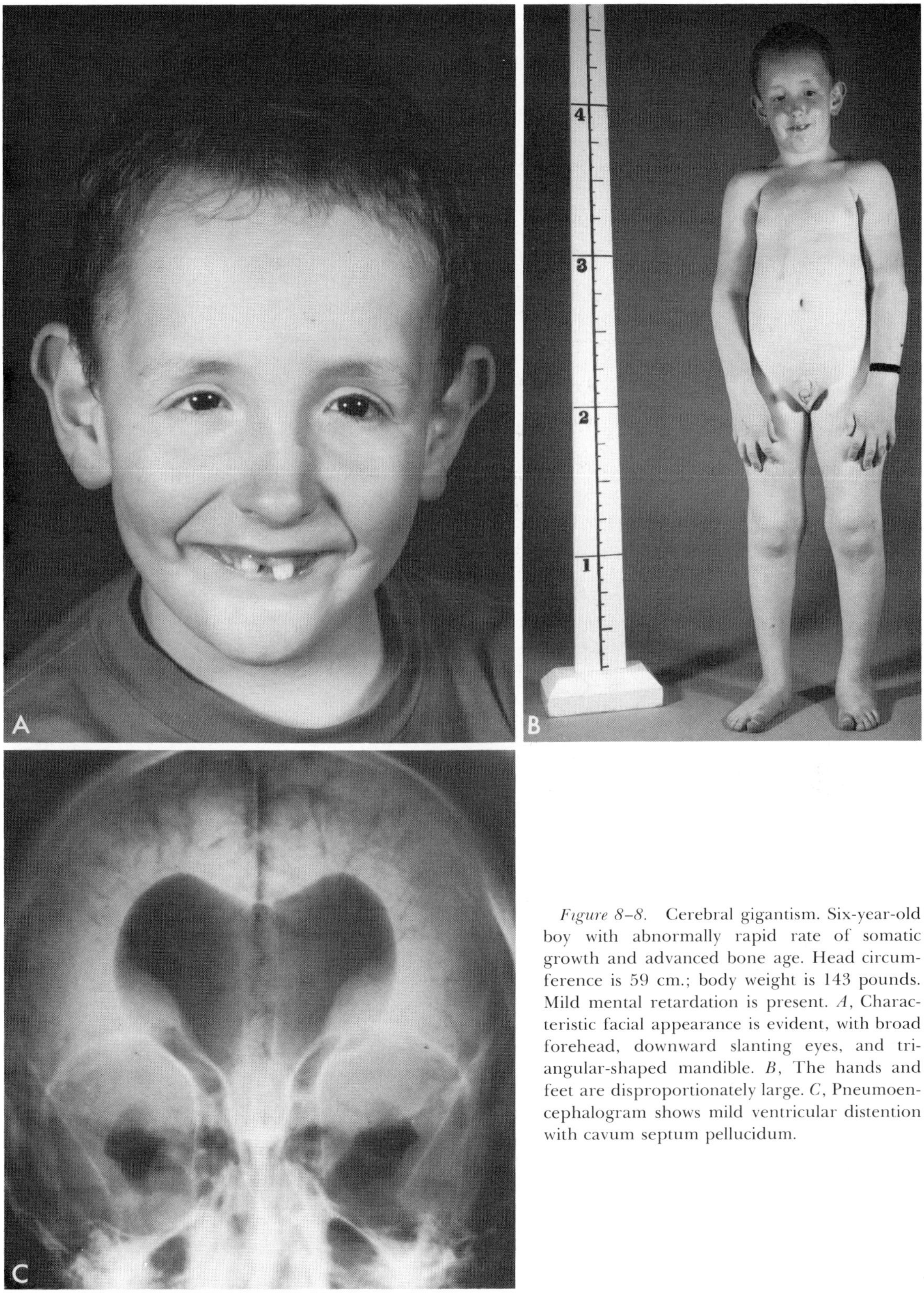

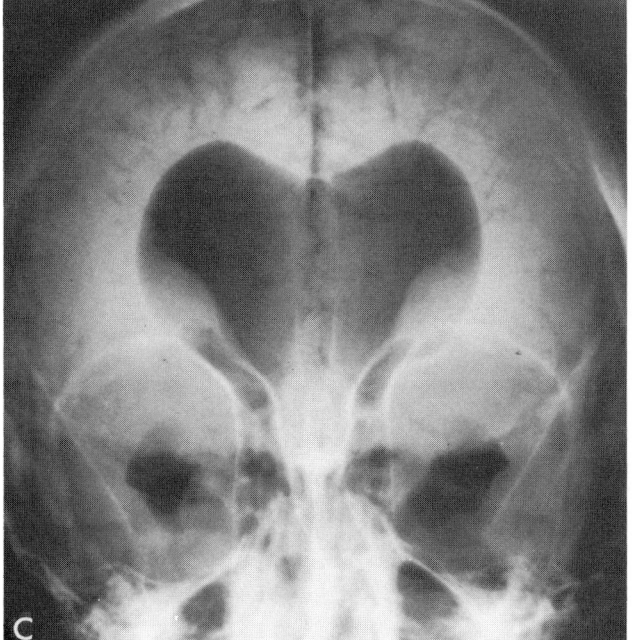

Figure 8–8. Cerebral gigantism. Six-year-old boy with abnormally rapid rate of somatic growth and advanced bone age. Head circumference is 59 cm.; body weight is 143 pounds. Mild mental retardation is present. *A*, Characteristic facial appearance is evident, with broad forehead, downward slanting eyes, and triangular-shaped mandible. *B*, The hands and feet are disproportionately large. *C*, Pneumoencephalogram shows mild ventricular distention with cavum septum pellucidum.

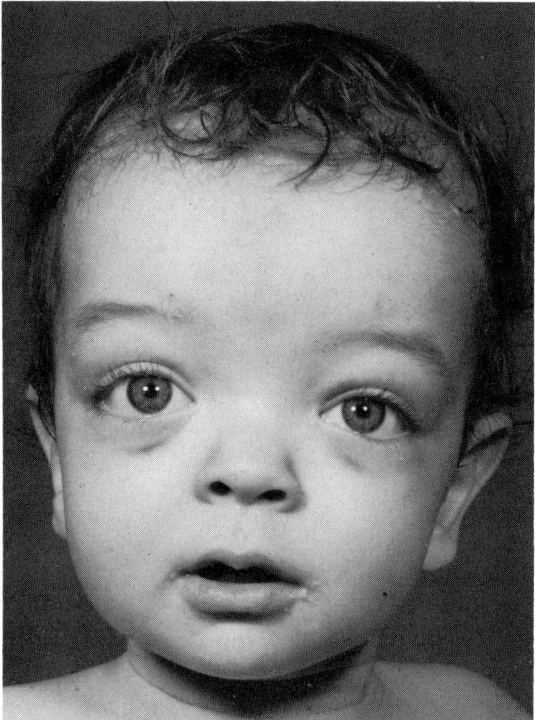

Figure 8-9. Eight-month-old boy referred for evaluation of "hydrocephalus." The child had a two-week illness with irritability and vomiting. Examination revealed head circumference of 50 cm., and tense and bulging fontanel. Edema of the eyelids, ecchymosis of the periorbital soft tissues and sedimentation rate of 108 per hour suggested neoplastic disease. Bone marrow examination revealed tumor cells, and mediastinal neuroblastoma subsequently was identified. Initial symptoms and signs suggestive of hydrocephalus were due to diffuse epidural infiltrates with metastatic neuroblastoma.

enlargement before other signs of the primary lesion become apparent (Fig. 8-9). Hydrocephalus may be erroneously assumed to be present in such cases unless anemia, high sedimentation rate, osteolytic bony lesions, neoplastic cells in the cerebrospinal fluid or an abdominal mass directs one to the true nature of the illness. Communicating hydrocephalus may also develop with other neoplastic diseases in childhood, including leukemic invasion of the meninges and histiocytosis X (Feinberg and Langer). Except in unusual cases, meningeal infiltration represents a relatively late stage of these disorders.

Finally, perhaps the most perplexing differential diagnostic consideration involves the seemingly normal child whose head is only slightly larger than expected for age but is continuing to expand at a greater than normal rate. One faces the dilemma of the undesirable aspects of pneumoencephalography opposed to the concern of permitting possible ventricular enlargement to proceed before recognition.

Many factors must be considered in such cases in order to make a logical decision regarding management. Reexamination at periodic intervals with serial head measurements plotted on a head circumference chart is of greatest help.

DIAGNOSTIC STUDIES

Head Measurement and Transillumination

The most important aspect of physical examination of an infant or young child who has or is believed to have hydrocephalus is accurate measurement of the occipitofrontal circumference of the head. A single measurement is useful and may strongly point to the existence of disease; however, serial determinations at periodic intervals with results plotted on a graph are often of greater value. Rate of change, especially precipitous change, of head size is frequently more informative than the results of any one particular measurement.

Head circumference is conveniently measured with the infant in the supine position. Paper tapes are desirable and steel tapes should be used with caution to avoid lacerations of the struggling infant's scalp or hands. The measurement should be from the most distant point in the occipital region to a point about 1 cm. above the eyebrows. Head circumference can be assumed to reflect intracranial volume reasonably well (Bray et al.) although exceptions occur when the head is

Table 8-2. Approximate Mean Head Circumference in Normal Male Term Infants from Birth to Age 18 Months (females average 1 cm. smaller)

Age	Circumference
Birth	35.0 cm. (± 1.5 cm.)
3 months	41.0 cm. (± 1.5 cm.)
6 months	44.0 cm. (± 1.5 cm.)
9 months	46.0 cm. (± 1.5 cm.)
12 months	47.0 cm. (± 1.5 cm.)
18 months	48.5 cm. (± 1.5 cm.)

markedly anomalous in shape. The significance of the head circumference, preferably recorded in centimeters, is judged in relation to many factors, including age of the child, birth weight, height and weight measurements, and the mean and standard deviation of head size expected from studies of normal children (Illingworth and Lutz, Nellhaus, O'Neill) (Fig. 8-10). Charts of normal head circumference are given in Figure 8-10.

From birth until the age of 12 months, the mean increment in head size is approximately 12 cm. The often quoted rule of expected enlargement of 1 cm. per month, however, is not accurate and should be discarded. During the first three months after birth, increments of head circumference of 2 cm. per month commonly occur while from three to six months of age the infant's head enlarges another 3 cm. From 6 to 12 months of age, the growth rate slows because the head normally grows another 3 cm. in circumference during this period. Thus, the most rapid growth rate of the head occurs in the first three months of life, reflecting the rapid growth of the brain during this period. Subsequent enlargement slows progressively, and by two years of age approximately two-thirds of total head growth from birth to adulthood has occurred (Nellhaus).

Transillumination of the skull is an additonal technique that should be performed whenever hydrocephalus is considered (Shurtleff, Mazur). The procedure is performed in a darkened room and the observer should delay until he is adequately adapted to the dark. A three-battery powered flashlight with a soft, rubber adapter permitting sealed contact with the infant's scalp is sufficient. In the normal infant, extension of the glow beyond the rim of the light source does not occur more than 2.5 cm. in the frontal region or beyond 1 cm. in the occipital region (Dodge and Porter). Abnormalities of transillumination in hydrocephalus indicate the cerebral mantle is less than 1 cm. in depth. The procedure is dependent on the relative thinness of the skull, and thus becomes of less value beyond 12 months of age.

In addition to advanced hydrocephalus or "hydranencephaly," abnormal transillumination may be observed in infants with subdural effusions, scalp edema, or porencephaly.

Arachnoid cysts over the convexity of the brain may also be demonstrable by transillumination (Anderson and Landing). The infant with the Dandy-Walker syndrome may exhibit abnormal transillumination adjacent to the dilated fourth ventricle. Caution is necessary in regard to overinterpretation of the findings with small premature babies because of the extreme thinness of the skull overlying the subarachnoid space of such infants (Horner et al.).

Ventricular Taps

Performance of a transfontanel tap of the lateral ventricle as an isolated procedure in an infant with an abnormally large head is usually not indicated, although exceptions do exist. As a general rule, if one is sufficiently concerned to do a ventricular tap, the child probably needs air ventriculography. Repeated needle passage through brain tissue may result in porencephalic cyst-formation at the needle tract site secondary to damage to the parenchyma of the brain (Salmon, Lorber and Emery) (Fig. 8-11).

Rapid head enlargement in the infant of a few weeks of age who appears disproportionately ill may warrant examination of the ventricular fluid to eliminate the possibility of meningitis. Precipitous head growth in the immediate postmeningitic period may be necessarily controlled by periodic ventricular taps, although placement of a ventricle-to-subcutaneous reservoir may provide a better means of ventricular decompression until a permanent shunt can be inserted.

Regardless of the circumstances, ventricular taps should be done by one knowledgeable and skillful at the procedure and under aseptic conditions. During the study, the subdural spaces should be inspected to exclude fluid collections therein as a cause of infantile head enlargement.

Matson has used combined placement of needles in one lateral ventricle and the lumbar subarachnoid space as a method to determine the patency of the system in hydrocephalic infants. With the infant lying on one side, simultaneous pressure measurement would be expected to be equal with communicating hydrocephalus and jugular compression should result in equivalent changes in the two manometers. Although the procedure is of physiological interest, the technical complexity restricts its value considerably.

Others have injected various dyes, such as phenolsulfonphthalein and indigo carmine,

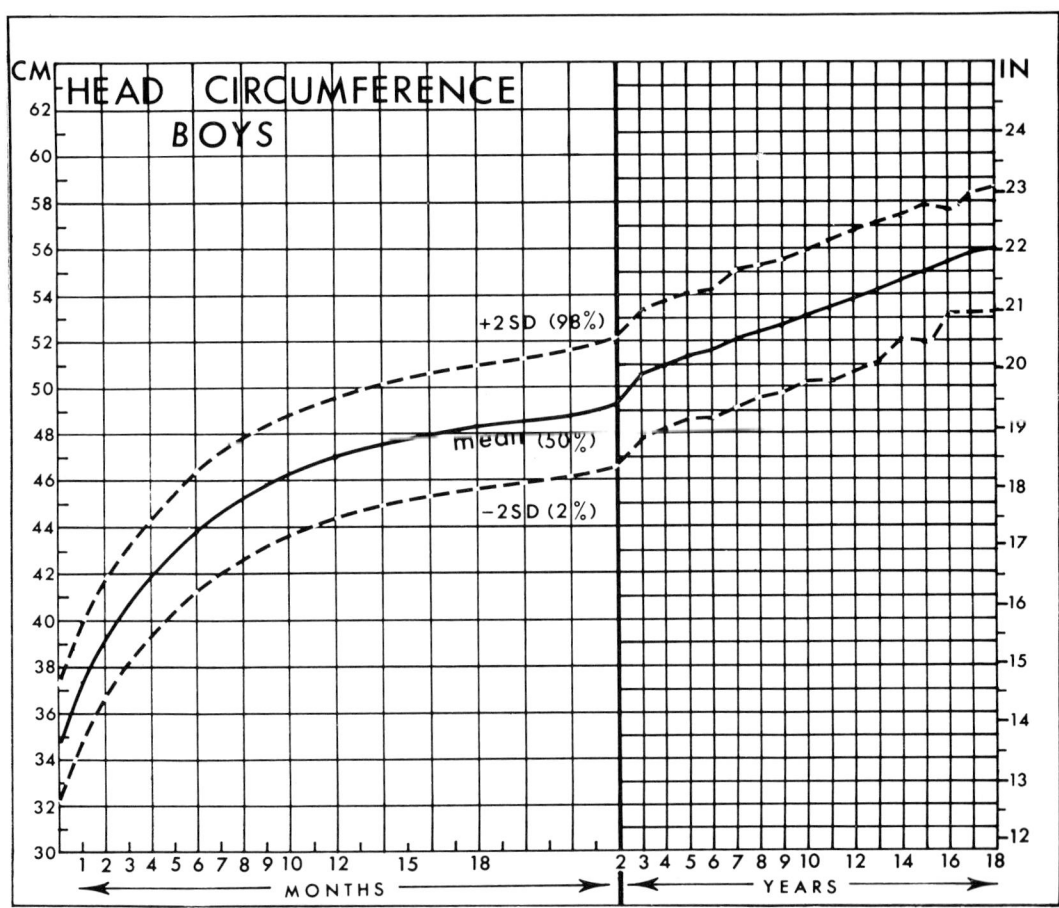

Figure 8-10. Head circumference charts from birth to age 18 years. (By permission of Gerhard Nellhaus, and *Pediatrics*, 41:106–114, 1968.)

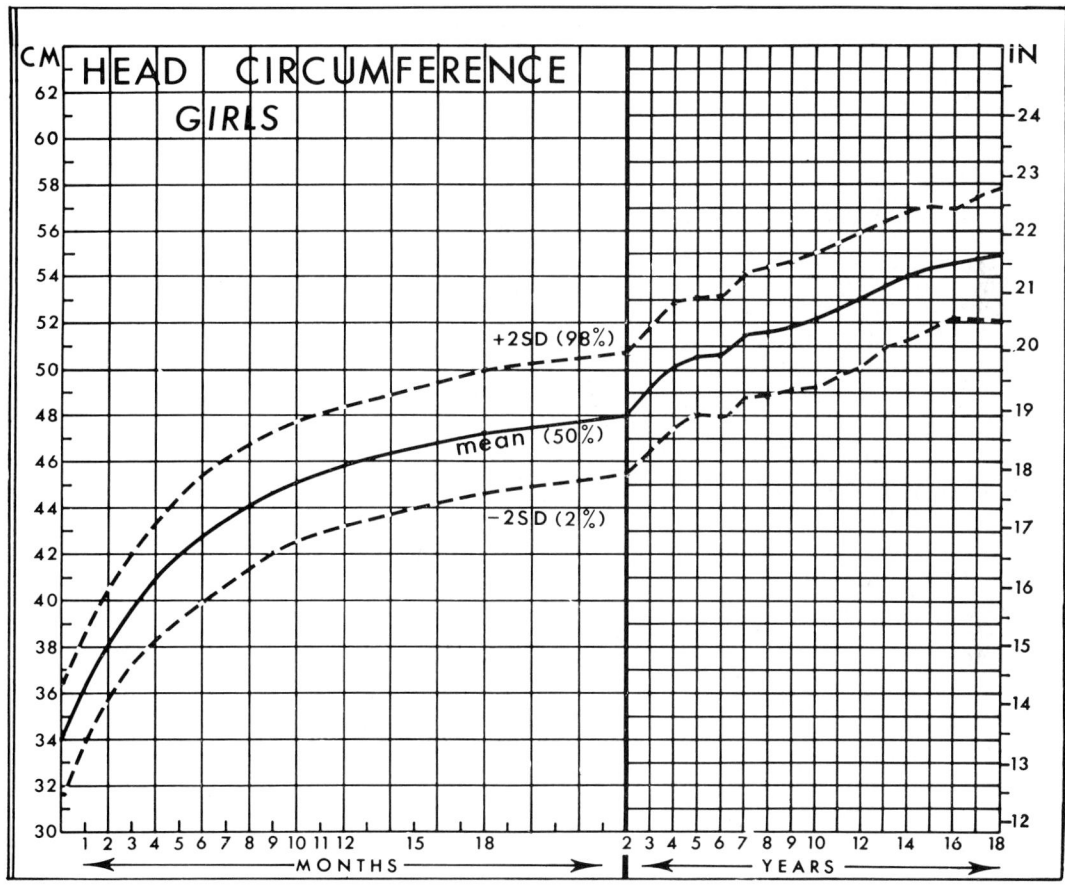

Figure 8–10. Continued.

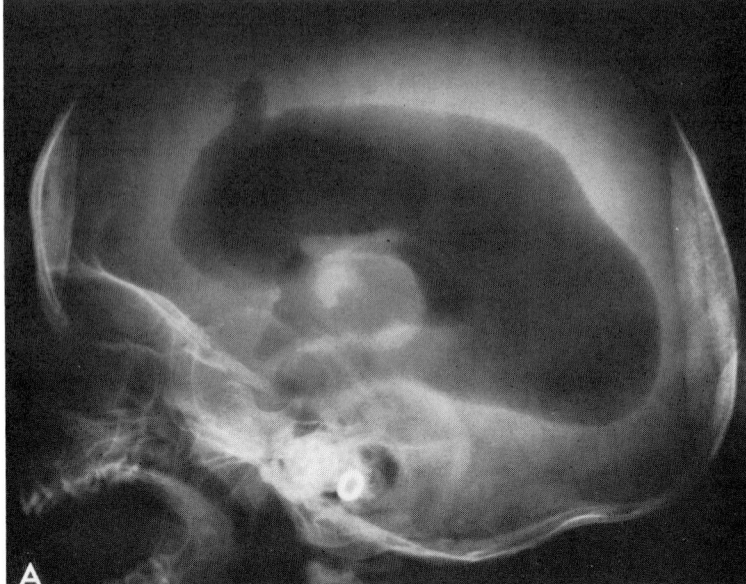
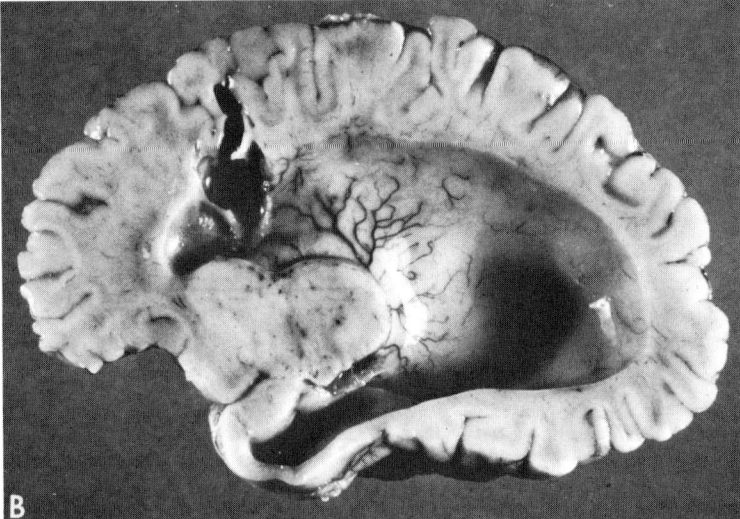

Figure 8-11. Porencephalic lesion secondary to ventricular taps ("puncture" porencephaly). *A*, Ventriculogram in a four-year-old child with hydrocephalus. Several ventricular taps had been done in early infancy. Note the air-filled porencephalic defect communicating with the roof of the anterior horn of the lateral ventricle. *B*, The defect in the white matter, which extends into the distended lateral ventricles, is evident.

into the ventricles as a method of examining the absorption capabilities of the cerebrospinal fluid pathways and the presence or absence of intraventricular obstructive lesions (Dandy and Blackfan, Bering, Laurence, 1957, 1959). The test is performed by injection of 1 ml. (6 mg.) of neutral phenolsulfonphthalein dye into one lateral ventricle followed by lumbar puncture 20 minutes later. Dye is observed in the lumbar fluid if communication is present but is absent if an intraventricular obstructive lesion exists.

Urine collected for 12 to 24 hours after the injection is examined for the percentage of dye excreted during this period. The normal child should excrete greater than 50 per cent of the phenolsulfonphthalein during the 12 hours after injection whereas one with communicating hydrocephalus would excrete 10 to 20 per cent. Less than 10 per cent excretion in 12 hours is expected with intraventricular obstructive hydrocephalus.

Many problems are evident with studies of this type, not the least of which is the ability to accomplish a lumbar puncture at precisely the desired time. Urine collections in infants and small children are also subject to numerous pitfalls unless an indwelling catheter is used. For these reasons, the phenolsulfonphthalein test has been little used in recent years and has been supplanted by other, more informative procedures.

Roentgen Studies

Radiologic abnormalities of the skull with increased intracranial pressure are discussed elsewhere and are not repeated here. In addition to the enlarged head and suture spread, numerous abnormalities may be observed on skull films in infantile hydrocephalus, depending on the cause and the degree of the process. The posterior fossa frequently is relatively small in those with hydrocephalus due to congenital aqueductal obstruction and is impressively enlarged when hydrocephalus is related to the Dandy-Walker syndrome. Congenital hydrocephalus secondary to toxoplasmosis may be associated with multiple and diffuse intracranial calcification.

The calvarium of the infant with a meningomyelocoele frequently has a honeycombed appearance, which is referred to as craniolacunia or lückenschadel. This pattern is temporary and does not resemble the increased digital markings observed in older children with increased intracranial pressure. Craniolacunia is probably a defect in membranous bone formation and occasionally is observed with cerebral anomalies other than meningomyelocoele. With uncontrolled communicating hydrocephalus of long duration, chronic pressure effects may be exerted in other areas. Scalloping of the posterior surface of the vertebral bodies at all levels has been described in such cases (Shealy et al.).

A variety of interesting radiographic changes of the skull may also occur in children with advanced hydrocephalus after successful shunt procedures. Certain cranial sutures may close prematurely following decompression, leading to a bizarre configuration of the shape of the head (Duggan et al., Andersson). Development of new bone along the inner table of the skull after relief of increased pressure can result in considerable reduction in the intracranial volume and may also be associated with reduction in the size of the sella (Griscom and Oh).

Definitive diagnosis, localization of the site of obstruction, and exclusion of a mass or

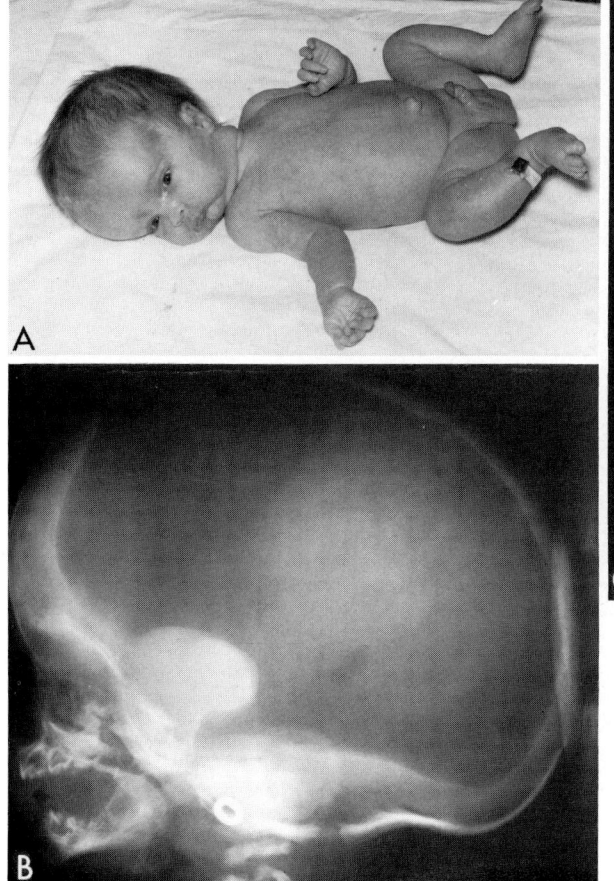
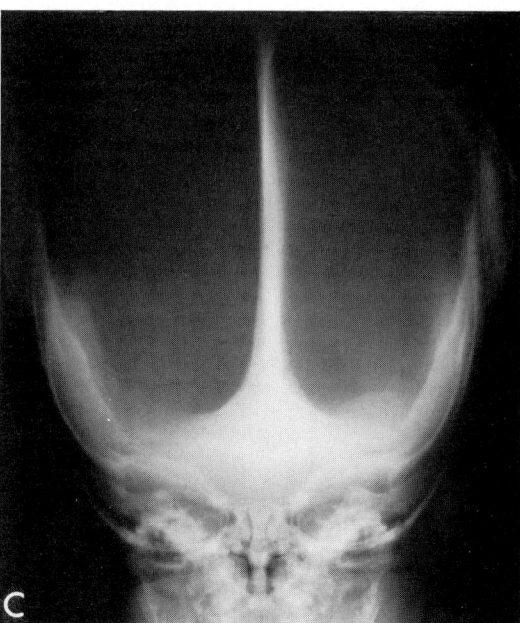

Figure 8-12. *A*, One-month-old infant with hydrocephalus due to aqueductal obstruction. Head circumference at birth was 38 cm. and at age one month 47 cm. *B*, Ventriculogram in lateral, and *C*, in anteroposterior projections, both illustrating profound ventricular distention despite only modest disproportion between head and body size.

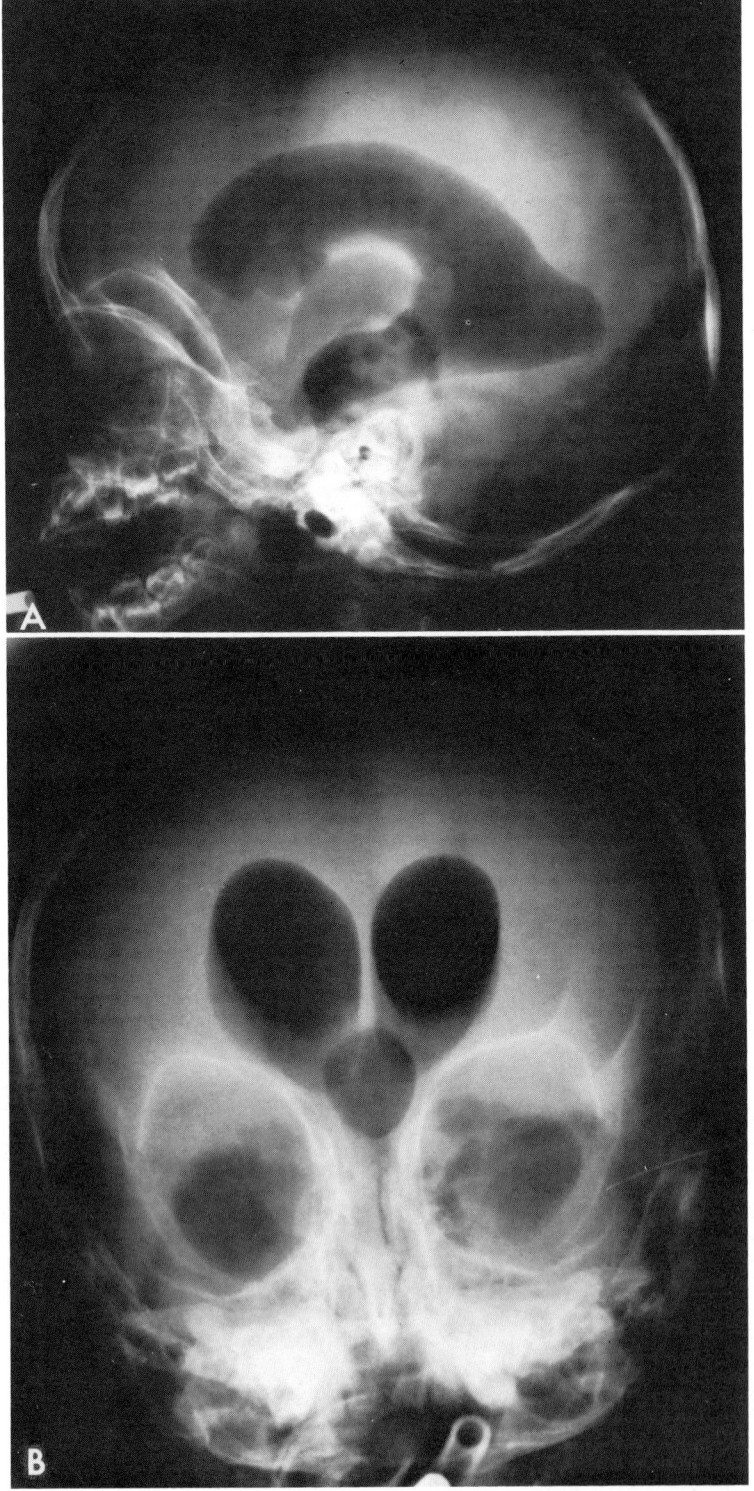

Figure 8–13. Pneumoencephalogram. Nine-month-old child with post-traumatic communicating hydrocephalus. Ventricular dilatation is at least partially secondary to communicating hydrocephalus rather than primary cerebral atrophy because of abnormal enlargement of the head circumference and suture spread on x-ray. Such pressure signs would not be expected with "passive" ventricular enlargement resulting from intrinsic cerebral atrophy.

compressive lesion are largely dependent on contrast procedures. Each case must be individualized to determine which procedure, or combination of procedures, offers the most useful information with the lowest possible risk. Infants with marked head enlargement are usually studied with air ventriculography by use of sufficient air to exclude a choroid plexus papilloma but not so much that it predisposes to collapse of the thinned cerebral mantle and massive intracranial bleeding (Fig. 8-12).

Proper positioning of the infant permits movement of air into the third ventricle and aqueduct, the site of frequent obstructive lesions. When air does not visualize this region, 2 ml. of Pantopaque may be injected into the lateral ventricle and subsequently moved to the aqueduct to demonstrate the precise level of obstruction. Because of possible adverse effects on the ependyma, positive contrast material should be used only when necessary (Clark et al.). The use of a water-soluble contrast medium, methylglucamine iothalamate 60 per cent (Conray 60), has achieved popularity for ventriculography (Heimburger et al, Handa and Handa). Advantages of this material are that the position of the head need not be altered to visualize various parts of the ventricular system and the meningeal reaction is usually less than that when air is used. However, the absorption is so rapid that films must be obtained almost immediately after injection into the ventricle. In addition, the positive contrast of the dilated lateral ventricles may obscure pathology at the level of the aqueduct.

Older infants with slowly progressive head enlargement believed to the due to communicating hydrocephalus may be studied by pneumoencephalography (Fig. 8-13). The fourth ventricle and aqueduct are more readily demonstrated by this method, which avoids needle passage through the brain. Lateral projections and tomograms during the initial phases of the study outline the posterior fossa ventricles before they become obscured by the temporal horns subsequently filled with air. In many instances, air must be injected from both above and below before conclusions can be made regarding the location of the obstructive lesion. This is especially the case in older children with aqueductal stenosis in whom ventriculography reveals distended lateral and third ventricles but does not provide further information.

Angiography is of greatest value when hydrocephalus is believed to be due to an an-

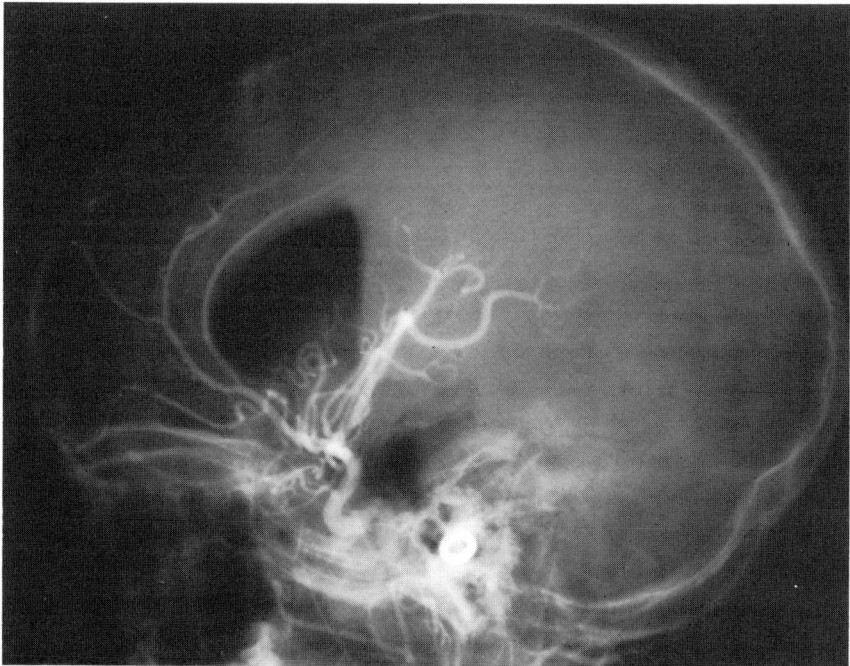

Figure 8–14. Carotid angiogram, lateral view. The anterior horn of the lateral ventricle is enlarged as outlined by air. Note the bowed course of the pericallosal branch of the anterior cerebral artery as it sweeps around the dilated ventricle. Note also the more vertical course of the middle cerebral artery complex, a normal characteristic of children as compared to adults.

eurysm of the vein of Galen suspected from a cranial bruit plus high-output cardiac failure. Angiographic features of aqueductal stenosis have been described by Huang et al. and include evidence of hydrocephalus, such as bowing of the pericallosal artery, (Fig. 8-14) and stretching with depression of the posterior cerebral artery on the lateral view. The internal cerebral vein is flattened and depressed and its tributary vessels are elongated. In the posterior circulation, the superior cerebellar artery is displaced downward while structures in the lower portion of the posterior fossa remain unaffected.

A variety of complex venous abnormalities in the posterior fossa have also been described by Huang and coworkers. Carotid angiography may also be required to distinguish so-called "hydranencephaly" with greatly dilated ventricular spaces from the infant with positive transillumination of the skull due to massive subdural collections of fluid, possibly secondary to intrauterine ventricular rupture.

Isotope Encephalography (Cisternography)

In 1964, DiChiro reported a scanning technique for evaluation of the cerebrospinal fluid dynamics utilizing the intrathecal injection of radioiodinated serum albumin (^{131}RISA). The procedure has been called cisternography; however, isotope encephalography would seem to be more descriptive and subject to less misinterpretation. Various radiopharmaceutical materials have been used for this purpose and injection sites have included the lumbar theca, the cisterna magna, and the lateral ventricle. Still, ^{131}RISA administered into the lumbar subarachnoid space has remained the preferred approach by most investigators. Movement or position of the patient following lumbar injection does not seem to affect dispersion of the radiopharmaceutical material.

The procedure appears to be safe, fairly simple, but requires complex and expensive scanning equipment. Because less than 1 ml. is injected into the system, it does not adversely affect cerebrospinal fluid dynamics. Reported side-effects have been rare, including mild temperature elevation and aseptic meningitis (Detmer and Blocker, Nicol). The radiation dose has been estimated to be 100 millirads to the total body and 1 rad to the nervous system (DiChiro et al).

Following instillation of the radioactive material into the lumbar subarachnoid space, scans of the head are made at periodic intervals, for example, at 2, 6, 24, and 72 hours. In the normal person radioactivity is detected in the basilar cisterns by two hours, in the Sylvian fissures by six hours, and over the convexity of the brain by 12 to 24 hours after injection (James et al). Radioactivity is largely dissipated by 48 hours and ventricular collection of the radioactive material does not occur in the normal person.

Isotope encephalography has many useful purposes but is of greatest value in patients with communicating hydrocephalus (Fig. 8-15). In this condition, isotope injected into the lumbar subarachnoid space can be demonstrated within the enlarged ventricles where it is retained in large quantity for 48 to 72 hours. When ventricular enlargement is secondary to primary cerebral atrophy, the isotope flow pattern follows normal pathways and lateral ventricular isotope collection either does not occur or is minimal (Bannister et al.). Thus, the procedure may provide critical information differentiating that group of patients with "normal pressure" hydrocephalus who might benefit from a shunt procedure from those with dementia due to intrinsic brain disease. Those with prolonged stasis of isotope within the ventricles are more likely to be clinically improved by shunting than are patients with hydrocephalus with less protracted ventricular stasis (McCullough et al.).

With intraventricular obstructive hydrocephalus, no isotope enters the ventricular system after the lumbar injection and the flow pattern is normal, unless an associated extraventricular block is present. The patency of a ventriculoatrial shunt can be assessed by intraventricular injection of the isotope (Glasauer et al.). Adequate shunt function is indicated by isotope movement in the ventricular fluid toward the shunt followed by its rapid clearing from the ventricles. Shunt failure leads to prolonged ventricular stasis of radioactivity.

Isotope encephalography provides the clinician with an additional method of evaluating cerebrospinal fluid physiology and flow, which undoubtedly will become more popular. With few exceptions, however, this technique should be employed in conjunction

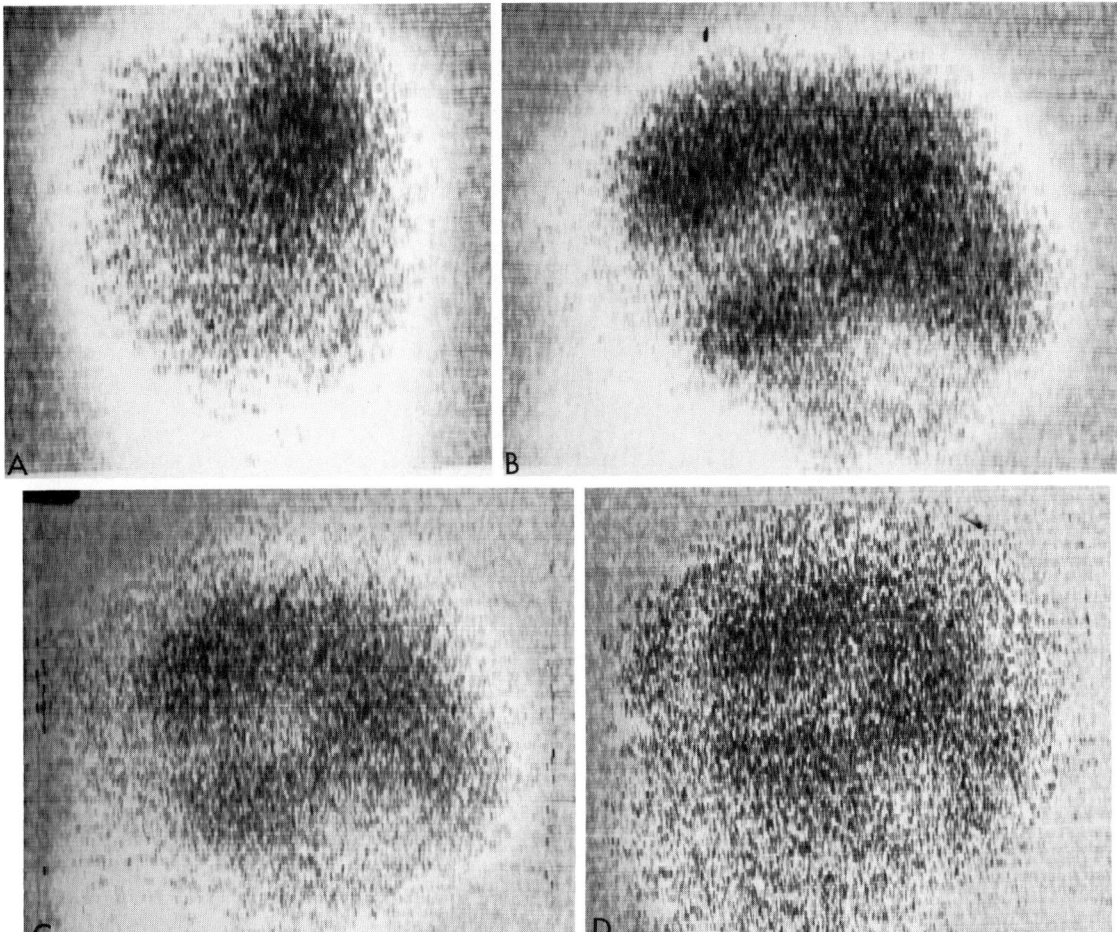

Figure 8–15. Isotope encephalogram (cisternogram) following intraspinal injection of I^{131} RISA in a two-year-old child with postmeningitic communicating hydrocephalus. *A*, Four-hour anterior scan with isotope outlining the lateral ventricles, the left being larger than the right. *B*, Four-hour lateral scan demonstrating dense accumulation of isotope within the dilated lateral ventricles, which are well delineated by the radioactive material. Persistence of isotope within the ventricles for 24 hours, *C*, and 48 hours, *D*, indicates disturbance of cerebrospinal fluid flow characteristic of communicating hydrocephalus.

with, and not instead of, conventional air contrast studies.

"Hydranencephaly"

Cruveilhier is generally credited with the first description of what is now referred to as "hydranencephaly," although Crome and Sylvester claimed it had been recognized before. Spielmeyer subsequently introduced the term hydranencephaly, one we consider to be ambiguous and to convey little meaning.

Hydranencephaly is a purely descriptive designation indicating that abnormal transillumination is observed if the patient is an infant and is associated with enormous ventricular enlargement with little or no cerebral mantle (Fig. 8-16). The basal ganglia, brain stem, and cerebellum are present in such patients but may reveal a variety of morphologic abnormalities. The causes are multiple and include any severe encephaloclastic insult that occurs in the prenatal period, during the birth process, or even postnatally. A small percentage of such cases are probably the result of a severe developmental anomaly in which normal formation of the cerebral mantle has not occurred (Yakovlov and Wadsworth). Thus, hydranencephaly should not be considered a diagnostic entity but the end result of one of many destructive processes.

An additional source of confusion in previously reported cases has been the lack of differentiation of infants who exhibit abnormal transillumination because of profound

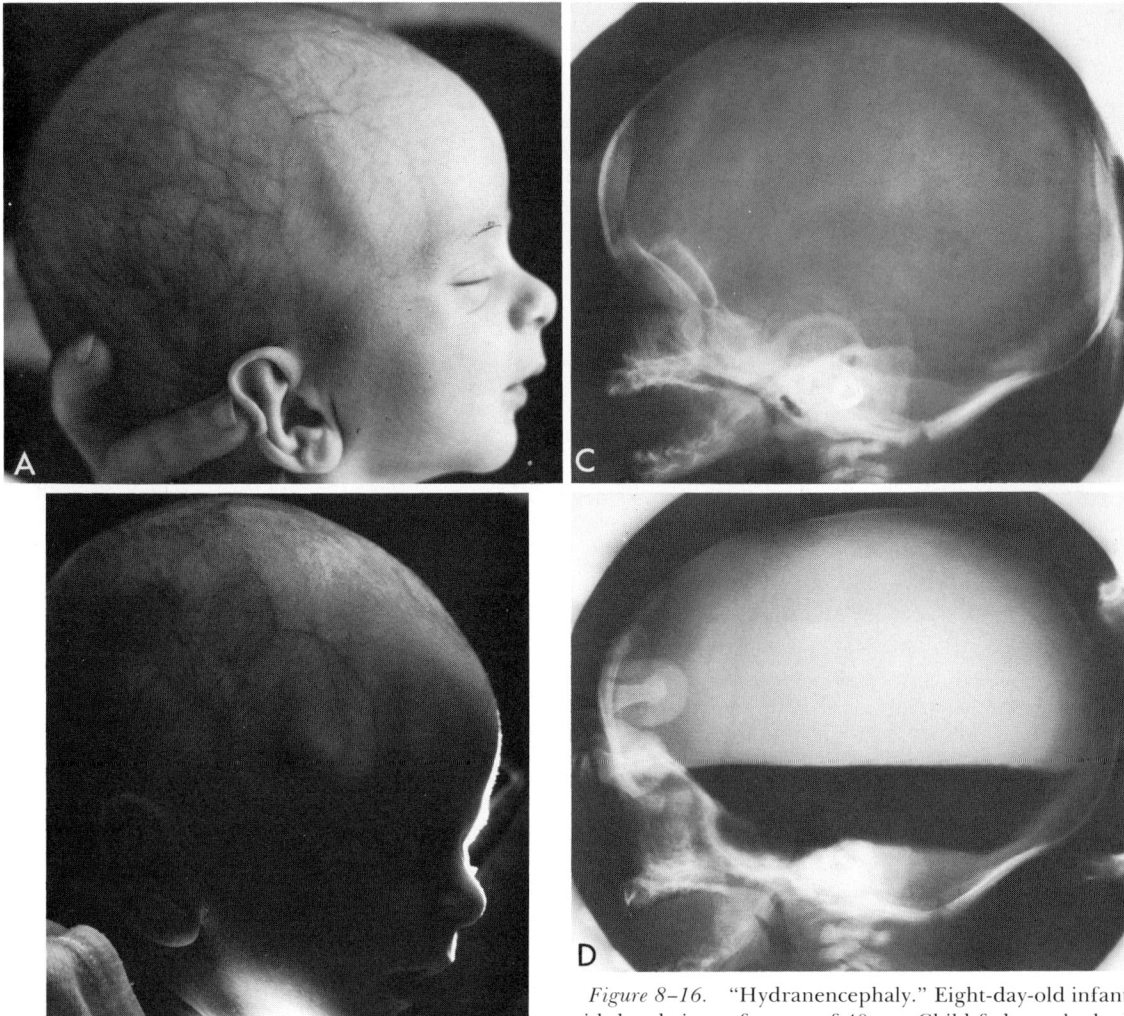

Figure 8–16. "Hydranencephaly." Eight-day-old infant with head circumference of 40 cm. Child fed poorly, had diffuse hyperreflexia, and exhibited marked inability to regulate body temperature despite absence of infection. Baby died at age three months. *A*, Only mild disproportion between size of head and facial structures. *B*, Positive transillumination with diffuse glow over entire scalp with light placed in left temporal region. *C*, Ventriculogram. Extreme dilatation of the ventricular system with virtual absence of the cerebral mantle. *D*, Hanging head view shows ventricular enlargement but with no air traversing the obstructed aqueduct.

ventricular distention, or "hydranencephaly," from those in whom the massive fluid collection is in the subdural spaces. Although the clinical signs may be similar, the latter group should not be categorized with the former. Patients with subdural effusions may be shown to have microcephalic brains by carotid angiography, even though the head size may be abnormally large. This group is apt to show fewer physical abnormalities, to live longer, and may be assumed to have "hydranencephaly" from transfontanel air studies unless angiography or pneumoencephalography is performed (Fig. 8-17). The case described by Poser et al. appears to have been of this type. The cause of the fluid collections external to the brain is unknown and in the past was referred to as "external" hydrocephalus.

Many types of injuries to the immature brain have been suggested as causes of near-total to total cerebral hemisphere destruction, several of which have been well documented. Courville has emphasized the pathology of successive gradations of oxygen deprivation extending from minimal laminar cortical neuronal changes to virtual total hemisphere destruction from severe insults. Carotid vas-

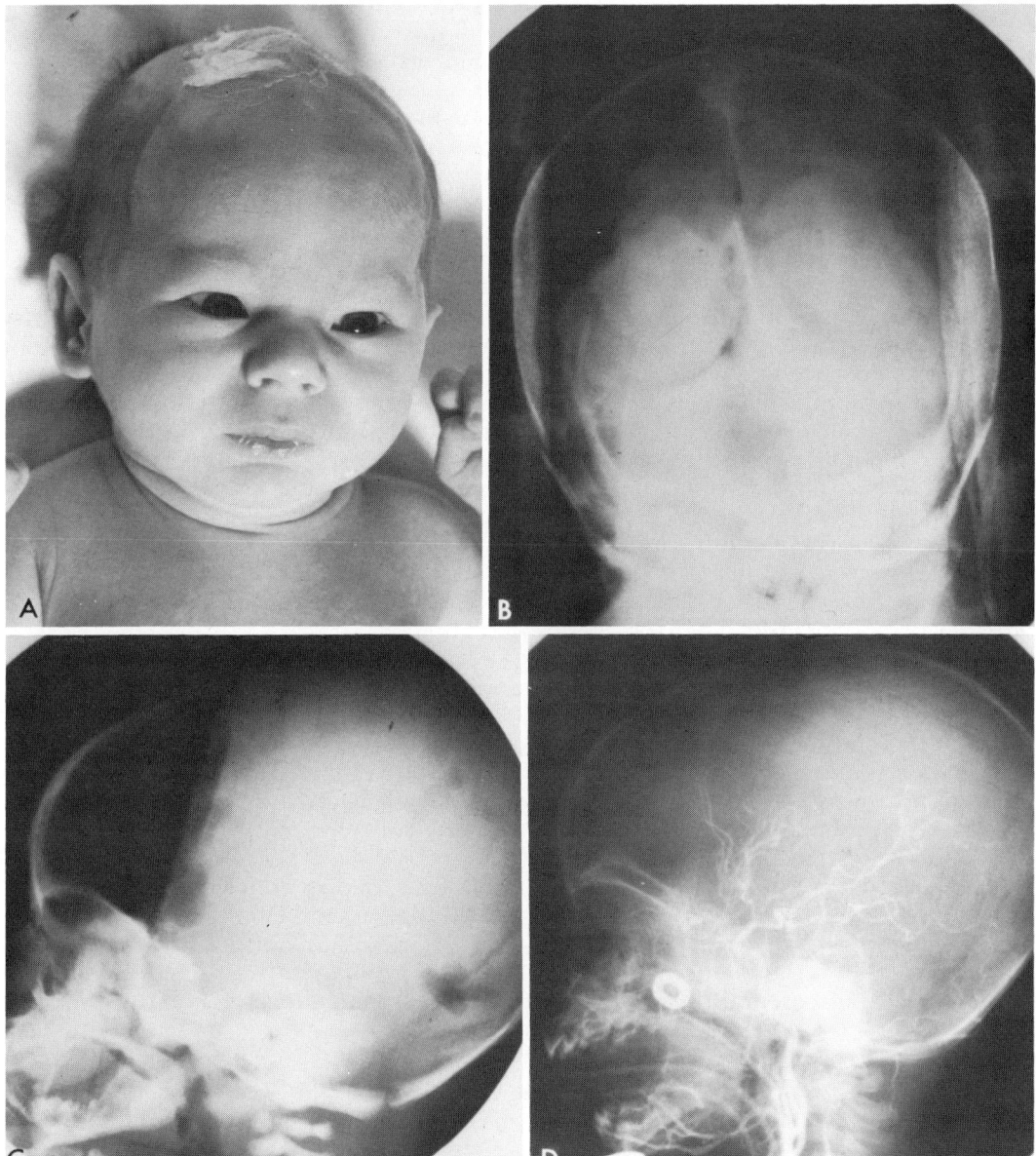

Figure 8–17. Massive subdural effusions in a 14-day-old infant initially assumed to have "hydranencephaly" because of positive transillumination. Birth weight was 6½ lb. and the child was apneic, requiring resuscitation. He fed poorly and was referred at age 14 days because of tremulousness, increased tone, and hyperreflexia. Head circumference at age 14 days was 33.5 cm. *A*, Facial appearance and head shape were not remarkable for a 14-day-old infant. *B*, Transfontanel air injection. Fluid obtained was xanthochromic with protein content of 960 mg. per 100 ml. Air outlines atrophic cerebral hemispheres well removed from the surface of the skull. *C* Lateral view of air study demonstrates depth of subdural space overlying the microcephalic brain. *D*, Carotid angiogram shows the vascular supply to the small brain. Vessels are displaced away from the surface of the skull by the large subdural fluid collection.

At age 13 months, the child had grown poorly and head circumference was 39 cm. He was last seen at 3½ years of age at which time he was severely retarded and had acquired few developmental skills and no speech. Such cases are distinguished from "hydranencephaly" by diagnostic contrast studies.

cular inadequacy has been suggested by some authors because of the sparing of portions of the inferior temporal and occipital lobes. Muir commented that the carotid arteries were often hypoplastic in these patients but pointed out that involution of these vessels could occur because of lack of need due to cerebral absence rather than as a causative factor.

Lindenberg and Swanson described five infants with postnatal, acquired disorders in whom bilateral hemisphere destruction was attributed to arterial compression at the base of the skull from severe brain swelling. In two cases, acute bacterial meningitis was the initiating illness, possibly also a factor leading to necrotizing cerebral changes. Massive destruction of brain tissue in the postnatal period has also been described by Weiss et al. Intracranial hemorrhage at two days of age was followed by progressive head enlargement requiring several shunt procedures. Death occurred at age two years and the cerebral mantle measured less than 2 mm.

Whether far-advanced hydrocephalus without an additional process affecting the brain can lead to the pattern referred to as "hydranencephaly" remains unproved. Halsey et al. (1971) considered the possibility but could find no documented example. Many of the reported cases with encephaloclastic insults to the cerebral parenchyma have exhibited associated hydrocephalus, which most likely accelerated the injurious effect of the primary insult to the brain.

It is not surprising that intraventricular or basilar cistern block should occur in such cases because rapid cerebral dissolution releases a considerable amount of foreign material into the ventricular system. Patients who develop an obstructive factor, or hydrocephalus, are probably those with progressive head enlargement. The absence of associated hydrocephalus in patients with severe encephaloclastic insults gives a picture with positive transillumination but with lack of head enlargement, and subsequently, an abnormally small head.

The clinical manifestations observed in infants with marked ventricular enlargement permitting transillumination are variable. The statement has often been made that such infants may behave in an entirely normal fashion for weeks or months after birth. The interpretation of what represents normal in the neonatal period is obviously dependent on the skill and experience of the one who makes the observations. Although children with these disorders may appear intact to the mother, careful examination by one familiar with neurologic activity of the neonate reveals abnormalities in the majority of such patients. The often stated concept that the newborn functions at the brain stem level without influence of the cerebral hemispheres is an exaggeration in our opinion and is in need of qualification.

Abnormalities usually recognized include excessive sleepiness or irritability manifested by continuous crying when awake. Feeding problems are usual, often because of lethargy and poor sucking, or manifested by vomiting. Tremulousness of limbs and increased muscle tone are frequently observed along with enhanced deep tendon reflexes. Nystagmus may be excessive and optic atrophy is common. The normal neonatal reflexes, such as the grasp, Moro, and stepping reflexes, can usually be elicited but become abnormal because of their persistence beyond the expected time of disappearance (Halsey et al., 1968).

If the child survives beyond three months, normal developmental landmarks are not achieved and the evidence of spasticity becomes more apparent. Autonomic dysfunction is sometimes manifested by extremes in body temperature, in part related to the environmental temperature (Appenzeller et al.). In most, electroencephalography reveals markedly depressed voltages or even a virtually flat tracing. Ventricular fluid may be clear and with a normal protein content or xanthochromic with a marked increase in protein, again, depending on the cause of the process.

Many infants with these disorders characterized by severe cerebral destruction die early in infancy, although a few survive for remarkably long periods of time. Of 28 children with "hydranencephaly" reviewed by Hunziker, only nine survived beyond three months of age.

OCCULT ("NORMAL PRESSURE") HYDROCEPHALUS

The observations that progressive hydrocephalus may exist without the conventional clinical manifestations of increased pressure or with "normal" spinal fluid pressure have necessitated revision of our earlier principles regarding anticipated benefit from shunt procedures. In 1956, Foltz and Ward described ten patients with communicating hydrocephalus following subarachnoid hemorrhage. They noted that several of these patients displayed symptoms and signs not typical of those usually attributed to increased intracranial pressure. They also observed that in certain cases the spinal fluid pressure was not elevated despite pneumographic evidence of hydrocephalus and that clinical improvement occurred after a ventriculomastoid shunt was performed. Even 20 years earlier, Riddoch had reported a patient with progressive dementia with intraventricular obstructive hydrocephalus in whom the spinal fluid pressure was only 160 mm. of water.

Little attention was directed to these remarkable observations until 1964, and 1965 when Hakim and DeDavila, Hakim and Adams, and Adams et al. published reports that established the concept of progressive hydrocephalus with pressure measurements in the range considered to be normal by conventional standards. Almost simultaneously, McHugh illustrated that hydrocephalus may remain asymptomatic, or occult, for many years to be identified unexpectedly at autopsy or abruptly to become decompensated, with signs of increased pressure then appearing. McHugh focused attention on spastic and ataxic gait disturbances exhibited by certain patients with occult hydrocephalus which could be readily confused with spinal cord disease.

Adams et al. placed emphasis on progressive dementia as the symptomatic hallmark of this disorder. In certain patients, only mild memory deficits are observed in the early phase of the illness. With progression, more advanced mentation abnormalities are evidenced by lack of spontaneity, mental confusion, and decline in span of interest and attention. Frank dementia, lethargy, or akinetic mutism may be associated with incontinence of urine, total inability to ambulate, and progressive visual loss with optic atrophy.

Most recorded examples of "normal pressure" hydrocephalus have been of the communicating type and the majority of reports have dealt with adults. The same principles are applicable to children, however, and especially to older children, in whom the clinical findings may be similar to those described in adults (Fig. 8-18). A child with previously identified and shunted hydrocephalus may manifest decompensation by worsening of gait with spastic lower limbs, deterioration of school performance, emotional lability, and progressive optic atrophy. Infants with hydrocephalus occasionally show progressive enlargement of the head despite reasonably "normal" ventricular pressure determinations. Although the latter is not totally analogous to adult-onset, "normal pressure" hydrocephalus, the mechanisms related to the pressure and ventricular size relationships are probably similar.

Benson et al. discussed the need for both pneumoencephalography and lumbar isotope encephalography to distinguish patients with "normal pressure" hydrocephalus who might improve with shunting from patients with primary cerebral atrophy. Pneumography is essential for diagnosis in this condition but must be viewed as a significant hazard. Rapid deterioration in the clinical status has been recorded in several patients following instillation of air. When the condition is suspected beforehand, a burr hole placed before the performance of the pneumogram would allow rapid decompression in case of worsening. Furthermore, removal of the air entrapped within the ventricles would seem logical before placement of a ventriculoatrial shunt.

The mechanism accounting for progressive ventricular enlargement in patients with a "normal" spinal fluid pressure has been widely disputed. Hakim and Adams and Adams et al. equated the ventricular system to an enclosed, fluid-filled container in which the force on the walls of the container is the result of the product of the pressure of the fluid and the surface area of the walls. They emphasized that evaluation of the significance of cerebrospinal fluid pressure must include consideration of the size, and thus surface area, of the ventricles. This explanation has not been entirely acceptable to some in that it does not take into consideration the structural properties of the periventricular tissues (Geschwind).

Although the theory proposed by Hakim and Adams probably only partially explains the mechanical factors involved, it undoubtedly adds new prospective to our concepts of what "normal" spinal fluid pressure represents. Much remains to be learned about this group of patients, but it is now apparent that progressive hydrocephalus may exist even though the spinal fluid or ventricular pressure is recorded at less than 180 mm. of water. Furthermore, the foregoing studies

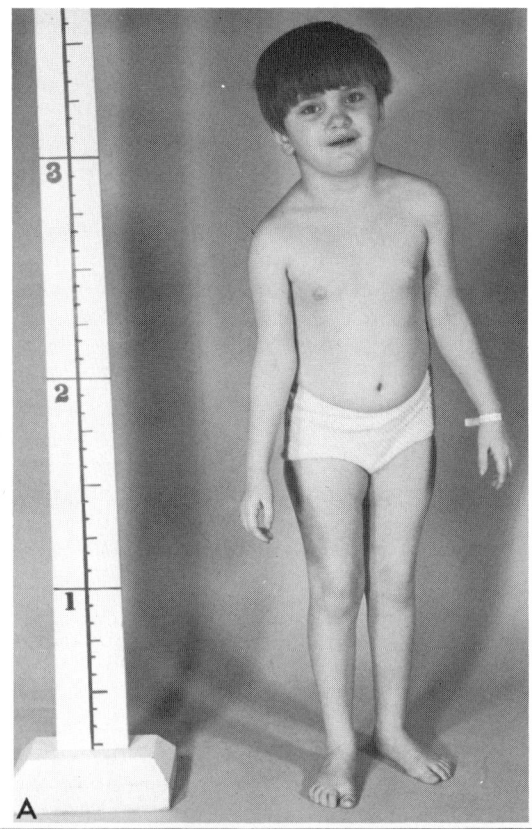
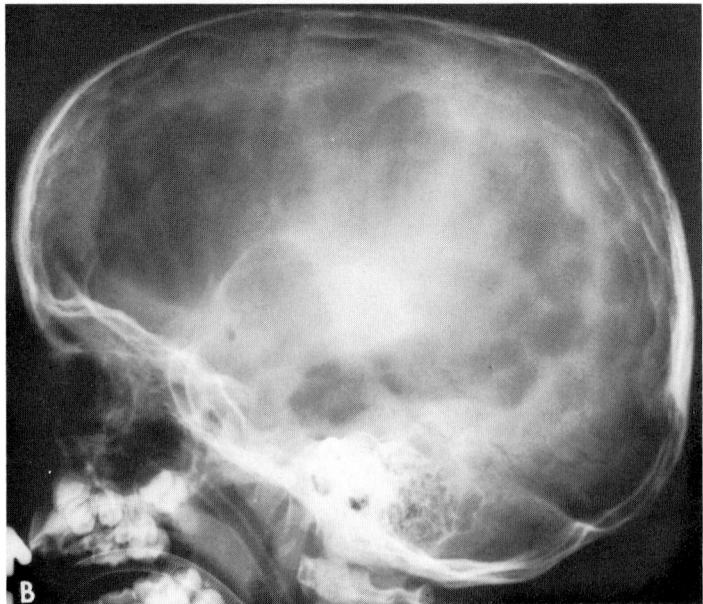

Figure 8–18. Occult ("normal-pressure") hydrocephalus, probably secondary to neonatal subarachnoid hemorrhage. Six-year-old girl with birth weight of 3 lb. and with evidence of subarachnoid bleeding in the neonatal period. Development was slow, but between five and six years of age she became ataxic, had speech regression, and developed loss of vision. *A*, Physical signs included head circumference of 54 cm., diffuse hyperreflexia, and primary optic atrophy. *B*, Pneumoencephalogram revealed communicating hydrocephalus with distention of the entire ventricular system but with no air over the convexity of the brain. The opening pressure at the time of the air study was normal. Note increased digital markings and changes in the sella turcica secondary to chronic increase in intracranial pressure.

have clarified the existence of progressive hydrocephalus, sometimes relieved by shunt procedures, with symptomatic deterioration that need not include headache, vomiting, or papilledema.

DANDY-WALKER SYNDROME

The pathogenesis of the Dandy-Walker syndrome has been a source of continued controversy since its description by Dandy and Blackfan in 1914 and 1917. These authors and many subsequent investigators attributed the cystic dilatation of the fourth ventricle characteristic of this malformation to atresia of the exit foramina of the fourth ventricle. In 1942, Taggart and Walker published an extensive review of the subject and also concluded that prenatal lack of development, or "atresia," of the foramina of Luschka and Magendie accounted for the morphologic abnormalities within the posterior fossa. Benda suggested the eponym Dandy-Walker syndrome in 1954, but departed from the earlier views on pathogenesis and considered the anomaly to be in the category of cleft formations or rachischisis at the level of the cerebellum.

Still another view was promoted by Brodal and Hauglie-Hanssen who suggested that the cerebellar anomalies observed in this syndrome develop at a fetal stage earlier than the formation of the foramina of Luschka and Magendie. They postulated increased intraventricular pressure of unknown origin as the cause of the cerebellar deformity and accepted outlet foramen atresia as a coexisting malformation in some cases.

Whether the total spectrum of abnormalities in the Dandy-Walker syndrome can be attributed to prenatal atresia of the foramina of Luschka and Magendie remains undetermined. There seems little doubt, however, that persistent embryonic and fetal obstruction of the outlet of the fourth ventricle is capable of production of most, if not all, of the morphologic features of this condition.

Certain authors have disputed the outlet obstruction theory on the basis of the occasional case in which air injected into the lumbar subarachnoid space gains free access to the lateral ventricles, which are not necessarily dilated. This would not seem incompatible with fetal outlet obstruction, however, because cystic distention of the fourth ventricle during the fetal period could produce irreparable changes of cerebellar development followed by the subsequent development of patency of the exit foramina (Matson, 1956, Taggart and Walker).

Distended lateral ventricles may diminish in size after alleviation of obstruction and thus might appear normal in the postnatal period in this syndrome. More often, infants with the Dandy-Walker syndrome have progressive hydrocephalus with lack of patency at the level of the foramina of Luschka and Magendie demonstrable by air studies.

The cardinal feature of the Dandy-Walker syndrome is profound cystic distention of the fourth ventricle. It is important to emphasize that the enormously dilated structure within the posterior fossa is, in fact, the fourth ventricle and not a cyst, as often referred to in prior literature. The enlarged fourth ventricle displaces the cerebellar hemispheres laterally and results in flattening of the brain stem with concavity of the posterior surface of the pons (Fig. 8-19).

The inferior vermis is not evident but its white matter is deployed as a thin sheet beneath the lining of the membrane roofing the distended fourth ventricle (Gibson). The anterior vermis is displaced rostrally and is flattened by the enlarged fourth ventricle. The status of the foramina of Luschka and Magendie is variable when examined in postnatal life but they are frequently atretic. In some reports, the lateral foramina have been patent but the foramen of Magendie is occluded (Sahs).

Because of the distended fourth ventricle and enlarged posterior fossa during fetal development, the normal posterior migration of the transverse sinuses and torcula is prevented, resulting in a remarkably high position of these structures in the postnatal period. The tentorium, likewise, occupies an elevated position because of the large posterior fossa and results in forward displacement of the occipital and temporal horns of the lateral ventricles (Fig. 8-20). Other anomalies may be present, including agenesis of the corpus callosum, porencephaly, and forking of the aqueduct (Juhl and Wesenberg).

Clinical Course

The clinical manifestations in patients with the Dandy-Walker syndrome are quite variable, in part depending on the degree of obstruction. Abnormal head enlargement is

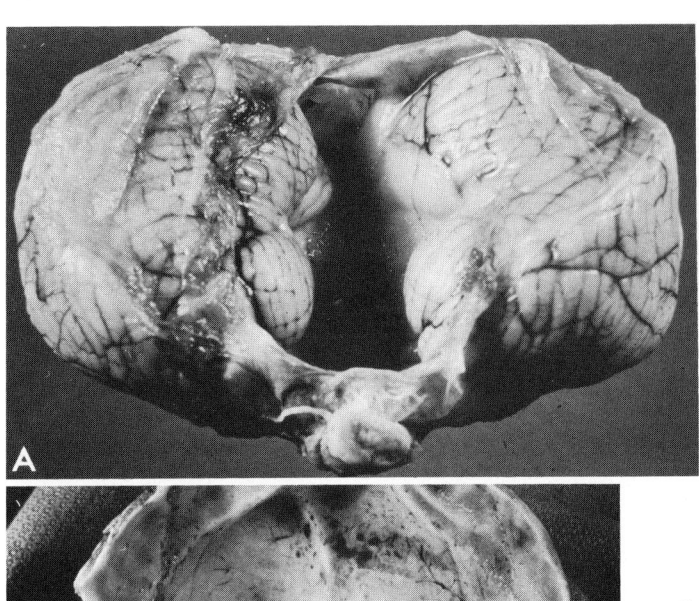
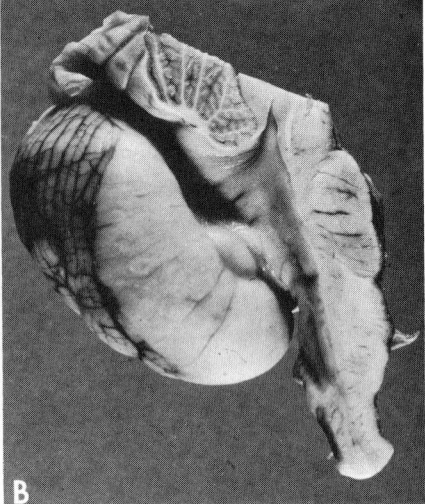
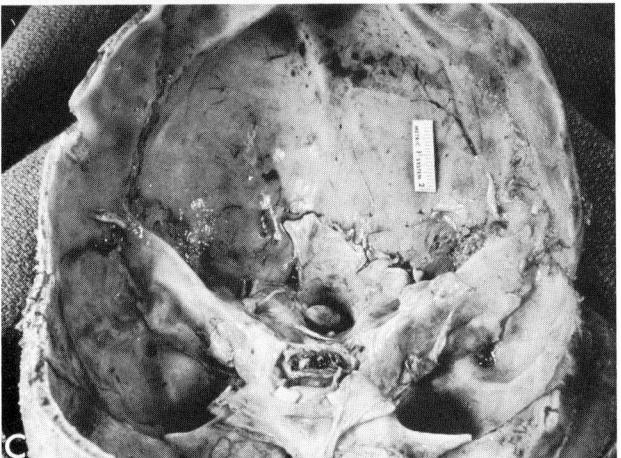

Figure 8–19. Dandy-Walker syndrome. *A*, Cystic distention of the fourth ventricle with partial absence of the cerebellar vermis and lateral displacement of the cerebellar hemispheres. *B*, Lateral view reveals flattening of the dorsal surface of the brain stem, absence of the inferior vermis, and rostal displacement of the anterior portion of the cerebellar vermis. *C*, View of base of the skull in a patient with Dandy-Walker syndrome. Note the enormous size of the posterior fossa, thinning of the skull in this region, and the abnormally high position of the grooves of the transverse sinuses.

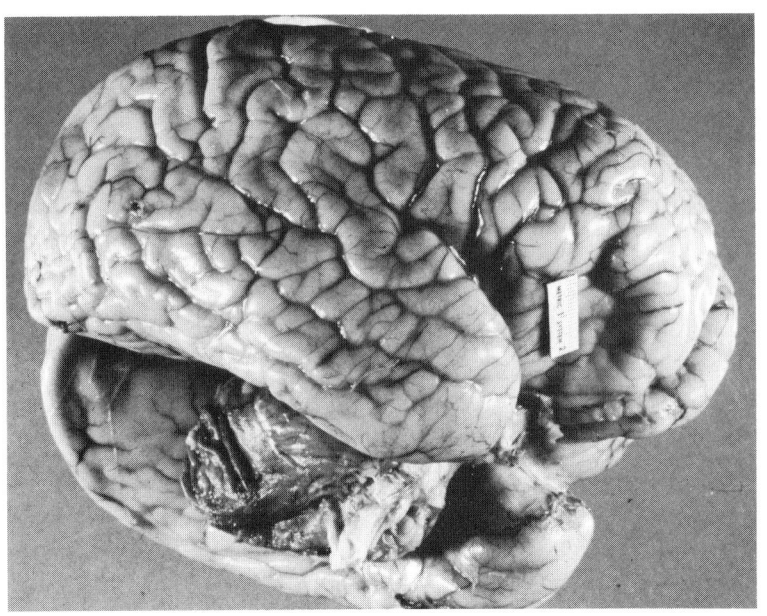

Figure 8–20. Dandy-Walker syndrome. View of the right cerebral hemisphere demonstrates elevation of the occipital and temporal lobes secondary to the abnormally high position of the tentorium.

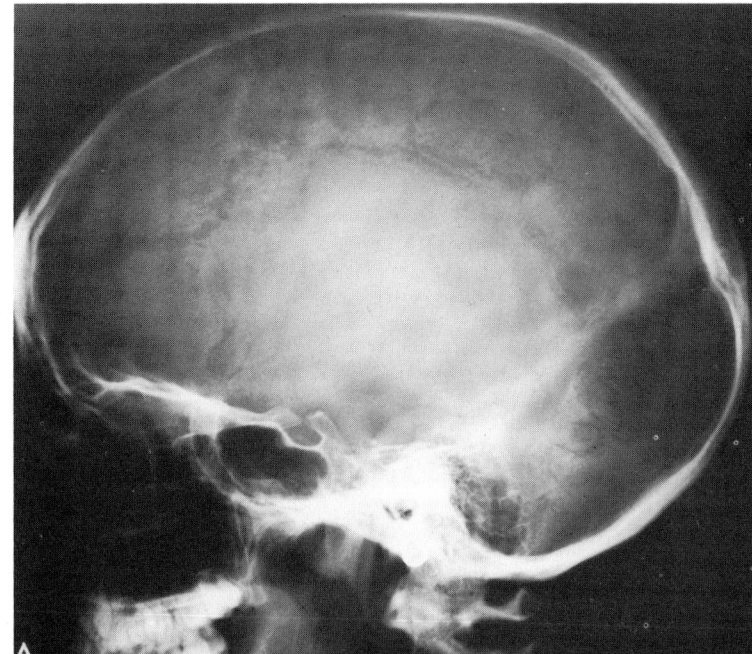

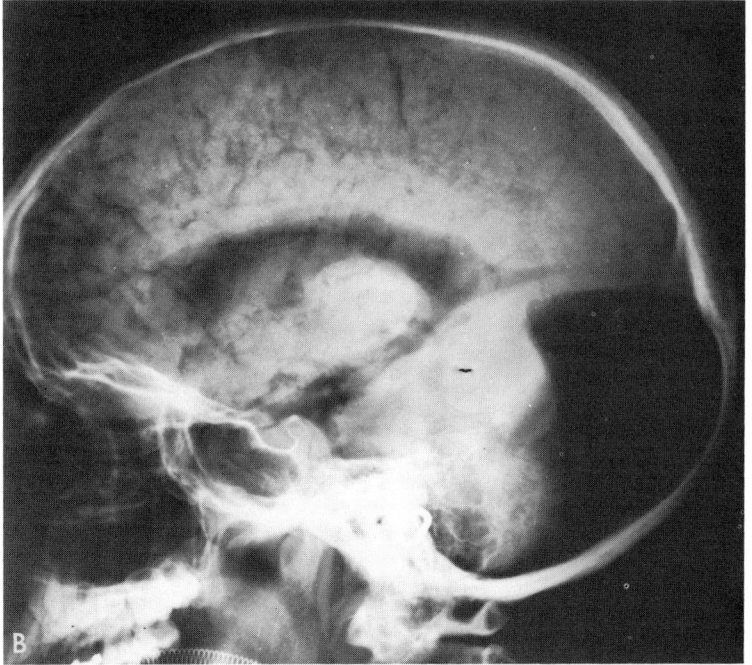

Figure 8–21. Dandy-Walker syndrome. Nine-year-old girl said to have been well until age seven years when she experienced repetitive episodes of vomiting, initially attributed to psychogenic factors. Vomiting persisted and the development of lethargy prompted further investigation. *A*, Skull film, lateral view. The posterior fossa is large, the tentorium and torcula are elevated, and the lambdoidal sutures are separated. *B*, Pneumoencephalogram shows free communication into the posterior fossa. The lateral ventricles are not enlarged and the profound cystic distention of the fourth ventricle is evident.

often present at birth and may rapidly increase as with other forms of hydrocephalus. The syndrome may be unsuspected in such instances until air studies identify the characteristic posterior fossa abnormalities.

In other infants, head enlargement is not initially present but proceeds slowly to become recognizable between the first and the second year. This slow evolution is explained on the basis of partial obstruction which can become accelerated at any time precipitating pressure symptoms of vomiting and irritability.

In the slowly progressive form, lumbar pneumography may result in filling of lateral ventricles that are only mildly dilated (Fig. 8-21). Even when no filling can be accomplished by pneumoencephalography,

Matson (1956) noted that tracers injected into the lateral ventricle can occasionally be recovered from the lumbar subarachnoid space. Thus, in some instances, the occlusive membranes in the posterior fossa may be sufficiently permeable to permit transmission of some fluid from the anatomically obstructed fourth ventricle providing a partial, but inadequate, compensating mechanism.

Certain children with the Dandy-Walker syndrome remain surprisingly well for several years after birth. Although it may not have been recognized, the head circumference in this group is usually greater than average and coordination is apt to be poor. Abrupt onset of vomiting, headache, ataxia, or vertigo may follow an infectious illness or head trauma, leading to the correct diagnosis. Sahs described a 16-year-old boy with a previously unrecognized Dandy-Walker syndrome who experienced headache, dizziness, and neck stiffness soon after engaging in a "neck-strengthening contest." The older child with an undiagnosed Dandy-Walker syndrome may develop symptoms in a precipitous fashion, which may be followed by respiratory arrest and death unless the process is identified and relieved expeditiously.

In addition to abnormal head enlargement, the infant with the Dandy-Walker syndrome presents a characteristic configuration of the head that suggests the diagnosis. The occipital region is prominent, with the distance from the external ear to the tip of the occiput far exceeding that present with other forms of hydrocephalus. An abnormal transillumination, restricted to the posterior fossa region in some cases, may also provide a diagnostic clue.

Roentgenographic Findings

Roentgenographic features of this disorder are specific and correlate with the morphologic aspects already discussed (Scarcella). Lateral skull films reveal marked enlargement of the occipital region with thinning of the lower occipital bones. When suture spread is present, it is often disproportionately marked at the lambdoid sutures, which are less severely spread with other forms of hydrocephalus. The grooves of the transverse sinuses are retained in an abnormally high position in the posterior parietal region rather than in normal location within the occipital bones (Fig. 8-22). This is the most suggestive roentgen sign of this condition on plain films; however, it is of little value in the infant period. The transverse sinus grooves are not roentgenographically apparent before one year of age. Between one and two years, the grooves can be visualized on x-ray in approximately 50 per cent of children and are almost always evident after two years of age (D'Agostino et al).

Air contrast studies provide the best delineation of the features of the Dandy-Walker

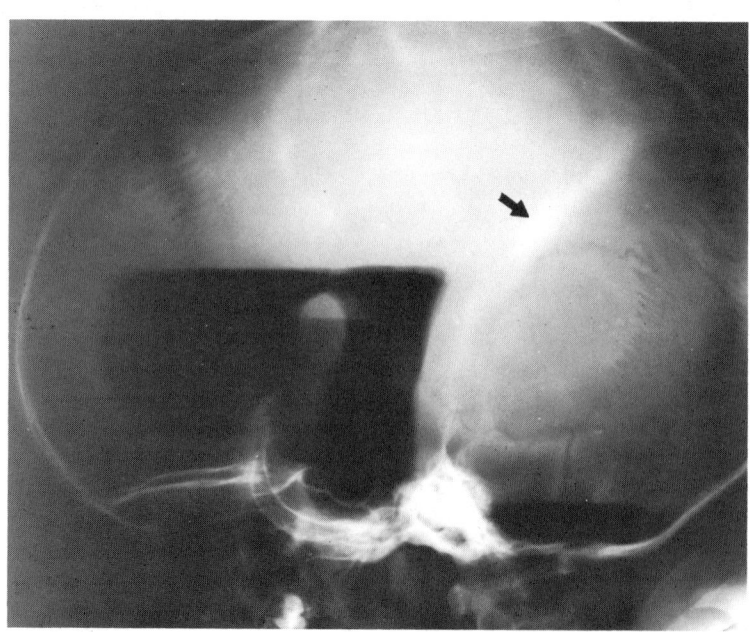

Figure 8–22. Dandy-Walker syndrome. Three-year-old girl with a history of delayed motor development and "large head" since birth. Head circumference was 61.5 cm. Lateral ventriculogram reveals ventricular dilatation, enormous posterior fossa beneath the elevated tentorium (arrow), and partially air-filled fourth ventricle. There is complete obstruction at the level of the outlet foramina of the fourth ventricle. The patient was treated by ventriculoatrial shunt, but the postoperative course was complicated by recurrent episodes of vomiting and coma with decerebrate rigidity.

syndrome, but the potential hazards of these procedures must be recognized in children with marked ventricular changes. Transfontanel ventriculography is usually chosen for infants with marked head enlargement (Fig. 8-23), although pneumoencephalography may be successful for older children with less profound enlargement of the head. As already mentioned, patients in whom the ventricles fill from below are less likely to have marked lateral ventricular distention than are those who are completely obstructed in

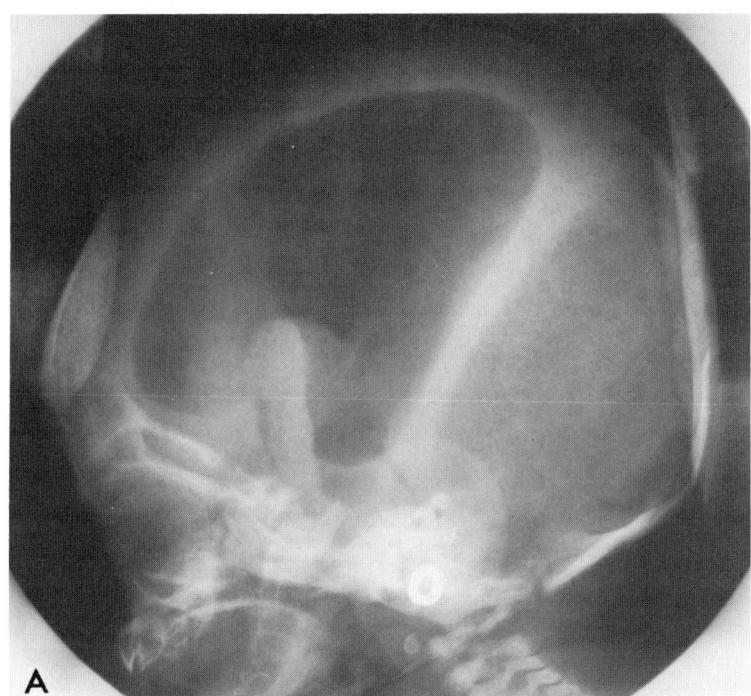

Figure 8-23. Dandy-Walker syndrome. Two-week-old boy with head circumference of 42 cm. *A*, Ventriculogram, lateral view. The lateral ventricles are enlarged and the cystic distention of the fourth ventricle occupies most of the posterior fossa. Note the abnormal elevation of the tentorium. *B*, Anteroposterior view. The septum pellucidum is absent.

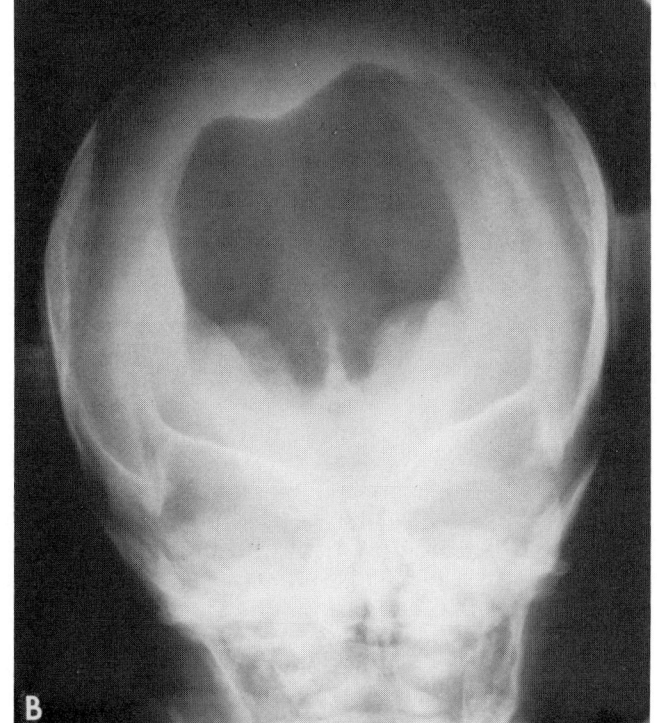

the posterior fossa. When ventriculography is done on the older child suspected of having the Dandy-Walker syndrome, burr holes should be placed higher than usual in order to permit needle passage above the elevated tentorium.

When ventricles become markedly enlarged, the septum pellucidum may reveal multiple perforations or even complete dissolution. The dilated aqueduct can be demonstrated to communicate with the hugely distended fourth ventricle, which may occupy the majority of the enlarged space inferior to the elevated tentorium. With the infant in the upside-down position, the obstructed fourth ventricle may be demonstrated to project from the posterior fossa into the upper cervical spinal canal.

Raimondi et al. expressed concern over the potential danger of air contrast studies in patients with the Dandy-Walker syndrome. These authors recommended confirmation of the diagnosis angiographically and postponement of air encephalography until after surgical treatment has alleviated the abnormal pressure relationships. Angiographic diagnosis is based on the demonstration of elevated transverse sinuses and a posterosuperior course of the posterior cerebral arteries. In addition, there is anterosuperior displacement of the superior cerebellar arteries and shortening of the course of the posterior inferior cerebellar arteries. Wolpert et al. have emphasized the value of angiography as a method to differentiate extra-axial cysts in the posterior fossa from the Dandy-Walker syndrome.

Treatment

Treatment of the Dandy-Walker syndrome is surgical, although the preferred method of approach has been debated. When complete obstruction is evident from air studies, many authorities have elected a suboccipital craniectomy and excision of the obstructing membranes as the initial step. This procedure alone, however, is not likely to be successful because healing may be followed by occlusion at the same site. Furthermore, in view of the prenatal origin of this disorder, dissection of the convexity subarachnoid pathways, and absorptive surfaces may have never occurred. Surgical opening of the posterior fossa obstruction may thus convert noncommunicating hydrocephalus to one of communicating type. For the same reason, a Torkildsen procedure, or ventriculocisternal shunt, may be of little benefit.

A lateral ventricular shunt to either the right atrium or the peritoneal space is needed in most such patients to arrest the hydrocephalic process. Raimondi and colleagues have called attention to the development of "functional" occlusion of the aqueduct following lateral ventricular shunts in patients with the Dandy-Walker syndrome. They postulate obstruction of the aqueduct after decompression of the lateral ventricle by superior displacement of the remaining vermis secondary to the persisting dilated fourth ventricle. Such children may have normal lateral ventricular pressures and exhibit progressive, multiple brain stem signs, including cranial nerve palsies, nystagmus, ataxia, and even decerebrate postures. For this reason, these authors have recommended combined lateral and fourth ventricular-peritoneal shunts as the initial treatment for the Dandy-Walker syndrome. Children managed by a lateral ventricle shunt only should be observed periodically for the possible development of signs of brain stem compression. If such signs occur and air injected into the lateral ventricle does not pass through the aqueduct despite proper positioning, a fourth ventricle-to-peritoneal shunt should be accomplished.

THE ARNOLD-CHIARI MALFORMATION

The Arnold-Chiari malformation consists of displacement of tissue derived from the inferior cerebellar vermis into the upper cervical canal in addition to caudal displacement of the medulla and fourth ventricle. The anomaly is usually associated with hydrocephalus and is found in most children with a meningomyelocoele (Fig. 8-24). Russell stated that from 1935 until her publication in 1949, she had examined no cases of meningomyelocoele that were not associated with an Arnold-Chiari malformation.

In 1891 and 1895, Chiari described the essential features of this condition, although Cleland had recognized many of the components years before. Arnold, in 1894, reported a single case with a sacrococcygeal tumor and spina bifida and mentioned downward displacement of the cerebellum into the spinal canal. Schwalbe and Gredig, students of Arnold, subsequently proposed that the anomaly be termed the "Arnold-Chiari malforma-

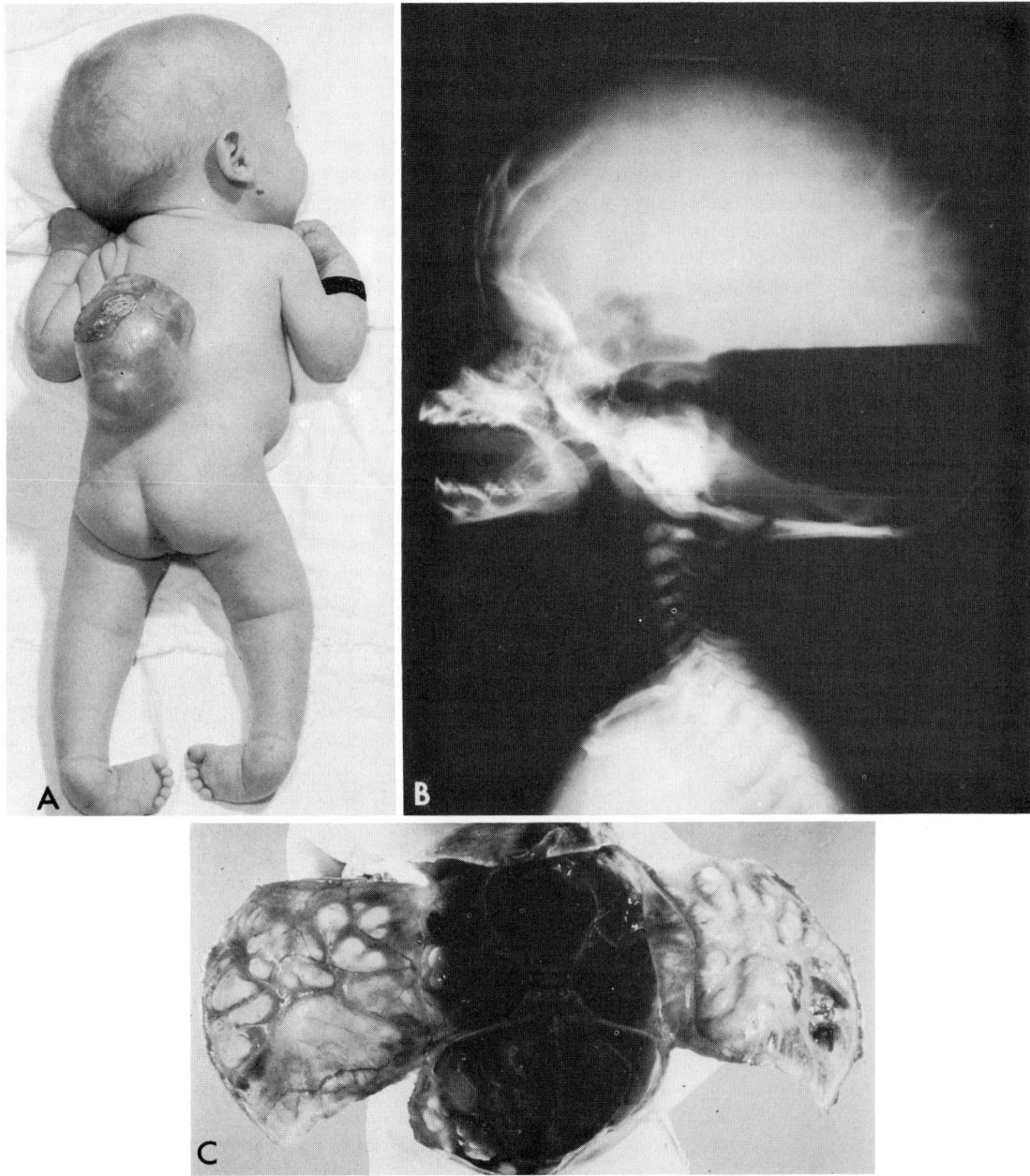

Figure 8–24. Arnold-Chiari malformation. *A*, Infant with large, thoracolumbar meningomyelocoele with partial paralysis and atrophy of the lower extremities, varus deformity of the feet, and hydrocephalus. The Arnold-Chiari malformation coexists in most infants with meningomyelocoeles associated with lower limb paralysis and hydrocephalus. *B*, Note the advanced degree of hydrocephalus even though the head is only mildly enlarged. Hydrocephalus in this child with a meningomyelocoele and Arnold-Chiari malformation resulted from obstruction within the aqueduct. Craniolacunia is evident. *C*, Craniolacunia. The dark, oval area represents the base of the skull with the skull convexities having been retracted laterally on either side. Note the weblike configuration of the inner surface of the skull, which results in the characteristic roentgenographic appearance with craniolacunia. This pattern is commonly observed in early infancy in children with meningomyelocoeles.

tion." Chiari had distinguished several forms of hindbrain malformations and referred to displacement of the cerebellar tonsils into the upper cervical canal without elongation of the medulla as type I. Chiari described 14 patients with this anomaly, all with congenital hydrocephalus and only one with meningomyelocoele. The Chiari type II anomaly included downward displacement of the cerebellar vermis plus the lower brain stem and corresponds to what is now referred to as the Arnold-Chiari malformation.

The most striking aspect of this malformation is the marked elongation and downward displacement of the brain stem (Fig. 8-25). The medulla and its contained fourth ventricle show the most marked changes but the pons is also involved. As the medulla extends into the cervical region, it overlaps and flattens the dorsal aspect of the cervical cord and presents a kinked appearance when viewed laterally. The displaced cerebellar vermis is usually partially bound to the adjacent medulla by fibrous tissue and may extend as low as the first thoracic vertebral level. The caudal displacement of the medulla and cervical cord causes the cervical nerve roots to take an ascending course to reach the foramina of

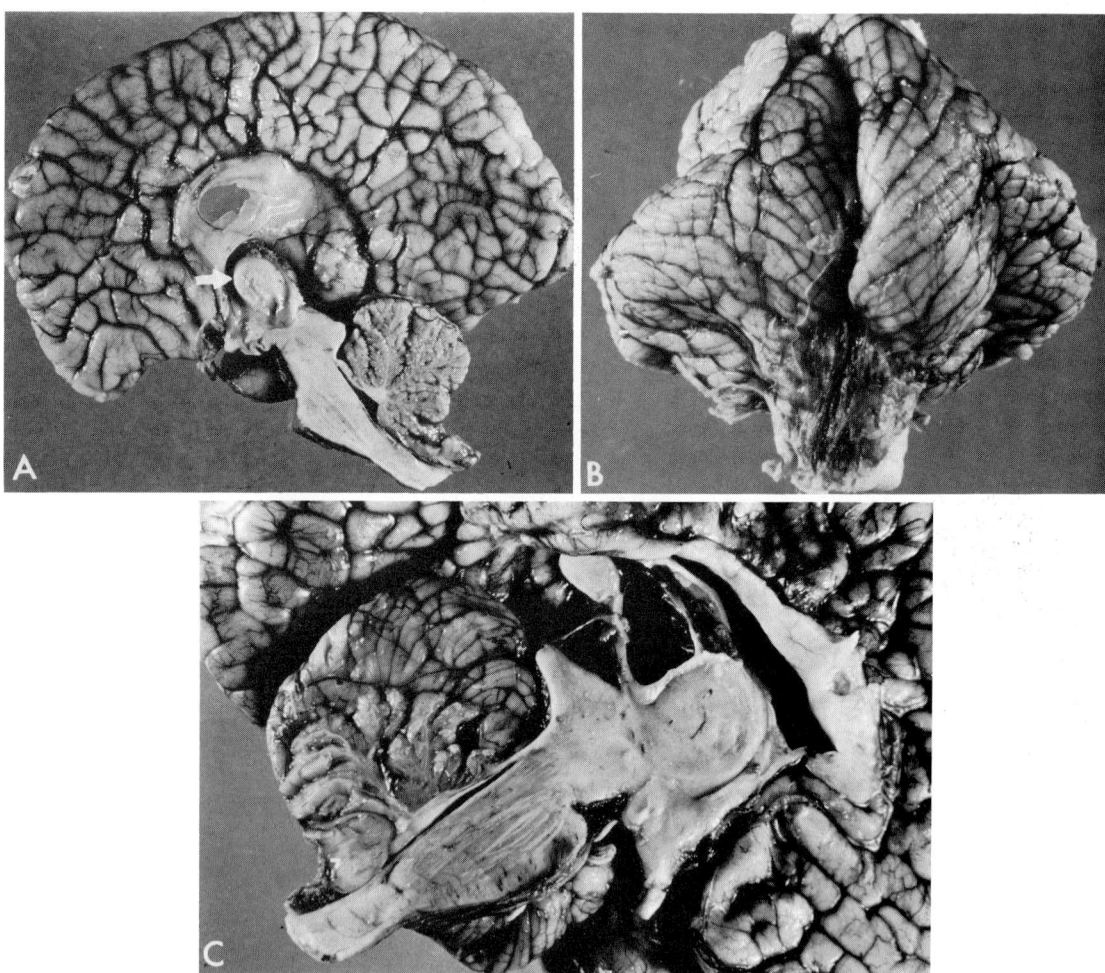

Figure 8–25. Arnold-Chiari malformation. *A*, There is elongation and downward displacement of the brain stem and the fourth ventricle. The cerebellar vermis also is displaced downward, extending inferior to the level of the foramen magnum, and is attached to the dorsal surface of the medulla. The aqueduct is nonpatent and the tectum shows the beaked appearance, characteristic of the Arnold-Chiari malformation. The massa intermedia is enlarged (arrow) and polymicrogyria is present. Note the perforation of the septum pellucidum, a common finding with any type of advanced hydrocephalus. *B*, View from the dorsal surface of the cerebellum and medulla. The inferior vermis is displaced caudally over the dorsal surface of the elongated medulla and has undergone hemorrhagic and necrotic changes. *C*, The brain stem is elongated, the inferior vermis is malformed, and the tectum of the midbrain is beak-shaped.

exit. A remarkable and nearly constant feature of this syndrome is the beak-shaped appearance of the tectum attributed to fusion of the superior and inferior colliculi (Daniel and Strich, Feigin).

The posterior fossa is much smaller than normal and the tentorium is attached abnormally low on the occipital bone. Marked enlargement of the massa intermedia is found in most cases (Peach) and many reveal generalized polymicrogyria as well as other cerebral anomalies. Hypoplasia of the falx cerebri, craniolacunia, and hydromyelia are additional common findings.

Most patients with the Arnold-Chiari malformation have hydrocephalus. In some cases, aqueductal anomalies account for obstruction, but in others the explanation for hydrocephalus is unclear. Russell suggested that communicating hydrocephalus in these children could result from obstruction to the reflux of cerebrospinal fluid into the cranial cavity because of plugging of the foramen magnum by the caudally placed cerebellomedullary tissue. She based this concept in part on the observation that purulent infection within the spinal canal would lead to little or no involvement at the base or over the surface of the brain but with extensive spread into the lateral ventricles.

Pathogenesis

Numerous theories have been designed to explain the Arnold-Chiari malformation, and to date, the exact cause and pathogenesis remain unestablished. Recent investigators have generally considered it to be an associated malformation developing in concert with spina bifida cystica and not secondary to it. Chiari assumed that the hindbrain anomalies characteristic of this disorder are secondary to caudal herniation from hydrocephalus above. This theory remains primarily a matter of historical interest since the occurrence of the anomaly in the absence of hydrocephalus has now been recorded. In addition, the herniated cerebellar tissue consists of portions of the inferior vermis rather than the tonsils, which are displaced with increased intracranial pressure.

The "traction" theory (van Houweninge Grafdijk, Penfield and Coburn, Lichtenstein) assumed that because of the attachment of the spinal cord at the site of vertebral defect, normal ascent of the cord relative to the vertebral canal could not occur and traction would displace hindbrain structures into the cervical canal. Lichtenstein also attributed the aqueductal occlusion observed in some cases to elongation of the midbrain secondary to the traction process. Many observations have established the inadequacy of traction as an explanation for this anomaly. The existence of the Arnold-Chiari malformation without a spine defect (Peach) and the beaked tectum, which resembles that of the normal embryo, provides the strongest evidence against this postulate.

From study of human embryos, Barry et al. suggested that the Arnold-Chiari malformation results from neural overgrowth beginning about the fourth week of development. Because of the excessive volume of the intracranial contents, these authors concluded that the posterior fossa contents were protruded through the foramen magnum into the cervical canal. Other investigators have attributed the elongation of the brain stem to failure of the pontine flexure to develop at approximately the sixth week of embryonic life because of a preceding developmental arrest (Daniel and Strich, Peach). According to this concept, the displaced cerebellar tissue represents a persistence of the embryonic portion of the intraventricular cerebellum, which is carried into the cervical canal because of lack of formation of the pontine flexure. Of the many postulated theories, that related to developmental arrest due to unknown causes is the most attractive.

Except for hydrocephalus, which may be secondary to the Arnold-Chiari malformation in some cases, the Arnold-Chiari malformation in most infants with meningomyelocoele remains relatively silent clinically. There have been several reports of this anomaly in older persons without associated spine defects with symptoms including headache, vertigo, cranial nerve palsies, and ataxia. In most such patients, however, the malformation identified at surgery appears to have been the Chiari type I anomaly and not the Arnold-Chiari malformation (Peach).

THE KLEEBLATTSCHÄDEL SYNDROME

This rare disorder consists of grotesque facial and skull deformities that result from the interaction of prenatal synostosis of multiple cranial sutures and congenital hydro-

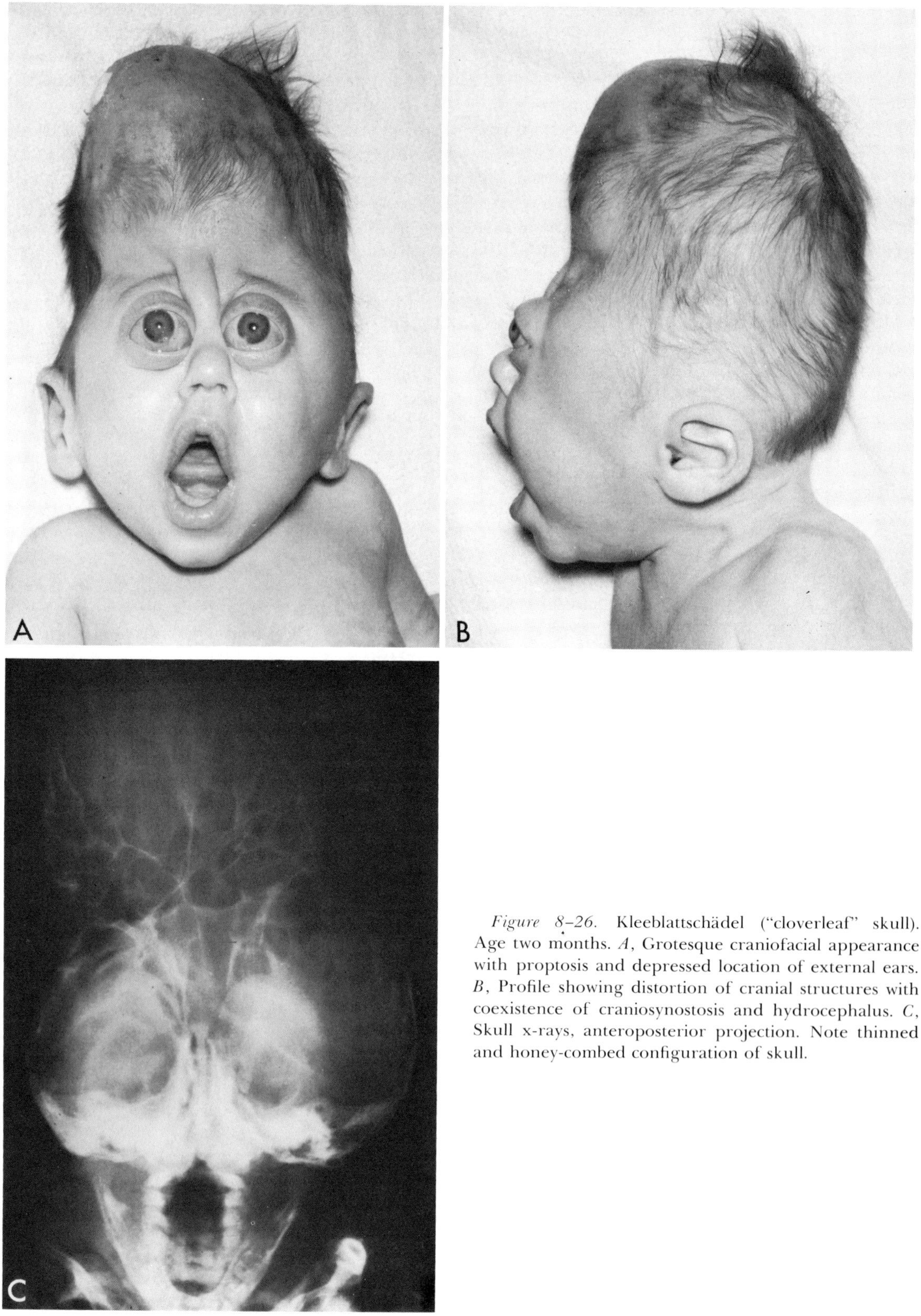

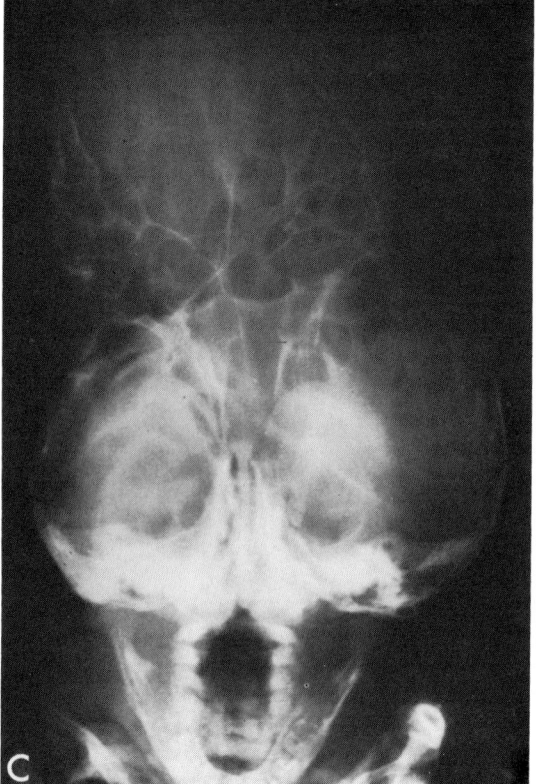

Figure 8–26. Kleeblattschädel ("cloverleaf" skull). Age two months. *A*, Grotesque craniofacial appearance with proptosis and depressed location of external ears. *B*, Profile showing distortion of cranial structures with coexistence of craniosynostosis and hydrocephalus. *C*, Skull x-rays, anteroposterior projection. Note thinned and honey-combed configuration of skull.

cephalus (Comings, Angle et al., Feingold et al.). Holtermüeller and Wiedemann in 1960 referred to this unfortunate combination of structural abnormalities as the "kleeblattschädel syndrome," or the cloverleaf skull.

Premature closure of the coronal and lambdoid sutures leads to a peculiar head shape, which is profoundly accentuated by increased pressure secondary to hydrocephalus (Fig. 8-26). The trilobed shape of the skull results from lateral expansion in the region of the squamosal sutures, which secondarily displaces the ears downward. Bilateral exophthalmos, wide-set eyes, and a depressed nasal bridge add to the unpleasant appearance of these infants.

Various types of deformities of long bones have occurred in several reported cases. Bony ankylosis of the elbows and abnormal shortening of long bones have been the skeletal anomalies most often observed. The cause of hydrocephalus in this syndrome has not been clarified, but it is believed to be secondary to basilar skull deformities reminiscent of those associated with achondroplasia. The prognosis has generally been considered poor, with early death expected in untreated patients. Feingold et al., however, reported a 14-year-old child with this syndrome.

TREATMENT OF HYDROCEPHALUS

Despite remarkable advances in the comprehension of the physiology and pathology of hydrocephalus, consistently successful treatment has not yet been achieved. Medical therapy has offered relatively little and the multiplicity of surgical procedures that have been developed are evidence of the lack of complete acceptance of any single approach. Although an attitude of total pessimism is unwarranted, the currently available surgical treatment of the infant with progressive hydrocephalus must be recognized as less than ideal and characterized by a variety of potentially frustrating and perplexing complications.

Hydrocephalus is most effectively managed when a primary lesion can be identified which, when removed, abolishes the cause of the process. Except for certain posterior fossa tumors, however, such lesions are infrequent and treatment of hydrocephalus must depend on the use of foreign materials inserted to bypass the site of obstruction or destructive procedures to alter the cerebrospinal fluid physiology. Rarely, one encounters a membranous obstruction of the inferior portion of the aqueduct that can be perforated reestablishing patency of the system (Turnbull and Drake).

The desirability of surgical treatment for congenital hydrocephalus in which the cause cannot be removed requires consideration of the expected benefits from treatment compared to the natural course of the illness. Laurence and Coates (1962) studied 182 untreated cases collected over 20 years and found that 89 (48 per cent) had died and 81 (44 per cent) were considered to have undergone spontaneous arrest. Of the "arrested" group, 38 per cent were judged to have IQ's of 85 or above. Yashon (1963) reported 58 patients with infantile hydrocephalus that had not been operated upon, 23 of whom had a fatal outcome. Of the survivors, in 31 the disorder was considered arrested.

The concept of spontaneous arrest of infantile hydrocephalus is subject to varied meanings, depending on how it is defined and what methods are used to demonstrate its occurrence. To have significant meaning, arrest of hydrocephalus should imply that further growth of the head does not occur, at least until the size of the rest of the body is proportional. Furthermore, arrest of the process should allow restoration of the ventricular size toward normal with reestablishment of the cerebral mantle. Assigning the designation of "arrested hydrocephalus" to a neurologically devastated child whose head has reached enormous proportions but then ceases to grow is artificial, is probably in error, and dilutes the potential meaning of "significant arrest."

If reasonably rigid criteria are adhered to, spontaneous and permanent arrest of progressive hydrocephalus in infancy appears to be an infrequent event (Foltz and Shurtleff, Lorber and Zachary). Comparing the outcome of patients with untreated infantile hydrocephalus with those managed surgically, there is little doubt that the results are better in the treated group in whom the immediate success rate for control of hydrocephalus is in the range of 70 per cent (Yashon).

Although the advantages of surgical treatment have been clearly demonstrated, all children with hydrocephalus are not necessarily candidates for such treatment. One must consider not only the probability of survival but also the quality of life that results from its prolongation. For example, the severely defective neonate with a large or infected meningomyelocoele, which cannot be attacked surgically, may be better managed by more conservative methods. Some have used the thickness of the cerebral mantle as an index for decisions regarding surgery but most now agree that the prognosis depends more on the nature of the associated cerebral lesions than on the degree of ventricular enlargement (Yashon et al., Lorber and Zachary, Hadenius et al.).

When treatment of the infant or child with progressive hydrocephalus is deemed necessary, the method selected depends on many factors, including the site of the obstruction, the characteristics of the ventricular fluid, and the surgeon's experience with different procedures. In some cases, temporary procedures are indicated when it is suspected that the more conventional shunt operations will be unsuccessful. For example, the child recovering from meningitis or subarachnoid hemorrhage complicated by communicating hydrocephalus can be maintained by the use of a ventriculostomy reservoir until a more permanent shunt can be inserted (Rickham and Penn). The high-protein ventricular fluid often present in such cases is likely to block the valve of the more permanent shunts, requiring repeated revisions. Regardless, treatment of infantile hydrocephalus must be assumed to be surgical in most cases because medical measures have not proved adequate.

Acetazolamide (Diamox) has controlled hydrocephalus in certain instances (Huttenlocher) but cannot be considered a satisfactory treatment method for most (Schain, Mealey and Barker).

"Physiologic" Procedures

Surgical treatment of progressive hydrocephalus in infancy has included either the so-called "physiologic" operations of third ventriculostomy or choroid plexectomy, or the more commonly used shunting procedures. Dandy devised third ventriculostomy for noncommunicating hydrocephalus in 1922 and introduced the concept of destruction of the choroid plexus for communicating hydrocephalus in 1918. Endoscopic cauterization of the choroid plexus was subsequently advanced by Putnam and still later by Scarff (1936).

In 1963 Scarff compared the results of third ventriculostomy and choroid plexectomy with the results of the shunt procedures. The initial success rate for control of hydrocephalus was approximately the same in both groups but late complications were 10 to 20 times greater after shunting operations that required mechanical valves and tubes. While the results reported by Scarff are impressive, great skill developed by a surgeon after the performance of an operation many times may have considerable bearing on the results in such a series.

Shunting Procedures

The first widely recognized shunting procedure for hydrocephalus was developed by Torkildsen in 1939 and is known as ventriculo-cisternostomy. The Torkildsen shunt drains fluid from one lateral ventricle to the cisterna magna and thus its use is restricted to noncommunicating hydrocephalus. It remains of value for the older child and adult with an obstructive process in the posterior fossa but, for technical reasons, it is not applicable to the infant and young child. Shunts from the ventricle or spinal subarachnoid space to almost every conceivable body cavity were subsequently designed. Most have now been abandoned except for the occasional use of a subarachnoid-ureteral shunt, the frequent use of the ventriculoperitoneal shunt, and the most popular ventriculoatrial (vascular) shunt.

Matson (1949, 1953) popularized the lumbar subarachnoid-ureteral shunt for communicating hydrocephalus and achieved results that compare favorably with other shunt procedures. Disadvantages of the operation include the need to sacrifice a normal kidney, the continous loss of salt via the urine, and the danger of meningitis if urinary tract infection is acquired.

Ventriculoperitoneal shunts are applicable to either communicating or noncommunicating hydrocephalus but have been plagued by the predisposition of the peritoneal end of the device to become repeatedly obstructed (Scott et al., Jackson and Snodgrass, Murtagh and Lehman). Except for the need for periodic revision, the peritoneal shunts are far less often beset by late complications than are the vascular shunts. Numerous modifications have improved the outlook for the ventriculoperitoneal shunt and some now prefer it to the ventriculoatrial shunt even though the need for revision remains great (Hammon). This procedure is especially valuable in children recovering from meningitis in whom the ventricular fluid may contain bacteria or has a high protein content which would readily obstruct the valve of a ventriculoatrial shunt.

Nulsen and Spitz introduced the Holter valve in 1952 and Pudenz et al. followed with the Heyer valve in 1957. In 1964, the Hakim valve became an additional system for vascular shunting. The development of these unidirectional valves paved the way for the use of the vascular system as a site for cerebrospinal fluid shunting from the lateral ventricle. The concept, however, had been devised many years before because Payr attempted ventriculovenous shunts as early as 1908. It was not until the design of valves that would prevent reflex of blood through the tube that vascular shunts were widely used.

The Holter system utilizies a right angle silicone rubber ventricular catheter. This is connected to a valve designed to allow evaluation of its patency by digital compression against the skull of the tubing of the valve mechanism. The Pudenz-Heyer valve system consists of a ventricular catheter connected to a circular flushing device located in a cranial burr hole and permits assessment of the patency of the system. The Heyer valve is contained within the cardiac end of the distal catheter.

The Hakim valve system is designed to permit autoclave sterilization and includes a ventricular catheter with a hook-shaped tip to prevent penetration into the brain. The valve, like the Holter valve, is placed over the mastoid process and consists of a ball-and-spring mechanism that regulates pressure required for flow. This system also can be tested for patency by external compression with the fingers.

As of 1963, Scarff had found reports on 345 cases of hydrocephalus treated with ventriculoatrial shunts with an operative mortality rate of 2 to 3 per cent and with an initial arrest of the process in 65 per cent of patients.

In keeping with all types of shunts used for treatment of hydrocephalus, one of the major problems has been obstruction of the catheter. This has been a problem of special importance when the shunt is inserted in the small infant in whom linear growth eventually results in retraction of the distal end of the tube from its position in the right atrium. It is generally recognized that placement of the end of the tube or retraction of the end into the neck vessels is followed by nonfunction within a short period of time. For this reason, periodic revision and lengthening of the tube is recommended by some (Tsingoglou and Forrest, Anderson).

One of the major problems with the Holter valve and ventriculoatrial shunt device is clinical assessment of its patency. The valve that can be easily collapsed but does not promptly refill suggests obstruction proximally, in the ventricular end of the tube. The valve that cannot be readily emptied by external pressure is probably obstructed distally. Although these guidelines seem reasonably sound, in practice one cannot always determine whether the shunt is patent by palpation and compression.

Go et al. (1970) proposed a method of evaluating cerebrospinal fluid flow through the shunt by using a thermosensitive apparatus containing two thermistors, while the valve is cooled by application of ice over its surface. Temperature changes recorded distal to the valve indicate patency of the lumen and cerebrospinal flow. An additional method of assessment of shunt patency consists of insertion of a 22-gauge needle into the Holter valve barrel followed by gentle aspiration. Continued withdrawal of cerebrospinal fluid suggests patency of the proximal segment. Injection of a small quantity of diatrizoate sodium (Hypaque) while observing the distal segment of tubing fluoroscopically permits evaluation of patency from the valve into the right atrium (Amador et al.). The disadvantage of this method is possible damage to the valve mechanism by the needle insertion.

Contraindications to ventriculoatrial shunts are infrequent and have not been clearly defined. The child with cyanotic congenital heart disease or with valvular abnormalities on the right side of the heart is a poor candidate, mainly because of the hazards of infection. A history of bacterial endocarditis or the presence of active intracranial infection also precludes the performance of a ventriculoatrial shunt. The presence of blood or a markedly elevated cerebrospinal fluid protein content within the ventricular fluid is not a specific contraindication but reduces the probability of success with a vascular shunt.

COMPLICATIONS OF TREATMENT

With any form of shunting procedure for hydrocephalus, the most disconcerting early complication is lack of function of the system because of obstruction or occlusion within the catheter. With ventriculoatrial shunts, this may occur within the ventricular end because of plugging of the tube by the choroid plexus or by material derived from white matter of the brain (Hakim). The distal segment becomes occluded by blood clot within its lumen or secondary to thrombosis of the superior vena cava if the end of the tube is within this vessel. In addition to obstruction of the tube, a valve in place for several years may develop increased resistance, impeding the flow of cerebrospinal fluid even though the system remains patent (Corkery and Zachary).

Complications of ventriculoatrial shunts previously mentioned include premature fusion of cranial sutures resulting in distortion of the shape of the head (Kloss, Roberts and Rickham), and diminution of the intracranial volume because of inward growth of the inner table of the skull (Griscom and Oh). Conversion of communicating hydrocephalus to occlusion of the aqueduct has also been described as a consequence of successful vascular shunts (Foltz and Shurtleff). Additional problems that have been described include perforation of the heart (Strenger) and penetration of the superior vena cava by the catheter (Hemmer). A misplaced catheter can lead to accumulation of the fluid in the pericardium with cardiac tamponade (Crome and Erdohazi).

Septicemia

Septicemia is one of the most significant and life-threatening complications of ventriculoatrial shunting and may be an important cause of malfunction and obstruction of the valve. The incidence of infection developing as a complication of vascular shunts is unknown but has been estimated to be as high as 20 per cent (Noonan and Ehmke). Among 183 shunted cases, Luthardt found septicemia in 9 per cent. Nicholas et al. observed that 7 per cent of Holter valves became colonized during the first year after insertion and a total of 12 per cent were infected during the first five years after the shunt procedure was performed.

The clinical manifestations of septicemia and shunt colonization vary remarkably, in part depending on the virulence of the organism. Evidence of infection may develop within days after the operation or may occur after several years of successful shunt function. In some, the symptoms are severe and fulminating with high, spiking fever, night sweating, and vomiting. This form of sepsis in children with vascular shunts is easily recognized as an infectious complication and is usually caused by *Staphylococcus aureus*. In others, the illness is chronic and smoldering with only subtle clinical manifestations suggesting a septic process.

Irritability, poor appetite, vomiting, recurrent low-grade fever, and progressive anemia are characteristic symptoms that usually result from persistent *Staphylococcus epidermidis (albus)* septicemia. The spleen may be enlarged, the sedimentation rate is usually elevated, and proteinuria may be present in these patients. Noble et al. described a child who appeared clinically well and without symptoms but with an enlarged spleen and petechial skin lesions. Staphylococcal sepsis was proved by blood culture.

Diagnosis of bacterial sepsis is dependent on isolating the organism from the blood, but several cultures may be necessary. Persistently negative cultures do not exclude the possibility of sepsis in a child with a vascular shunt, especially if antibotics have been previously administered. Blood is best obtained for culture during a febrile spike or after the valve has been manually pumped several times (Bruce et al.). In infants suspected of sepsis with shunt colonization, ventricular tap with examination and culture of the fluid may also be of diagnostic importance. Although staphylococcal sepsis is most common, other organisms, including *Escherichia coli* and *Serratia marcescens* may occur in patients with vascular shunts (Bruce et al.).

Bacterial colonization of the valve of a vascular shunt can rarely be obliterated with antibiotics. Most authors have indicated that an infected shunt must be removed, although there are many opinions regarding how the child should be managed once this has been accomplished (Nicholas et al., Perrin and McLaurin, Bruce et al., Luthardt). Some replace the infected shunt with a new prosthesis utilizing the same vein; others prefer to delay replacement of the shunt until antibiotics have been given for two to four weeks. Still another method, which seems most reasonable, is removal of the infected device and immediate replacement with a ventriculoperitoneal shunt.

Medical treatment of children with bacterial sepsis complicating vascular shunting requires four to six weeks of antibiotics in large dosage, preferably given by the intravenous route. The choice of antibiotic depends on the in vitro sensitivity studies but is usually either penicillin or a semisynthetic penicillinase-resistant penicillin derivative. When therapy is started before the organism is isolated, either methicillin or oxacillin is used until one has determined the organism is sensitive to penicillin.

A recently recognized complication of ventriculoatrial shunts infected with coagulase-negative staphylococci is progressive glomerulonephritis (Black et al., Stickler et al., Stauffer, Rames et al.). The onset of renal disease in these patients has varied from one month to several years after insertion of the shunt. Hematuria is a common early finding but several reported cases have had manifestations of the nephrotic syndrome, including edema, proteinuria, hypoproteinemia, hypercholesterolemia, and azotemia. Hypertension has been noted in some. Serum complement may be reduced and immunofluorescent staining of renal tissue reveals immune globulin and complement within glomeruli (Rames et al.). Although the pathogenesis of renal involvement remains unclear, investigators have postulated an immunologic process secondary to persistent bacterial sepsis (Stickler et al., Rames et al.). Improvement has occurred in certain patients following removal of the vascular shunt.

Pulmonary Thromboembolism

Pulmonary vascular occlusive changes have become well known in children with ventriculoatrial shunts (Friedman et al., Sperling et al., Erdohazi et al., Nugent et al., Noonan and Ehmke, Rao et al.). Thromboembolism of pulmonary vessels has often been found at autopsy even though symptoms had not been observed in life. In some children, pulmonary hypertension with cor pulmonale has led to recognizable symptoms and signs.

There have been many postulates as to the pathogenesis of this condition and it is probable that several factors are of importance. Repeated embolization of microthrombi from the tube or the right atrium accounts for many of the vascular occlusive abnormalities. Sepsis may play an important role, especially in the formation of thrombi within the right atrium. Emery and Hilton suggested the possibility of an autoimmune response of pulmonary vessels to some component of cerebrospinal fluid. The relatively high incidence of pulmonary vascular occlusive disease secondary to ventriculoatrial shunts warrants chest x-ray and electrocardiogram at periodic intervals in these patients.

REFERENCES

Adams, R. D., Fisher, C. M., Hakim, S., Ojemann, R., and Sweet, W. H.: Symptomatic occult hydrocephalus with "normal" cerebrospinal fluid pressure. *New Eng. J. Med.*, **273**:117–126, 1965.

Adeloye, A., Singh, S. P., and Odeku, E. L.: Stridor, myelomeningocele, and hydrocephalus in a child. *Arch. Neurol.*, **23**:271–273, 1970.

Alexander, W. S.: Progressive fibrinoid degeneration of fibrillary astrocytes associated with mental retardation in a hydrocephalic infant. *Brain*, **72**:373–381, 1949.

Amador, L. V., Jara, O., and Porras, C. L.: Valvulography. A test for patency of Holter valve shunts. *Amer. J. Dis. Child.*, **117**:190–193, 1969.

Anderson, F. M.: A method for revision of ventriculocardiac shunts. *J. Neurosurgery*, **34**:796–799, 1971.

Anderson, F. M.: and Landing, B. H.: Cerebral arachnoid cysts in infants. *J. Pediat.*, **69**:88–96, 1966.

Andersson, H.: Craniosynostosis as complication after operation for hydrocephalus. *Acta Pediat. Scandinav.*, **55**:192–196, 1966.

Angle, C. R., McIntire, M. S., and Moore, R. C.: Cloverleaf skull: Kleeblattschädel-deformity syndrome. *Amer. J. Dis. Child.*, **114**:198–202, 1967.

Appenzeller, O., Snyder, R., and Kornfeld, M.: Autonomic failure in hydrencephaly. *J. Neurol. Neurosurg. Psychiat.*, **33**:532–543, 1970.

Arnold, J.: Myelocyste, transposition von gewebskeimen und sympodie. *Beitr. path. Anat. u. allg. Path.*, **16**:1–28, 1894.

Bakwin, H., Golden, A., and Fox, S.: Familial osteoectasia with macrocranium. *Amer. J. Roentgen.*, **91**:609–617, 1964.

Bannister, R., Gilford, E., and Kocen, R.: Isotope encephalography in the diagnosis of dementia due to communicating hydrocephalus. *Lancet*, **2**:1014–1017, 1967.

Barry, A., Patten, B. M., and Stewart, B. H.: Possible factors in the development of the Arnold-Chiari malformation. *J. Neurosurg.*, **14**:285–301, 1957.

Bejar, R. L., Smith, G. F., Park, S., Spellacy, W. N., Wolfson, S. L., and Nyhan, W. L.: Cerebral gigantism. Concentrations of amino acids in plasma and muscle. *J. Pediat.*, **76**:105–111, 1970.

Benda, C. E.: *Developmental Disorders of Mentation and Cerebral Palsies*. New York, Grune and Stratton, 1952.

Benda, C. E.: The Dandy-Walker syndrome or the so-called atresia of the foramen of Magendie. *J. Neuropath. Exper. Neurol.*, **13**:14–29, 1954.

Benson, D. F., LeMay, M., Patton, D. H., and Rubens,

A. B.: Diagnosis of normal-pressure hydrocephalus. *New Eng. J. Med.*, **283**:609–615, 1970.

Benton, J. W., Nellhaus, G., Huttenlocher, P. R., Ojemann, R. G., and Dodge, P. R.: The bobble-head doll syndrome. Report of a unique truncal tremor associated with third ventricular cyst and hydrocephalus in children. *Neurology*, **16**:725–729, 1966.

Bering, E. A., Jr.: Choroid plexus and arterial pulsation of the cerebrospinal fluid. *Arch. Neurol. Psychiat.*, **73**:165–172, 1955.

Bering, E. A., Jr.: The use of phenolsulphonphthalein in the clinical evaluation of hydrocephalus. *J. Neurosurg.*, **13**:587–595, 1956.

Bering, E. A., Jr.: Circulation of the cerebrospinal fluid. *J. Neurosurg.*, **19**:405–413, 1962.

Bickers, D. S., and Adams, R. D.: Hereditary stenosis of the aqueduct of Sylvius as a cause of hydrocephalus. *Brain*, **72**:246–262, 1949.

Black, J. A., Challacombe, D. N., and Ockenden, B. G.: Nephrotic syndrome associated with bacteraemia after shunt operations for hydrocephalus. *Lancet*, **2**:921–924, 1965.

Bowsher, D.: *Cerebrospinal Fluid Dynamics in Health and Disease*. Springfield, Ill., Charles C Thomas, 1960.

Bray, P. F., Shields, W. D., Wolcott, G. J., and Madsen, J. A.: Occipitofrontal head circumference—an accurate measure of intracranial volume. *J. Pediat.*, **75**:303–305, 1969.

Brodal, A., and Hauglie-Hanssen, E.: Congenital hydrocephalus with defective development of the cerebellar vermis (Dandy-Walker syndrome). *J. Neurol. Neurosurg. Psychiat.*, **22**:99–108, 1959.

Bruce, A. M., Lorber, J., Shedden, W. I. H., and Zachary, R. B.: Persistent bacteraemia following ventriculocaval shunt operations for hydrocephalus in infants. *Develop. Med. Child. Neurol.*, **5**:461–470, 1963.

Canavan, M. M.: Schilder's encephalitis periaxialis diffusa. *Arch. Neurol. Psychiat.*, **25**:299–308, 1931.

Carter, L. P., and Pittman, H. W.: Posterior fossa subdural hematoma of the newborn. *J. Neurosurg.*, **34**:423–426, 1971.

Chiari, H.: Ueber veränderungen des kleinhirns infolge von hydrocephalie. *Deutsche Med. Wchnschr.*, **17**: 1172–1175, 1891.

Chiari, H.: Ueber veränderungen des kleinhirns, des pons, und der medulla oblongata infolge von congenitaler hydrocephalie des grosshirns. *Denkschr. d. Akad. Wissensch. Math—naturw.*, **63**:71–116, 1895.

Clark, R. G., Milhorat, T. H., Stanley, W. C., and DiChiro, G.: Experimental Pantopaque ventriculography. *J. Neurosurg.*, **34**:387–395, 1971.

Cleland, J.: Contribution to the stury of spina bifida, encephalocoele and anencephalus. *J. Anat. Physiol.*, **17**:257–292, 1883.

Cohen, M. E., Rosenthal, A. D., and Matson, D. D.: Neurological abnormalities in achondroplastic children. *J. Pediat.*, **71**:367–376, 1967.

Comings, D. E.: The Kleeblattschädel syndrome—a grotesque form of hydrocephalus. *J. Pediat.*, **67**: 126–129, 1965.

Cooper, E. R. A.: An anatomical study of hydrocephalus. *Acta Anat.* (Basel), **52**(Suppl. 48–2):1–48, 1963.

Corkery, J. J., and Zachary, R. B.: Increased resistance developing in Holter valves. *Lancet*, **2**:1331–1334, 1967.

Courville, C. B.: Etiology and pathogenesis of laminar cortical necrosis. *Arch. Neurol. Psychiat.*, **79**:7–30, 1958.

Crome, L., and Erdohazi, M.: Main pathological findings in hydrocephalic children treated by ventriculoatrial shunt. *Arch. Dis. Childh.*, **41**:179–182, 1966.

Crome, L., and Sylvester, P. E.: Hydranencephaly (hydrencephaly). *Arch. Dis. Childh.*, **33**:235–245, 1958.

Cruveilhier, J.: *Anatomie Pathologique du Corps Humain.* Vol. 2. Paris, Bailliere, 1829.

Cushing, H.: Studies on the cerebrospinal fluid. *J. Med. Res.*, **31**:1, 1914.

Cutler, R. W. P., Page, L., Galicich, J., and Watters, G. V.: Formation and absorption of cerebrospinal fluid in man. *Brain*, **91**:707–720, 1968.

D'Agostino, A. N., Kernohan, J. W., and Brown, J. R.: The Dandy-Walker syndrome. *J. Neuropath. Exper. Neurol.*, **22**:450–470, 1963.

Dandy, W. E.: Extirpation of the choroid plexus of the lateral ventricles in communicating hydrocephalus. *Ann. Surg.*, **68**:569, 1918.

Dandy, W. E.: Experimental hydrocephalus. *Ann. Surg.*, **70**:129–142, 1919.

Dandy, W. C.: The cause of so-called idiopathic hydrocephalus. *Bull. Johns Hopk. Hosp.*, **32**:67, 1921.

Dandy, W. E.: Cerebral ventriculoscopy. *Bull. Johns Hopk. Hosp.*, **33**:189, 1922.

Dandy, W. E., and Blackfan, K. D.: An experimental and clinical study of internal hydrocephalus. *J.A.M.A.*, **61**:2216–2217, 1913.

Dandy, W. C., and Blackfan, K. D.: Internal hydrocephalus. An experimental, clinical and pathological study. *Amer. J. Dis. Child.*, **8**:406–482, 1914.

Dandy, W. E., and Blackfan, K. D.: Internal hydrocephalus. *Amer. J. Dis. Child.*, **14**:424–443, 1917.

Daniel, P. M., and Strich, S. J.: Some observations on the congenital deformity of the central nervous system known as the Arnold-Chiari malformation. *J. Neuropath. Exper. Neurol.*, **17**:255–266, 1958.

Dennis, J. P., Rosenberg, H. S., and Alvord, E. C., Jr.: Megalencephaly, internal hydrocephalus and other neurological aspects of achondroplasia. *Brain*, **84**: 427–445, 1961.

Detmer, D. E., and Blocker, H. M.: A case of aseptic meningitis secondary to intrathecal injection of I-131 human serum albumin. *Neurology*, **15**:642–643, 1965.

DiChiro, G.: New radiographic and isotopic procedures in neurosurgical diagnosis. *J.A.M.A.*, **188**:524–529, 1964.

DiChiro, G., Reames, P. M., and Matthews, W. B.: RISA—ventriculography and RISA—cisternography. *Neurology*, **14**:185–191, 1964.

Dodge, P. R., and Porter, P.: Demonstration of intracranial pathology by transillumination. *Arch. Neurol.*, **5**:594–605, 1961.

Dorff, G. B., and Shapiro, L. M.: A clinicopathologic study of sexual precocity with hydrocephalus. *Amer. J. Dis. Child.*, **53**:481–499, 1937.

Drachman, D. A., and Richardson, E. P., Jr.: Aqueductal narrowing, congenital and acquired. *Arch. Neurol.*, **5**:552–559, 1961.

Duggan, C. A., Keener, E. B., and Gray, B. B., Jr.: Secondary craniosynostosis. *Amer. J. Roentgen.*, **109**: 277–293, 1970.

Dyggve, H., and Tygstrup, I.: Megalencephaly. *Develop. Med. Child Neurol.*, **6**:581–584, 1964.

Edwards, J. H.: The syndrome of sex-linked hydrocephalus. *Arch. Dis. Childh.*, **36**:486–493, 1961.

Edwards, J. H., Norman, R. M., and Roberts, J. M.: Sex-linked hydrocephalus: report of a family with 15 affected members. *Arch. Dis. Childh.*, **36**:481–485, 1961.

Elmore, S. M.: Pycnodysostosis. A review. *J. Bone & Joint Surg.*, **49-A**:153–162, 1967.

Emery, J. L., and Hilton, H. B.: Lung and heart complications of treatment of hydrocephalus by ventriculo-auriculostomy. *Surgery*, **50**:309–314, 1961.

Erdohazi, M., Eckstein, H. B., and Crome, L.: Pulmonary embolization as a complication of ventriculo-atrial shunts inserted for hydrocephalus. *Develop. Med. Child Neurol.*, Suppl. **11**:36–44, 1966.

Feigin, I.: Arnold-Chiari malformation with associated analogous malformation of the midbrain. *Neurology*, **6**:22–31, 1956.

Feinberg, S. B., and Langer, L. O.: Roentgen findings of increased intracranial pressure and communicating hydrocephalus as insidious manifestations of chronic histiocytosis-X. *Amer. J. Roentgen.*, **95**:41–47, 1965.

Feingold, M., O'Conner, J. F., Berkman, M., and Darling, D. B.: Kleeblattschädel syndrome. *Amer. J. Dis. Child.*, **118**:589–594, 1969.

Fishman, R. A., and Greer, M.: Experimental obstructive hydrocephalus. *Arch. Neurol.*, **8**:156–161, 1963.

Fitzsimmons, J. S.: Laryngeal stridor and respiratory obstruction associated with meningomyelocele. *Arch. Dis. Childh.*, **40**:687–688, 1965.

Foltz, E. L., and Shurtleff, D. B.: Five-year comparative study of hydrocephalus in children with and without operation (113 cases). *J. Neurosurg.*, **20**:1064–1079, 1963.

Foltz, E. L., and Shurtleff, D. B.: Conversion of communicating hydrocephalus to stenosis or occlusion of the aqueduct during ventricular shunt. *J. Neurosurg.*, **24**:520–529, 1966.

Foltz, E. L., and Ward, A. A., Jr.: Communicating hydrocephalus from subarachnoid bleeding. *J. Neurosurg.*, **13**:546–566, 1956.

Forland, M.: Cleidocranial dysostosis. *Amer. J. Med.*, **33**:792–799, 1962.

Friedman, S., Zita-Gozum, C., and Chatten, J.: Pulmonary vascular changes complicating ventriculo-vascular shunting for hydrocephalus. *J. Pediat.*, **64**:305–314, 1964.

Fuleihan, D. S., Vazken, M., Der Kaloustian, and Najjar, S. S.: The Russell-Silver syndrome. Report of three siblings. *J. Pediat.*, **78**:654–657, 1971.

Gardner, W. J.: Hydrodynamic mechanism of syringomyelia: its relation to myelocoele. *J. Neurol. Neurosurg. Psychiat.*, **28**:247–259, 1965.

Geschwind, N.: The mechanism of normal pressure hydrocephalus. *J. Neurol. Sci.*, **7**:481–493, 1968.

Gibson, J. B.: Congenital hydrocephalus due to atresia of the foramen of Magendie. *J. Neuropath. Exper. Neurol.*, **14**:244–262, 1955.

Glasauer, F. E., Alker, G. J., Jr., and Leslie, E. V.: Isotope cisternography and ventriculography. Evaluation of hydrocephalus in children. *Amer. J. Dis. Child.*, **120**:109–114, 1970.

Go, K. G., Van Der Veen, P. H., and Van Der Berg, J. W.: Detection of CSF flow in ventriculo-atrial shunts by cold transfer. *Develop. Med. Child Neurol.*, **12**, Suppl. 22:69–72, 1970.

Griscom, N. T., and Oh, K. S.: The contracting skull. Inward growth of the inner table as a physiologic response to diminution of intracranial content in children. *Amer. J. Roentgen.*, **110**:106–110, 1970.

Gubbay, S. S.: Derangement of temperature control in hydrocephalus. *Develop. Med. Child Neurol.*, Suppl. 13:125–132, 1967.

Guillame, J., and Roge, R.: Troubles neuro-endocriniens et hydrocephalie chronique. *Rev. Neurol.*, **82**:424, 1950.

Hadenius, A. M., Hagberg, B., Hyttnas-Bensch, K., and Sjögren, I.: The natural prognosis of infantile hydrocephalus. *Acta Paediat. Scand.*, **51**:117–118, 1962.

Hakim, S.: Observations on the physiopathology of the CSF pulse and prevention of ventricular catheter obstruction in valve shunts. *Develop. Med. Child Neurol.*, Suppl. **20**:42–48, 1969.

Hakim, S., and Adams, R. D.: The special clinical problem of symptomatic hydrocephalus with normal cerebrospinal fluid pressure. *J. Neurol. Sci.*, **2**:307–327, 1965.

Hakim, S., and De Davila, O.: Algunas observaciones sobre la presion del L. C. R. dindrome hydrocefalico en al adulto con presion "normal" del L. C. R. Tesis de grado. Facultad de Medicina, Universidad Javeriana, Bogota, 1964.

Halsey, J. H., Jr., Allen, N., and Chamberlin, H. R.: Chronic decerebrate state in infancy. Neurologic observations in long surviving cases of hydranencephaly. *Arch. Neurol.*, **19**:339–346, 1968.

Halsey, J. H., Jr., Allen, N., and Chamberlin, H. R.: The morphogenesis of hydranencephaly. *J. Neurol. Sci.*, **12**:187–217, 1971.

Hammon, W. H.: Evaluation and use of the ventriculoperitoneal shunt in hydrocephalus. *J. Neurosurg.*, **34**:792–795, 1971.

Handa, J., and Handa, H.: Methylglucamine iothalamate 60 per cent for cerebral ventriculography. *Amer. J. Roentgen.*, **107**:631–636, 1969.

Hassen, G. B.: Hydrocephalus. Studies of the pathology and pathogenesis with remarks on the cerebrospinal fluid. *Arch. Neurol. Psychiat.*, **24**:1164–1186, 1930.

Hays, R. M., McHugh, P. R., and Williams, H. E.: Absence of thirst in association with hydrocephalus. *New Eng. J. Med.*, **269**:227–231, 1963.

Heimburger, R. F., Kalsbeck, J. E., Campbell, R. L., and Mealey, J., Jr.: Positive contrast cerebral ventriculography using water-soluble media. *J. Neurol. Neurosurg. Psychiat.*, **29**:281–290, 1966.

Hemmer, R.: Complications relating to ventricularvenous shunts: a five-year study. *Develop. Med. Child. Neurol.*, Suppl. **13**:108–112, 1967.

Hogan, P. A., and Woolsey, R. M.: Polydipsia associated with occult hydrocephalus. *New Eng. J. Med.*, **277**:639–640, 1967.

Holden, J. D.: The Russell-Silver's dwarf. *Develop. Med. Child Neurol.*, **9**:457–459, 1967.

Holtermüeller, K., and Wiedemann, H. R.: Kleeblattschädel syndrom. *Med. Mschr.*, **14**:439–446, 1960.

Holtz, A., Borman, G., and Li, C. P.: Hydrocephalus in mice infected with polyoma virus. *Proc. Soc. Exper. Biol. Med.*, **121**:1196–1200, 1966.

Hook, E. B., and Reynolds, J. W.: Cerebral gigantism. Endocrinological and clinical observations of six patients including a congenital giant, concordant monozygotic twins, and a child who achieved gigantic size. *J. Pediat.*, **70**:900–914, 1967.

Horner, F. A., Webb, N. C., Jr., and Welch, K.: Diagnosis of collection of subdural fluid by transillumination. (Abstr.) *Amer. J. Dis. Child.*, **96**:594–595, 1958.

Huang, Y. P., Wolf, B. S., Antin, S. P., Okudera, T., and Kim, I. H.: Angiographic features of aqueductal stenosis. *Amer. J. Roentgen.*, **104**:90–108, 1968.

Hunziker, K.: Über einen fall von hydranencephalie. *Mschr. Psychiat. Neurol.*, **114**:129, 1947.

Huttenlocher, P. R.: Treatment of hydrocephalus with acetazolamine. *J. Pediat.*, **66**:1023–1030, 1965.

Illingworth, R. S., and Lutz, W.: Head circumference of infants related to body weight. *Arch. Dis. Childh.*, **40**:672–676, 1965.

Jackson, I. J., and Snodgrass, W.: Peritoneal shunts in the treatment of hydrocephalus, 4 year study of 62 patients. *J. Neurosurg.*, **12**:216–222, 1955.

James. A. E., Jr., DeLand, F. D., Hodges, F. J., and Wagner, H. N., Jr.: Normal pressure hydrocephalus. Role of cisternography in diagnosis. *J.A.M.A.*, **213**:1615–1622, 1970.

Johnson, R. T., and Johnson, K. P.: Hydrocephalus following viral infection: The pathology of aqueductal stenosis developing after experimental mumps virus infection. *J. Neuropath. Exper. Neurol.*, **27**:591–606, 1968.

Johnston, C. C., Jr., Lavy, N., Lord, T., Vellios, F., Merritt, A. D., and Deiss, W. P., Jr.: Osteopetrosis. *Medicine*, **47**:149–167, 1968.

Juhl, J. H., and Wesenberg, R. L.: Radiological findings in congenital and acquired occlusions of the foramina of Magendie and Luschka. *Radiology*, **86**:801–813, 1966.

Keats, T. E.: Cleidocranial dysostosis: Some atypical roentgen manifestations. *Amer. J. Roentgen.*, **100**:71–74, 1967.

Key, A., and Retzius, G.: *Studien in der anatomie des nervensystems und des bindegewebes.* Stockholm, Samson and Wallin, 1875.

Kirsch, W. M., Duncan, B. R., Black, F. O., and Stears, J. C.: Laryngeal palsy in association with myelomeningocoele, hydrocephalus, and the Arnold-Chiari malformation. *J. Neurosurg.*, **28**:207–214, 1968.

Kloss, J. L.: Craniosynostosis secondary to ventriculoatrial shunt. *Amer. J. Dis. Child.*, **116**:315–317, 1968.

Kruyff, E.: Paracollicular plate cysts. *Amer. J. Roentgen.*, **95**:899–916, 1965.

Laurence, K. M.: The urinary phenolsulphonphthalein (phenol red) excretion test in hydrocephalus. *Arch. Dis. Childh.*, **32**:413–416, 1957.

Laurence, K. M.: Some applications of the urinary phenolsulphonphthalein excretion test in hydrocephalus and related conditions. *Brain*, **82**:551–565, 1959.

Laurence, K. M.: The pathology of hydrocephalus. *Ann. Roy. Coll. Surg. Engl.*, **24**:388–401, 1959.

Laurence, K. M.: A case of unilateral megalencephaly. *Develop. Med. Child Neurol.*, **6**:585–590, 1964.

Laurence, K. M.: Megalencephaly. *Develop. Med. Child Neurol.*, **6**:638–640, 1964.

Laurence, K. M., and Coates, S.: The natural history of hydrocephalus. Detailed analysis of 182 unoperated cases. *Arch. Dis. Child.*, **37**:345–362, 1962.

Laurence, K. M., Hoare, R. D., and Till, K.: The diagnosis of the choroid plexus papilloma of the lateral ventricle. *Brain*, **84**:628–641, 1961.

Li, C. P., and Jahnes, W. G.: Hydrocephalus in suckling mice innoculated with SE polyoma virus. *Virology*, **9**:489–492, 1959.

Lichtenstein, B. W.: Distant neuroanatomic complications of spina bifida (spinal dysraphism)—hydrocephalus, Arnold-Chiari deformity, stenosis of the aqueduct of Sylvius, etc.—pathogenesis and pathology. *Arch. Neurol. Psychiat.*, **47**:195–214, 1942.

Lindenberg, R., and Swanson, P. D.: "Infantile hydranencephaly"—a report of five cases of infarction of both cerebral hemispheres in infancy. *Brain*, **90**:839–850, 1967.

Lorber, J.: Systematic ventriculographic studies in infants born with meningomyelocele and encephalocele. The incidence and development of hydrocephalus. *Arch. Dis. Childh.*, **36**:381–389, 1961.

Lorber, J., and Bassi, U.: The aetiology of neonatal hydrocephalus. *Develop. Med. Child Neurol.*, **7**:289–294, 1965.

Lorber, J., and De, N. C.: Family history of congenital hydrocephalus. *Develop. Med. Child Neurol.*, **12**, Suppl. 22:94–100, 1970.

Lorber, J., and Emery, J. L.: Intracerebral cysts complicating ventricular needling in hydrocephalic infants. A clinico-pathologic study. *Develop. Med. Child Neurol.*, **6**:125–139, 1964.

Lorber, J., and Zachary, R. B.: Primary congenital hydrocephalus. *Arch. Dis. Childh.*, **43**:516–527, 1968.

Lorenzo, A. V., Page, L. K., and Vatters, G. V.: Relationships between cerebrospinal fluid formation, absorption and pressure in human hydrocephalus. *Brain*, **93**:679–692, 1970.

Lourie, H., and Berne, A. S.: A contribution on the etiology and pathogenesis of congenital communicating hydrocephalus. *Neurology*, **15**:815–822, 1965.

Luthardt, T.: Bacterial infections in ventriculo-auricular shunt systems. *Develop. Med. Child Neurol.*, **12**, Suppl. 22:105–109, 1970.

Magendie, F.: *Recherches Philosphiques et Cliniques sur le Liquide Cephalorachidien ou Cerebro-spinal.* Paris, Mcquignon-Marvis, 1842.

Margolis, G., and Kilham, L.: Experimental virus-induced hydrocephalus. *J. Neurosurg.*, **31**:1–9, 1969.

Maroteaux, P., and Lamy, M.: Etude radiologique de trois nouvelles affections osseuses constitutionnelles. *Ann. de radiol.*, **5**:551–563, 1963.

Matson, D. D.: New operation for treatment of communicating hydrocephalus: report of case secondary to generalized meningitis. *J. Neurosurg.*, **6**:238–247, 1949.

Matson, D. D.: Hydrocephalus treated by arachnoid-ureterostomy: report of 50 cases. *Pediatrics*, **12**:326–334, 1953.

Matson, D. D.: Prenatal obstruction of the fourth ventricle. *Amer. J. Roentgen.*, **76**:499–506, 1956.

Matson, D. D., and Crofton, F. D. L.: Papilloma of the choroid plexus in childhood. *J. Neurosurg.*, **17**:1002–1027, 1960.

Mazur, R.: Transillumination of the skull in the diagnosis of intracranial disease in children up to 3 years. *Develop. Med. Child Neurol.*, **7**:634–642, 1965.

McCullough, D. C., Harbert, J. C., DiChiro, G., and Ommaya, A. K.: Prognostic criteria for cerebrospinal fluid shunting from isotope cisternography in communicating hydrocephalus. *Neurology*, **20**:594–598, 1970.

McHugh, P. R.: Occult hydrocephalus. *Quart. J. Med.*, **33**:297–308, 1964.

Mealey, J., Jr., and Barker, D. T.: Failure of oral acetazolamide to avert hydrocephalus in infants with myelomeningocoele. *J. Pediat.*, **72**:257–259, 1968.

Milhorat, T. H.: Choroid plexus and cerebrospinal fluid production. *Science*, **166**:1514–1516, 1969.

Milhorat, T. H.: Acute hydrocephalus. *New Eng. J. Med.*, **283**:857–859, 1970.

Milhorat, T. H., and Hammock, M. K.: Isotope ventriculography. Interpretation of ventricular size and configuration in hydrocephalus. *Arch. Neurol.*, **25**:1–8, 1971.

Milhorat, T. H., Clark, R. G., Hammock, M. K., and McGrath, P. P.: Structural, ultrastructural, and permeability changes in the ependyma and surrounding brain favoring equilibration in progressive hydrocephalus. *Arch. Neurol.*, **22**:397–407, 1970.

Milhorat, T. H., Hammock, M. K., and Chandra, R. S.: The subarachnoid space in congenital obstructive hydrocephalus. Part 2. Microscopic findings. *J. Neurosurg.*, **35**:7-15, 1971.

Milhorat, T. H., Hammock, M. K., and Di Chiro, G.: The subarachnoid space in congenital obstructive hydrocephalus. Part 1. Cisternographic findings. *J. Neurosurg.*, **35**:1-6, 1971.

Milhorat, T. H., Mosher, M. B., Hammock, M. K., and Murphy, C. F.: Evidence for choroid-plexus absorption in hydrocephalus. *New Eng. J. Med.*, **283**: 286-289, 1970.

Milunsky, A., Cowie, V. A., and Donoghue, E. C.: Cerebral gigantism in childhood. *Pediatrics*, **40**: 395-402, 1967.

Morgagni, G. B.: The seats and causes of diseases investigated by anatomy. Trans. Benjamin Alexander, 1761, Miller and Cadell, London.

Morley, A. R.: Laryngeal stridor, Arnold-Chiari malformation and medullary hemorrhages. *Develop. Med. Child Neurol.*, **11**:471-475, 1969.

Muir, C. S.: Hydranencephaly and allied disorders. *Arch. Dis. Childh.*, **34**:231-246, 1959.

Murtagh, F., and Lehman, R.: Peritoneal shunts in the management of hydrocephalus. *J.A.M.A.*, **202**:1010-1014, 1967.

Needleman, H. L., and Root, A. W.: Sex-linked hydrocephalus. *Pediatrics*, **31**:396-399, 1963.

Nellhaus, G.: The bobble-head doll syndrome. A "tic" with a neuropathologic basis. *Pediatrics*, **40**:250-253, 1967.

Nellhaus, G.: Head circumference from birth to eighteen years. *Pediatrics*, **41**:106-114, 1968.

Nicholas, J. L., Kamal, I. M., and Eckstein, H. B.: Immediate shunt replacement in the treatment of bacterial colonization of Holter valves. *Develop. Med. Clild Neurol.*, **12**, Suppl. 22:110-113, 1970.

Nicol, C. F.: A second case of aseptic meningitis following isotope cisternography using I-131 human serum albumin. *Neurology*, **17**:199-200, 1967.

Noble, T. C., Lassman, L. P., Urguhart, W., and Aherne, W. A.: Thrombotic and embolic complications of ventriculo-atrial shunts. *Develop. Med. Child Neurol.*, **12**, Suppl. 22:114-122, 1970.

Noonan, J. A., and Ehmke, D. A.: Complications of ventriculovenous shunts for control of hydrocephalus. *New Eng. J. Med.*, **269**:70-74, 1963.

Nugent, G. R., Lucas, R., Judy, M., Bloor, B. M., and Warden, H.: Thrombo-embolic complications of ventriculo-atrial shunts. Angiographic and pathologic correlations. *J. Neurosurg.*, **24**:34-42, 1966.

Nulsen, F. E., and Spitz, E. B.: Treatment of hydrocephalus by direct shunt from ventricle to jugular vein. *Surg. Forum*, **2**:399-403, 1952.

O'Neill, E. M.: Normal head growth and the prediction of head size in infantile hydrocephalus. *Arch. Dis. Childh.*, **36**:241-252, 1961.

Ott, J. E., and Robinson, A.: Cerebral gigantism. *Amer. J. Dis. Child.*, **117**:357-368, 1969.

Payr, E.: Drainage der hirnventrikel mittelst frei transplantirter blutgefässe; bemerkungen über hydrocephalus. *Arch. Klin. Chir.*, **87**:801-885, 1908.

Peach, B.: Arnold-Chiari malformation with normal spine. *Arch. Neurol.*, **10**:497-501, 1964.

Peach, B.: Arnold-Chiari malformation. Anatomic features of 20 cases. *Arch. Neurol.*, **12**:613-621, 1965.

Peach, B.: The Arnold-Chiari malformation. Morphogenesis. *Arch. Neurol.*, **12**:527-535, 1965.

Penfield, W., and Coburn, D. F.: Arnold-Chiari malformation and its operative treatment. *Arch. Neurol. Psych.*, **40**:328-336, 1938.

Perrin, J. C. S., and McLaurin, R. L.: Infected ventriculoatrial shunts. *J. Neurosurg.*, **27**:21-26, 1967.

Pollock, L. J.: Hypopituitarism in chronic hydrocephalus. *J.A.M.A.*, **64**:395-398, 1915.

Poser, C. M., Walsh, F. C., and Scheinberg, L. C.: Hydranencephaly. *Neurology*, **5**:284-289, 1955.

Pudenz, R. H., Russell, F. E., Hurd, A. H., and Shelden, C. H.: Ventriculo-auriculostomy. A technique for shunting cerebrospinal fluid into the right auricle. Preliminary report. *J. Neurosurg.*, **14**:171-179, 1957.

Putnam, T. J.: Treatment of hydrocephalus by endoscopic coagulation of the choroid plexus. Description of a new instrument and preliminary report of results. *New Eng. J. Med.*, **210**:1373-1376, 1934.

Raimondi, A. J., Samuelson, G., Yarzagaray, L., and Norton, T.: Atresia of the foramina of Luschka and Magendie: The Dandy-Walker cyst. *J. Neurosurg.*, **31**:202-216, 1969.

Rames, L., Wise, B., Goodman, J. R., and Piel, C. F.: Renal disease with *Staphylococcus albus* bacteremia. *J.A.M.A.*, **212**:1671-1677, 1970.

Rao, P. S., Molthan, M. E., and Lipow, H. W.: Cor pulmonale as a complication of ventriculoatrial shunts. *J. Neurosurg.*, **33**:221-225, 1970.

Rickham, P. P., and Penn, I. A.: The place of the ventriculostomy reservoir in the treatment of myelomeningocoeles and hydrocephalus. *Develop. Med. Child Neurol.*, **7**:296-301, 1965.

Riddoch, G.: Progressive dementia, without headache or changes in the optic discs due to tumors of the third ventricle. *Brain*, **59**:225-233, 1936.

Riley, H. D., Jr., and Smith, W. R.: Macrocephaly, pseudopapilledema and multiple hemangiomata. *Pediatrics*, **26**:293-300, 1960.

Roberts, J. R., and Rickham, P. P.: Craniostenosis following Holter valve operation. *Develop. Med. Child Neurol.*, **12**, Suppl 22:145-149, 1970.

Russell, A.: A syndrome of "intra-uterine" dwarfism recognizable at birth with cranio-facial dysostosis, disproportionately short arms, and other anomalies (5 examples). *Proc. Roy. Soc. Med.* **47**:1040-1044, 1954.

Russell, D. S.: Observations on the pathology of hydrocephalus. Medical Research Council Report No. 265. London, 1949.

Sahs, A. L.: Congenital anomaly of the cerebellar vermis. *Arch. Path.*, **32**:52-63, 1941.

Salmon, J. H.: Puncture porencephaly. *Amer. J. Dis. Child.*, **114**:72-79, 1967.

Scarcella, G.: Radiologic aspects of Dandy-Walker syndrome. *Neurology*, **10**:260-266, 1960.

Scarff, J. E.: Endoscopic treatment of hydrocephalus. Description of a ventriculoscope and preliminary report of cases. *Arch. Neurol. Psychiat.*, **35**:853-860, 1936.

Scarff, J. E.: Treatment of hydrocephalus: An historical and critical review of methods and results. *J. Neurol. Neurosurg. Psychiat.*, **26**:1-26, 1963.

Schain, R. J.: Carbonic anhydrase inhibitors in chronic infantile hydrocephalus. *Amer. J. Dis. Child.*, **117**: 621-625, 1969.

Schaltenbrand, G., and Putnam, T.: Untersuchungen zum kreislauf des liquor cerebrospinalis mit hilfe intravenöser fluoresineinspritzungen. *Dtsch. Z. Nervenheilk*, **96**:123, 1927.

Schochet, S. S., Lampert, P. W., and Earle, K. M.:

Alexander's disease: A case report with electron microscopic observations. *Neurology,* **18**:543–549, 1968.

Schwalbe, E., and Gredig, M.: Ueber entwicklungsstörungen des kleinhirns hirnstamms und halsmarks bei spina bifida (Arnold'sche und Chiari'sche missbildung). *Beitr. path. Anat. u. allg. Path.,* **40**:132–194, 1907.

Scott, M., Wycis, H. T., Murtagh, F., and Reyes, U.: Observations on ventricular and lumbar subarachnoid peritoneal shunts in hydrocephalus in infants. *J. Neurosurg.,* **12**:165–175, 1955.

Shealy, C. N., Lemay, M., and Haddad, F. S.: Posterior scalloping of vertebral bodies in uncontrolled hydrocephalus. *J. Neurol. Neurosurg. Psychiat.,* **27**:567–573, 1964.

Sherwin, R. M., and Berthrong, M.: Alexander's disease with sudanophilic leukodystrophy. *Arch. Path.,* **89**:321–328, 1970.

Shurtleff, D. B.: Transillumination of skull in infants and children. *Amer. J. Dis. Child.,* **107**:14–24, 1964.

Smith, J. L., Walsh, T. J., and Shipley, T.: Cortical blindness in congenital hydrocephalus. *Amer. J. Ophth.,* **62**:251–257, 1966.

Sotos, J. F., Dodge, P. R., Muirhead, D., Crawford, J. D., and Talbot, N. B.: Cerebral gigantism in childhood. A syndrome of excessively rapid growth with acromegalic features and a nonprogressive neurologic disorder. *New Eng. J. Med.,* **271**:109–116, 1964.

Sperling, D. R., Patrick, J. R., Anderson, F. M., and Fyler, D. C.: Cor pulmonale secondary to ventriculoauriculostomy. *Amer. J. Dis. Child.,* **107**:308–315, 1964.

Spielmeyer, W.: Ein hydranencephales zwillingspaar. *Arch. Psychiat. Nervenkr.,* **39**:807, 1904–1905.

Stauffer, U. G.: Shunt nephritis. Diffuse glomerulonephritis complicating ventriculo-atrial shunts. *Develop. Med. Child Neurol.,* **12**, Suppl. 22:161–164, 1970.

Stickler, G. B., Shin, M. H., Burke, E. C., Holley, K. E., Miller, R. H., and Segar, W. E.: Diffuse glomerulonephritis associated with infected ventriculoatrial shunt. *New Eng. J. Med.,* **279**:1077–1082, 1968.

Strenger, L.: Complications of ventriculovenous shunts. *J. Neurosurg.,* **20**:219–224, 1963.

Szalay, G. C.: Pseudohydrocephalus in dwarfs. The Russell dwarf. *J. Pediat.,* **63**:622–633, 1963.

Taggart, J. K., Jr., and Walker, A. E.: Congenital atresia of the foramens of Luschka and Magendie. *Arch. Neurol. Psychiat.,* **48**:583–612, 1942.

Timmons, G. D., and Johnson, K. P.: Aqueductal stenosis of hydrocephalus after mumps encephalitis. *New Eng. J. Med.,* **283**:1505–1507, 1970.

Torkildsen, A.: A new palliative operation in cases of inoperative occlusion of the Sylvian aqueduct. *Acta chir. scandinav.,* **82**:117–124, 1939.

Tsingoglou, S., and Forrest, D. M.: Therapeutic and prophylactic lengthening of distal catheter of the Holter ventriculo-atrial shunt. *Develop. Med. Child Neurol.,* Suppl. **16**:35–43, 1968.

Turnbull, I. M., and Drake, C. G.: Membranous occlusion of the aqueduct of Sylvius. *J. Neurosurg.,* **24**:24–33, 1966.

van Houweninge Grafdijk, C. J.: Over hydrocephalus. Dissertation, Leiden, 1932.

Volk, B. W.: *Tay-Sachs' disease.* New York, Grune and Stratton, 1964.

von Luschka, H.: Die adergeflechte des menschlichen gehirns. Berlin, G. Reimer, 1855.

Warren, M. C., Lu, A. T., and Ziering, W. H.: Sex-linked hydrocephalus with aqueductal stenosis. *J. Pediat.,* **63**:1104–1110, 1963.

Weed, L. H.: Studies on cerebrospinal fluid. The pathways of escape from the subarachnoid spaces with particular reference to the arachnoid villi. *J. Med. Res.,* **31**:51–113, 1914.

Weed, L. H.: The development of the cerebrospinal fluid spaces in pig and in man. *Carnegie Contrib. to Embryol.,* **5**:3–116, 1917.

Weiss, M. H., Young, H. F., and McFarland, D. E.: Hydrancephaly of postnatal origin. *J. Neurosurg.,* **32**:715–720, 1970.

Welch, K., and Friedman, V.: The cerebrospinal fluid valves. *Brain,* **83**:454–469, 1960.

Whytt, R.: *Observations on the Dropsy of the Brain.* Edinburgh, Balfour, Auld and Smellie, 1768.

Wilson, C. B., and Bertan, V.: Interruption of the anterior choroidal artery in experimental hydrocephalus. *Arch. Neurol.,* **17**:614–619, 1967.

Wolpert, S. M., Haller, J. S., and Rabe, E. F.: The value of angiography in the Dandy-Walker syndrome and posterior fossa extra-axial cysts. *Amer. J. Roentgen.,* **109**:261–272, 1970.

Yakovlev, P. I.: Paraplegias of hydrocephalus (clinical note and interpretation). *Amer. J. Ment. Deficiency,* **51**:561–576, 1947.

Yakovlev, P., and Wadsworth, R. C.: Schizencephalies. A study of the congenital clefts in the cerebral mantle. Part I. *J. Neuropath. Exper. Neurol.,* **5**:116–168, 1946.

Yakovlev, P., and Wadsworth, R. C.: Schizencephalies. A study of the congenital clefts in the cerebral mantle. *J. Neuropath. Exper. Neurol.,* **5**:169–206, 1946.

Yashon, D.: Prognosis in infantile hydrocephalus. *J. Neurosurg.,* **20**:105–111, 1963.

Yashon, D., Jane, J. A., and Sugar, O.: The course of severe untreated infantile hydrocephalus. *J. Neurosurg.,* **23**:509–516, 1965.

Ylppö, A.: Das wachstum der fruhgebarenen von der geburt bis zum schulalter (growth of prematures from birth to school age). *Atschr. Kinderh.,* **24**:111, 1919.

Chapter Nine

BENIGN INTRACRANIAL HYPERTENSION (PSEUDOTUMOR CEREBRI)

Benign intracranial hypertension refers to a syndrome of unknown etiology that is characterized by the manifestations of increased intracranial pressure in the absence of focal neurologic abnormalities. Quincke is generally given credit for the initial recognition of this disorder, and Nonne introduced the name pseudotumor cerebri in 1914. Quincke described 10 cases under the designation of "serous meningitis" and made reference to the normal spinal fluid findings except for the elevated pressure.

In 1936, Davidoff and Dyke demonstrated that the disorder occurred with a ventricular system that is normal based on encephalographic studies. One year later, Dandy reported 22 patients with this condition and pointed out that in some, air encephalographic studies revealed the ventricular system to be actually smaller than normally expected. He therefore postulated that if excessive fluid was present, its location must be within the substance of the brain.

Sahs and Hyndman soon thereafter described additional cases suggesting that the syndrome was one of brain swelling of unknown cause. Subsequent histologic studies on tissue obtained from biopsy have demonstrated cerebral edema to be present in some patients with this syndrome (Sahs and Joynt). Others have remained skeptical of the brain edema concept as the cause of increased intracranial pressure with this disorder.

Argument opposing cerebral edema as the cause of increased pressure has been based partly on the common observation that patients with this condition remain strikingly alert and may look quite well, despite the marked degree of intracranial hypertension. In addition, observations occasionally made at the time of therapeutic subtemporal decompressive procedures have been less than entirely compatible with cerebral edema as a cause.

Davidoff, among others, pointed out the appearance of large amounts of clear cerebrospinal fluid welling up from deepened subarachnoid spaces at the time of operation. This led to the term "hypertensive meningeal hydrops." The advocates of parenchymal edema in turn have challenged this concept on the basis of the small ventricular system often seen on pneumoencephalography. If excessive fluid were to collect in the surface subarachnoid space, one might expect ventricular enlargement, as occurs in communicating hydrocephalus.

A possible alternative explanation that might reconcile both groups is that the cause of increased pressure in this syndrome may not be an either/or problem. One might postulate the presence of excess fluid in both locations, within the brain and the subarachnoid space, in proportions that may vary considerably from case to case. The variable observations in regard to the site of excess fluid described in the foregoing need not be mutually exclusive. Because of the lack of certainty of these factors, the term benign intracranial hypertension, suggested by Foley in 1955, remains the most descriptive and noncommittal designation for this syndrome.

The etiology of this syndrome remains unestablished, although there is much to suggest endocrine imbalance. The propensity for the disorder to occur in obese, young adult females has been used as evidence of this. Although endocrine disturbances are considered etiologically related, Greer (1965) was unable to demonstrate laboratory evidence of adrenal insufficiency or estrogen excess in a group of obese females with pseudotumor cerebri. The development of pseudotumor cerebri in women with preexisting menstrual dysfunction also suggests a hormonal basis for the disorder (Greer, 1964). Whether the neurologic syndrome in such cases results from an effect of ovarian hormones or from adrenal insufficiency has not been clarified.

The increased incidence of pseudotumor cerebri associated with corticosteroid therapy in children adds further support for endocrine derangement. In addition to the relationship with steroid therapy, the syndrome of benign intracranial hypertension has been described in patients with Addison's disease (Walsh), adding further impetus to the endocrine concept. In a series of 17 females with pseudotumor cerebri, Paterson et al remarked on the frequency of obesity, the common association of menstrual irregularity or pregnancy, the occasional association of galactorrhea, and the relationship of other endocrine diseases with this disorder. These authors proposed that physiologic hyperpituitarism might be expected in many of the conditions now recognized to be related to pseudotumor cerebri and may be etiologically related to the genesis of this disorder.

Other conditions with which the syndrome of benign intracranial hypertension has been related have been mentioned earlier. These include hypoparathyroidism, vitamin A intoxication or deficiency, tetracycline administration in infancy, and iron deficiency anemia in adolescent girls. Intracranial venous sinus obstruction has long been recognized as a cause of increased intracranial pressure without focal neurologic signs.

Symonds described increased intracranial pressure secondary to otitis media in 1931 and introduced the term "otitic hydrocephalus." The following year, Ohnacker presented two cases with this syndrome with venous sinus thrombosis demonstrated at autopsy. Following Gardner's demonstration of the absence of ventricular enlargement in this disorder, Symonds (1956) agreed that the term "otitic hydrocephalus" was a misnomer. The disorder secondary to otitis media or mastoiditis is now recognized to be mainly the result of lateral sinus thrombosis with brain swelling due to venous engorgement.

Symonds (1956) has pointed out the strikingly high incidence of ipsilateral sixth nerve palsy in patients with lateral sinus thrombosis. It has been suggested that, in some instances, abducens paresis in this disorder is caused by extension of the thrombus to the inferior petrosal sinus with compression of the sixth nerve. Extension of the clot from the lateral sinus to the jugular bulb may cause paralysis of the ninth, tenth, or eleventh cranial nerves.

Symptoms and Signs

The syndrome of benign intracranial hypertension of unknown cause may occur at any age in childhood. The presenting symptoms are uniform and consist primarily of the manifestations of increased intracranial pressure. Headaches, nausea, vomiting, diplopia, and papilledema are usually present but in varying combinations. One often is impressed by how well the child may look generally, despite evidence of high-grade increased intracranial pressure. The clinical manifestations of this disorder may become apparent a few days or up to two weeks following a mild systemic infectious illness or soon after head trauma. In other children, the onset cannot be related to any medical event. The duration of symptoms existent when the child is first seen in medical consultation may be a few days or as long as several months.

Younger children with this condition may become irritable and listless, perhaps because of a combination of headache and vomiting. As a rule, the only overt signs on examination are papilledema and perhaps lateral rectus palsy. Seizures are ordinarily not described and signs indicative of focal neurologic involvement are absent.

Pseudotumor cerebri in childhood is now recognized to be a complication of chronic corticosteroid therapy in some cases (Greer, 1963; Walker and Adamkiewicz). In most instances, symptoms have become evident at the time of reduction or discontinuation of steroids or shortly after substitution of one steroid preparation for another. In 1959, Dees and McKay described three asthmatic children who developed symptoms and signs of increased intracranial pressure coincident with reduction in steroid dosage. Similar instances have subsequently been noted in patients receiving steroids for eczema, nephrosis, arthritis, and congenital adrenal hyperplasia. In most cases, the steroids have been given orally; however, even topical use has resulted in the pseudotumor cerebri syndrome (Benson and Pharoah). A number of steroid preparations have been associated with this disorder. Triamcinolone and prednisone have been most commonly related but perhaps only because of their greater general use.

Diagnostic Studies

Diagnosis of benign intracranial hypertension in childhood cannot be established until proper studies have excluded an intracranial tumor. Midline tumors especially may produce clinical and laboratory findings identical to those with pseudotumor. Contrast studies must be used to exclude such lesions before the diagnosis of pseudotumor cerebri can be accepted. There are certain exceptions in which air studies can be avoided. For example, the abrupt development of papilledema unequivocally related to therapeutic reduction of steroids may be sufficient for diagnosis if other findings are consistent.

Skull x-rays in children with pseudotumor cerebri are normal, except for manifestations of increased pressure. Suture spread may be evident in young patients. The lumbar puncture is usually entirely normal, except for the elevation of the opening pressure. The electroencephalogram in patients with this disorder has often been said to be normal.

Sidell and Daly reviewed the electroencephalographic findings of 16 patients, three of whom were children. Eleven of the 16 patients had normal electroenocephalographic tracings. In the others, excessive theta activity was present. In only two patients was the electroencephalogram unequivocally abnormal. An additional series included 16 children with benign intracranial hypertension with electroencephalographic studies (Rose and Matson). In this group, only three patients had entirely normal electroencephalograms. The most frequently observed abnormality was paroxysmal bursts of high-voltage, slow activity, especially anteriorly located. In five childhood patients with benign intracranial hypertension associated with steroid therapy, Greer (1963) described generalized slowing on electroencephalography in all.

These plus other observations suggest that electroencephalographic abnormalities are more common in children with pseudotumor cerebri than in adults.

As already mentioned, definitive contrast studies in most instances are required before a diagnosis of benign intracranial hypertension can be established. Because a posterior fossa tumor is often suspected from the clinical data, air ventriculography may be elected as the procedure of choice. If successful, the procedure demonstrates normal or small lateral ventricles without shift or distortion, thus being consistent with the diagnosis of pseudotumor cerebri. The surgeon may find difficulty entering the lateral ventricle with the needle, a finding alone that suggests small ventricles. The drawback of ventriculography in such cases is that several attempts may be required to enter the ventricle.

In some cases, transient, bilateral visual loss has followed ventriculography, presumably because of occipital lobe involvement due to the needle passage (Greer, 1965). When ventriculography is attempted but is unsuccessful, it is usually advisable to proceed with fractional positive-pressure pneumoencephalography. An occasional observation in patients with pseudotumor cerebri is the marked diminution of symptoms and signs or total resolution of the illness following pneumoencephalography.

An alternative approach may be used diagnostically if one strongly suspects pseudotumor cerebri from the clinical findings. Carotid angiography may be performed initially and, if normal markedly reduces the probability of ventricular enlargement (Fig. 9-1). In patients with ventricular enlargement due to intraventricular obstructive hydrocephalus, angiography reveals upward displacement and bowing of the curve of the pericallosal artery in addition to elevation and straightening of branches of the middle

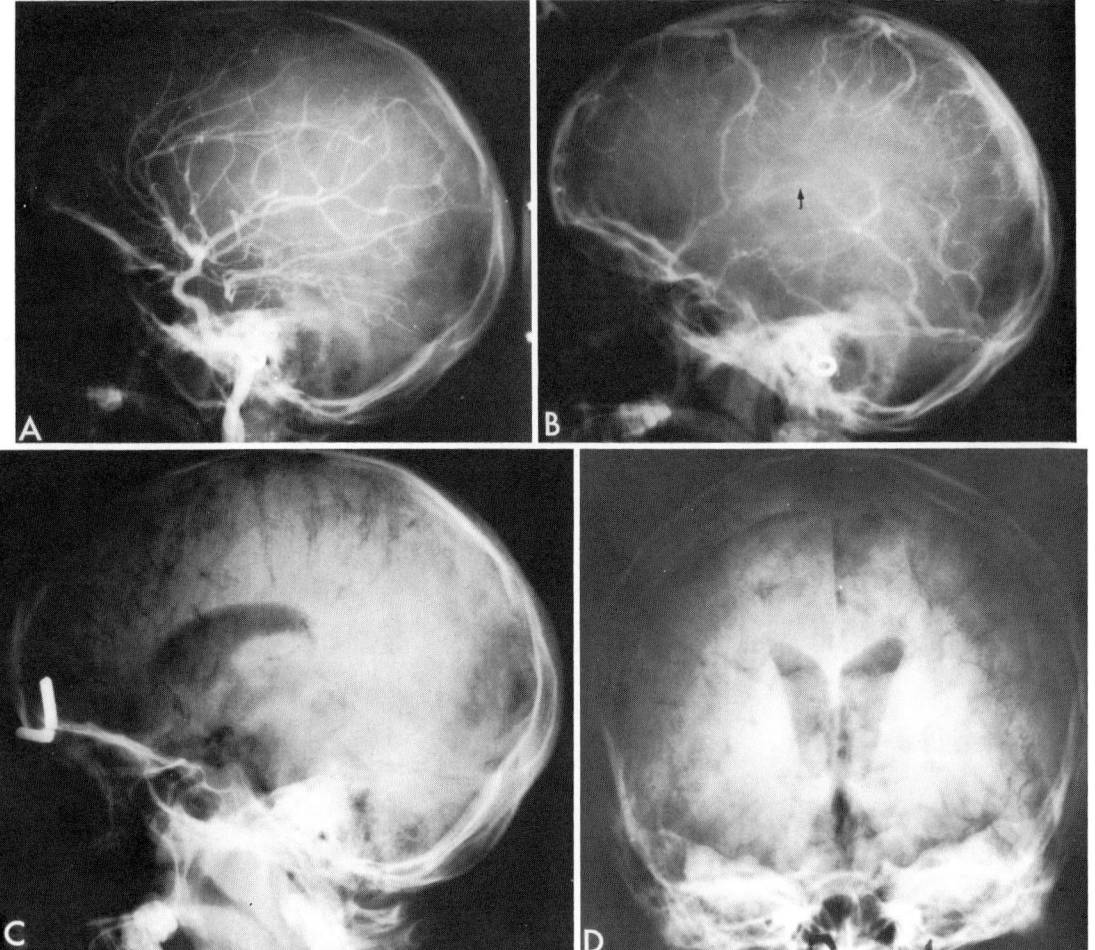

Figure 9–1. Diagnostic contrast studies in a 14-year-old girl with pseudotumor cerebri. The patient had a two-week history of headaches and vomiting. A, Carotid angiogram shows normal curve of the anterior cerebral system, indicating that the lateral ventricles are not distended. B, Venous phase reveals a normal internal cerebral vein (arrow) rather than one depressed and flattened as would occur with ventricular enlargement. The negative findings on angiography in a patient with papilledema and clinical suspicion of pseudotumor cerebri indicate pneumoencephalography can be done with reasonable safety. C and D, The pneumoencephalogram outlines a normal ventricular system.

cerebral artery on the lateral view. The lateral venous phase may show downward displacement or flattening of the internal cerebral vein.

The absence of these angiographic findings decreases the likelihood of a posterior fossa tumor with associated hydrocephalus and renders pneumoencephalography relatively safe. In this fashion, the difficulties and hazards of ventriculography can be avoided. In addition, if the venous phase satisfactorily demonstrates the superior longitudinal and lateral sinuses, thrombosis in these venous tributaries as a cause of increased pressure is excluded.

After studies have adequately established a diagnosis of pseudotumor cerebri, further examinations should be accomplished to exclude the disorders associated with this syndrome. Thus, hemoglobin, hematocrit, serum calcium and phosphorus, serum electrolytes, and urine 17-ketosteroid determinations should be obtained. If the patient is markedly obese, vital capacity, pCO_2, and blood pH will help exclude papilledema secondary to respiratory acidosis. Visual fields and acuity should be recorded and determinations repeated at periodic intervals, until the disorder has subsided.

Treatment

Treatment of pseudotumor cerebri in childhood is designed to relieve symptoms and, most important, to prevent loss of vision due to secondary optic atrophy. In some patients, spontaneous remission appears to follow air contrast studies and no further treatment is necessary. In obese adolescents with this disorder, weight reduction and salt restriction comprise part of the therapeutic approach. Periodic lumbar puncture, perhaps at daily intervals, often suffices to maintain the pressure at normal levels until remission occurs. The fluid is removed slowly and cautiously but in sufficient quantity to reduce the closing pressure to 180 mm. or less of water.

Certain patients with pseudotumor cerebri of unknown etiology respond to corticosteroid therapy. The response is variable, however, and steroids are totally without benefit in other patients. In those in whom increased pressure results from steroid reduction when used for other systemic illnesses, the initial therapeutic approach should be to return to the original steroid dosage.

If the syndrome develops after substitution of one steroid preparation for another, the original agent should be reinstituted. If symptoms do not promptly abate, periodic lumbar puncture should then be undertaken. Slowly, the steroid dose can be reduced gradually. Glycerol administered orally may have a place in long-term treatment of pseudotumor cerebri, but experience with this agent for this illness is lacking.

When none of the foregoing conservative measures is successful, or decline of visual acuity becomes evident, more radical measures should be considered. Vander Ark et al. have utilized a lumbar subarachnoid-peritoneal shunt and observed good results in a small series of patients. Right subtemporal decompression was done for intractable cases in past years but is no longer a recommended treatment approach.

The prognosis of the syndrome of benign intracranial hypertension in children is generally regarded as excellent. Recurrences are unusual. If the syndrome is managed skillfully, residual visual deficits should be infrequent. In some instances, the disorder is short-lived and responds promptly to therapy. In others, the total duration of the process may be measured in months or even over a year.

REFERENCES

Benson, P. F., and Pharoah, P. O. D.: Benign intracranial hypertension due to adrenal steroid therapy. *Guy's Hosp. Rep.*, **109**:212–218, 1960.

Dandy, W. E.: Intracranial pressure without brain tumor. Diagnosis and treatment. *Ann. Surg.*, **106**:492–513, 1937.

Davidoff, L. M.: Pseudotumor cerebri. *Neurology*, **6**:605–615, 1956.

Davidoff, L. M., and Dyke C. G.: A presentation of a series of cases of serous meningitis. *J. Nerv. Ment. Dis.*, **83**:700–705, 1936.

Dees, S. C., and McKay, H. W.: Occurrence of pseudotumor cerebri (benign intracranial hypertension) during treatment of children with asthma by adrenal steroids. *Pediatrics*, **23**:1143–1151, 1959.

Foley, J.: Benign forms of intracranial hypertension. "Toxic" and "otitic" hydrocephalus. *Brain*, **78**:1–41, 1955.

Gardner, W. J.: Otitic sinus thrombosis causing intracranial hypertension. *Arch. Otolaryng.*, **30**:253–268, 1939.

Greer, M.: Benign intracranial hypertension. II. Following corticosteroid therapy. *Neurology*, **13**:439–441, 1963.

Greer, M.: Benign intracranial hypertension. V. Menstrual dysfunction. *Neurology*, **14**:668–673, 1964.

Greer, M.: Benign intracranial hypertension. VI. Obesity. *Neurology*, **15**:382–388, 1965.

Nonne, M.: Der pseudotumor cerebri. *Neue Dtsch. Chir.*, **10**:107, 1914.

Ohnacker, P.: Zirkulatorisch bedingte hirnerscheinungen im anschluss an sinus und jugularisausschaltung. *Arch. Otr. Nas. u. Kehlk. Heilk.*, **131**:1–12, 1932.

Paterson, R., DePasquale, N., and Mann, S.: Pseudotumor cerebri. *Medicine*, **40**:85–99, 1961.

Quincke, H.: Ueber meningitis serosa und verwandte zustande. *Deutsche Ztschr. Nervenh.*, **9**:149–168, 1897.

Sahs, A. L., and Hyndman, O. R.: Intracranial hypertension of unknown cause. Cerebral edema. *Arch. Surg.*, **38**:428–442, 1939.

Sahs, A. L., and Joynt, R. J.: Brain swelling of unknown cause. *Neurology*, **6**:791–803, 1956.

Shenkin, H. A., and Bouzarth, W. F.: Clinical methods of reducing intracranial pressure. *New Eng. J. Med.*, **282**:1465–1471, 1970.

Sidell, A. D., and Daly, D. D.: The electroencephalogram in cases of benign intracranial hypertension. *Neurology*, **11**:413–417, 1961.

Symonds, C. P.: Otitic hydrocephalus. *Brain*, **54**:55–71, 1931.

Symonds, C. P.: Otitic hydrocephalus. *Neurology*, **6**:681–685, 1956.

Vander Ark, G. D., Kempe, L. G., and Smith, D. R.: Pseudotumor cerebri treated with lumbar-peritoneal shunt. *J.A.M.A.*, **217**:1832–1834, 1971.

Walker, A. E., and Adamkiewicz, J. J.: Pseudotumor cerebri associated with prolonged corticosteroid therapy. *J.A.M.A.*, **188**:779–784, 1964.

Walsh, F. B.: Papilledema associated with increased intracranial pressure in Addison's disease. *Arch. Ophthal.*, **47**:86, 1952.

Chapter Ten

LEAD ENCEPHALOPATHY

Lead intoxication (plumbism) in children is commonly associated with a severe encephalopathy with brain swelling as opposed to peripheral motor nerve dysfunction more characteristic in adults. Although peripheral neuropathy due to lead has been described in children (Seto and Freeman), it has been greatly overshadowed by the more frequent and more devastating effects on the central nervous system. Lead encephalopathy occurs predominantly in the age group between 18 months and five years. It has been recognized more often in the summer months than in the winter and occurs far more often in families of lower socioeconomic status living in larger cities. It must be considered a serious disease with a significant mortality and morbidity rate and is fatal in approximately 25 per cent of cases (Greengard et al.). Of those who survive, there is a high incidence of seizures, behavioral abnormalities, and mental retardation.

Children with mild, nondescript symptoms of lead poisoning may not be identified unless the physician maintains a high index of diagnostic suspicion. The early stages of intoxication with this heavy metal are characterized by subtle complaints and may occur without basophilic stippling of red blood cells or abnormalities of long bones on x-ray. Thus, a history of pica plus growth failure, constipation, vomiting, or irritability is an indication for a blood lead analysis and other studies used as indicators of lead poisoning.

Identification of a single case of lead poisoning in a family requires an epidemiologic study of the home to remove the source of lead, if possible, and to prevent exposure of other children. If other young children are present in the family, it is advisable that blood and urine studies of each one be done, regardless of the presence or absence of overt symptoms.

The child may be exposed to various sources of lead, including the ingestion of water passing through old lead-containing pipes, or the consumption of liquids stored in earthenware containers (Klein et al.). Inhalation of lead fumes from the burning of abandoned storage battery casings for heat may cause acute intoxication. In the past, infants have been poisoned with lead as a result of the use of lead-containing nipple shields or subsequent to the application of lead-containing powders to the mother's breast.

The most common source of lead is by direct oral ingestion and results from the habit referred to as pica. Pica is an abnormal tendency to eat nonfood materials, such as dirt, clay, plaster, painted wood and other materials. Certain children may chew on woodwork, painted walls, window sills, or the crib siding and acquire large amounts of lead over a lengthy period of time. The child may eat through the recent coats of lead-free paint, eventually gaining access to paint applied years before that contained lead in large quantities.

Paint designated for dwelling interiors is now largely lead-free. However, the financially deprived may buy cheaper paint containing lead designed for housing exteriors and apply it within the house, thereby exposing the child. Children who acquire large amounts of lead by eating foreign materials may develop other medical problems therefrom. The habit of dirt ingestion may result in intestinal parasites and should be searched for in any child with manifestations of lead toxicity due to oral ingestion. Moore described a fatal case of *Toxocara canis* encephalitis and lead encephalopathy in a child due to such indiscriminate dietary habits.

Symptoms and Signs

There is a great deal of variability in the historical data and the physical signs in children with lead encephalopathy. The first signs of the disease may become apparent with the development of what seems to be a mild systemic infection. The child may abruptly become irritable with vomiting and fever, experience what is initially interpreted as a febrile convulsion. Rapid progression of neurologic deficits and recurrent seizures give evidence of a more serious nervous system insult. With this type of presentation, it is common that the child is believed to have encephalitis or bacterial meningitis until the appropriate studies establish the diagnosis of acute lead encephalopathy. Other children are seemingly entirely well and asymptomatic until the illness is precipitated by a mild head injury. Vomiting, seizures, and progressive decline of responsiveness follow soon thereafter.

Unless one recognizes the generalized manifestations of the encephalopathy, an unnecessary search for a tumor or subdural or epidural hematoma may be made in such cases. Children three to five years of age with chronic, low-grade lead poisoning may have recurrent seizures and not be recognized to be ill between episodes. Others may exhibit aggressive or hyperkinetic behavior problems, or be labeled as retarded without more obvious manifestations of a toxic encephalopathy (Chisolm and Kaplan).

A more characteristic history in a child with lead encephalopathy is one beginning with an insidious onset. Nonspecific signs of illness are followed by progressive deterioration generally and with either abrupt or gradually developing evidence of increased intracranial pressure and signs of diffuse cerebral involvement. Lassitude, irritability, and anorexia are frequently the first observed abnormalities associated with intermittent abdominal pain, episodic vomiting, and constipation.

With progression of the illness, weight loss develops and pallor becomes evident. The child becomes clumsy and often is markedly ataxic. Convulsions may occur of either a generalized or focal type, or a combination of the two. Convulsions may become intractable in children with lead encephalopathy and can lead to respiratory failure unless controlled by appropriate therapy.

Signs of increased intracranial pressure due to severe cerebral edema become more profound as the process advances. Over a period of several days or two to three weeks, ease of fatigue proceeds to lethargy and finally to coma. Children with a progressively worsening course over one to three weeks are often considered to have either an intracranial tumor or tuberculous meningitis.

Posterior fossa neoplasm is commonly entertained in differential diagnosis because of the combination of signs of increased intracranial pressure and ataxia. Important points differentiating lead poisoning from the neoplasm include other evidence of diffuse cerebral involvement and urine abnormalities to be described later.

Tuberculous meningitis may be more difficult to distinguish from lead encephalopathy because of similarities of the clinical picture and spinal fluid findings. The reduced amount of cerebrospinal fluid sugar with tuberculous meningitis is not expected in lead poisoning. A point favoring lead in this circumstance is evidence in the history of exposure of the child to the heavy metal. History of pica is usually available if the parents are properly questioned about the child's eating habits. They are not likely to volunteer information in this regard because parents frequently do not recognize it as a medically significant problem.

If cerebral edema has become marked by the time the child is first seen, signs of increased pressure are apt to be striking, including papilledema and lateral rectus palsy. Fever is often present in addition to signs of dehydration resulting from vomiting plus inadequate oral intake. Pupillary abnormalities are variable. Anisocoria may be noted or both pupils may be dilated and react poorly to light.

Lateralizing long tract signs are often encountered, superimposed on signs of more diffuse cerebral dysfunction. One side of the body may be spastic while the opposite side appears limp. The signs may fluctuate and alternate from one side to the other on repeated examinations as the hours pass.

The state of the physical signs in the extremities is altered by recurrent seizures because postictal weakness may persist for hours following focal motor convulsions. Cervical rigidity is frequently noted on examination and, like other neurologic signs, may fluctuate, depending on the degree of stupor. One should observe the gums for a lead line; however, although this is frequently observed in adults with lead poisoning, its presence in children is unusual. In rare instances, children with chronic lead poisoning show evidence of myocarditis (Freeman). The mechanism by which lead affects the myocardium remains unestablished.

Diagnostic Studies

Laboratory and roentgenographic studies in lead poisoning provide important diagnostic evidence of involvement of organ systems other than the brain. The identification of hematologic, renal, and skeletal abnormalities points to the generalized nature of the disease and at once becomes inconsistent with a disorder limited to the nervous system.

A significant degree of hypochromic microcytic anemia is usually present and is believed to be due to an interruption of the conversion of protoporphyrin into heme (Chisolm). Diminished red cell survival may also play a role because basophilic-stippled cells have been shown to be removed from the circulation at an accelerated rate by the reticuloendothelial system (McFadzean and Davis). Basophilic stippling of red blood cells due to lead poisoning is less commonly identified in children than generally believed. Some have indicated that its occurrence may be as low as 30 to 40 per cent (Greengard). Red cell stippling has been ascribed to the injurious effect of lead on the ribonucleic acid of erythrocyte precursors. Basophilic stippling is not limited to lead poisoning, because it may occur in other types of anemia. The combination of hypochromic anemia and basophilic stippling observed in thalassemia major may resemble closely the peripheral blood findings in lead poisoning.

Urine abnormalities with lead intoxication may include glycosuria, proteinuria, and aminoaciduria. Chisolm has pointed out the resemblance of glycosuria, aminoaciduria, and hypophosphatemia in lead poisoning to those occurring in the proximal renal tubular dysfunction syndrome described by Fanconi. These abnormalities occur in the acute phase of lead poisoning and are generally believed to be reversible with proper therapy and cessation of exposure. Some investigators believe that with long-term exposure to lead, one may eventually develop a chronic nephritis with interstitial fibrosis leading to progressive renal insufficiency and hypertension (Morgan et al.). Emmerson and Thiele have suggested that certain cases of chronic nephritis in adults may stem from prolonged exposure to lead in childhood.

An additional urinary abnormality that may be used as a screening test for lead intoxication is the presence of coproporphyrin III. This substance appears in the urine in excessive quantities because of the interference of heme synthesis by the toxic effects of lead. The normal urinary excretion of coproporphyrins is approximately 60 to 280 micrograms per day. Quantitative determinations in a 24-hour urine specimen are more reliable; however, a qualitative estimate of the presence of coproporphyrins in a random urine specimen may be of immediate diagnostic help.

Urine excretion of delta-aminolevulinic acid has been considered to be a sensitive indicator of intoxication in industrial workers exposed to lead (Haeger-Aronsen). The serum level of delta-aminolevulinic acid has also been useful as a screening test for lead poisoning in children (Feldman et al.). Markedly elevated levels in the serum are believed to be due to the effect of lead on the heme biosynthetic pathway. Weissberg et al. suggested that reduced content of erythrocyte delta-aminolevulinic acid dehydratase, an enzyme required for the conversion of delta-aminolevulinic acid to porphobilinogen, could be used as an indicator for the detection of lead poisoning.

More definitive laboratory diagnosis of lead intoxication depends on the determination of lead content in the blood and urine. The lead content of hair is also elevated with chronic ingestion and may add confirmation in conjunction with other tests (Kopito et al.). The blood lead determination is the most reliable laboratory means for diagnosis of this disease. A blood level of 0.06 mg. or more per 100 ml. of blood is considered abnormal (Jacobziner). However, children may be encountered with overt symptoms of lead encephalopathy with lower blood levels. Blood for lead analysis should be drawn in a lead-free syringe and placed into a lead-free tube before transfer to the laboratory.

Urine lead determinations are considered less reliable. Levels may be disproportionately low in severe intoxication because of impairment of renal function resulting from the toxic effects of lead. Normal urine levels in children range from 0 to 400 micrograms per liter. When the disease is suspected but the urine lead values are not diagnostic, the versinate stimulation test should be attempted (Whitaker et al.).

After the first 24-hour urine collection for lead is completed, the child is given calcium disodium edetate, 75 mg. per kilogram of body weight per day intramuscularly, divided into three doses. A second 24-hour urine specimen is collected during administration of the drug. The excretion of lead at a rate exceeding 500 micrograms per liter in the second specimen is considered to be evidence that there has been excessive ingestion of lead-containing substances.

When one is considering a diagnosis of lead poisoning in childhood, roentgenographic examination should include chest and skull films, a flat plate of the abdomen, and certain long bones. If increased intracranial pressure is marked in the younger child, skull suture separation will be present. Lead may be apparent as a radiopaque density on the abdominal flat plate if it was ingested. Recognition of the presence of lead within the gastrointestinal tract may be helpful diagnostically and also important therapeutically. Efforts should be made to free the bowel of lead if chelation therapy is to be utilized, but initiation of treatment should not be delayed while this is being accomplished.

With chronic intake of lead, deposition of the material within rapidly growing bone may provide another valuable diagnostic finding. Transverse bands of increased density in the metaphyseal region of long bones may be present roentgenographically (Fig. 10-1). For lead to be deposited in the bony metaphysis, prerequisites include rapid bone growth and available calcium salts for deposition within bone. Thus, ricketic children are not likely to develop lead lines on x-ray until healing and mineral deposition begins.

Lead deposition in children is most apparent in the more rapidly growing bones, including the anterior ends of the ribs and the iliac crests. With continued chronic exposure, lines high-lighting the superior and inferior margins of the vertebral bodies may be visua-

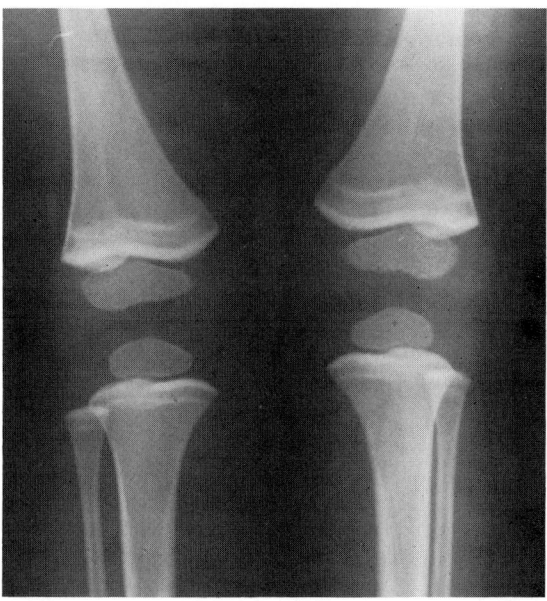

Figure 10–1. Lead lines, distal femur and proximal tibia, in two-year-old child with lead encephalopathy. (Courtesy of Drs. Gerald Kuhn and Peter Vlad, Buffalo Children's Hospital.)

lized on the lateral spine film. For diagnostic purposes, x-rays of the distal femur, including the proximal portion of the tibia, and of the wrist are usually adequate.

Roentgen evidence of bony deposition of lead is of obvious diagnostic importance when present. The absence of skeletal abnormalities on x-ray, however, does not exclude the possibility of lead poisoning (Sartain et al.). One occasionally finds transverse bands of increased density in the terminal segments of long bones in normal young children. These may be confused with the lines due to lead and adds another potential diagnostic pitfall. In addition, metaphyseal densities of the type seen with lead deposition may occur in other conditions, including exposure to bismuth and phosphorus.

Lumbar puncture in children with lead encephalopathy usually shows a very high opening pressure because of diffuse cerebral edema. For this reason, the procedure should be cautiously performed, if at all. After the subarachnoid space is entered, the needle stylet should be slowly removed, preventing spurting of fluid from the needle. The fluid is clear and the spinal fluid protein level is usually mildly to moderately elevated. The glucose content is not decreased, as it is in most cases of bacterial meningitis. In some cases, the spinal fluid glucose level may be significantly elevated. The spinal fluid cell count in lead encephalopathy is variable, but the usual case shows a mild lymphocytic pleocytosis with 10 to 20 mononuclear cells per cubic millimeter. Less common findings include the total absence of cells or the presence of a polymorphonuclear pleocytosis. Because the diagnosis of lead encephalopathy is usually not established at the time the lumbar puncture is done, the fluid should be examined for bacteria by smear and culture.

Cerebral Pathology

The gross cerebral pathology in lead encephalopathy includes marked cerebral edema evidenced by flattening of the cerebral gyri and narrowing of the sulci. Petechial hemorrhages may be present and dural sinus thrombosis may occur in some cases. Microscopic abnormalities depend in part on the severity and duration of the process. Parenchymal destructive changes involve both gray and white matter. Marked neuronal loss may be evident in the cerebral cortex and thalamus in addition to astrocytic and phagocytic proliferation. The white matter may be more edematous but generally shows less destructive changes than are seen in the cortical areas.

A significant effect of lead intoxication is an alteration of the small vessels in the brain, including endothelial proliferation of capillaries and venules, contributing to the edema (Popoff et al.). Vascular abnormalities occur in both cerebral gray and white matter. Both large and small veins may be affected, with thickening of the vessel wall and collagen disorganization. Perivascular cellular cuffing and perivenous edema are also commonly noted in the brain in this disease.

Treatment

Several agents are available for use in the treatment of lead encephalopathy. However, the outcome is often poor, regardless of therapy. Thus, preventive measures must continue to be stressed. The initial step is to remove the child from the source of lead and to begin therapeutic measures as rapidly as possible.

With severe lead intoxication, convulsions may be frequent and represent a life-threatening hazard. Continuous seizures are most effectively controlled by the use of diazepam (Valium), which can be administered intravenously in a dose of one to 10 mg., depending on the body weight of the child. The drug should be injected by direct push but done so over a minute or two while the respiratory pattern is closely observed. It may be repeated several times during the course of the day if seizures recur.

Paraldehyde may be used alternatively, because it may control seizures without causing significant respiratory depression. If time is available, paraldehyde may be given rectally in a dose of 0.2 ml. per pound of body weight. If a more rapid response is needed, paraldehyde may be given intramuscularly in a dose of 0.1 ml. per pound of body weight. Paraldehyde may be repeated in these doses in 30 to 60 minutes if seizures recur. At the onset of therapy, diazepam or paraldehyde is supplemented with diphenylhydantoin (Dilantin) in a dosage of 6 mg. per kilogram of body weight per day intramuscularly in three divided doses.

Barbiturates are preferably avoided because of the anticipated respiratory depression resulting from their use. However, if seizures persist despite the foregoing regimen, control may be achieved by very slow intravenous administration of amobarbital sodium (Amytal). In children one to three years of age the drug may be given intravenously by slow injection of 30 mg. while the respiratory pattern is monitored. If no respiratory suppression occurs, this amount may be repeated until seizures cease. Seizures usually cease after 60 to 120 mg. have been given. One should be prepared to intubate the child and temporarily support respiration if intravenous amobarbital sodium is used. Morphine should not be given.

The seriously ill child with lead encephalopathy may have renal and cardiac involvement in addition to cerebral edema. Furthermore, Chisolm (1968) has suggested that inappropriate antidiuretic hormone secretion may occur in this disease, adding to the metabolic derangements. Fluid management is therefore critical and must be carefully designed if the child is to survive. Unless the patient is obviously markedly dehydrated, intravenous fluids should be limited to an amount equal to insensible loss plus urine output per day. Insensible fluid loss may be estimated at 400 ml. per square meter of body surface area per day. An indwelling catheter is usually necessary, because the urine volume must be measured and because the child is apt to be sufficiently ill that urine retention is likely. Salt-free fluids should be avoided in order to prevent additional cerebral edema.

Respiratory care includes proper nontraumatic suctioning, endotracheal intubation if respiration suddenly ceases and tracheotomy if respirator care becomes necessary. If aspiration occurs or if intubation is required, antibiotics should be given because of the hazard of bacterial pneumonitis.

After an airway has been assured and convulsions controlled, efforts to reduce cerebral edema should be initiated. In the past, surgical subtemporal decompression was utilized to manage brain swelling in this disease. This procedure has becomes less popular and may now be considered to be contraindicated in view of the development of more effective measures.

Agents now used to reduce cerebral edema include mannitol, dexamethasone, and urea. Urea is less beneficial in lead poisoning because of its cellular effects and its tendency to produce a rebound increase in pressure following an initial decrease. Dexamethasone may reduce cerebral edema but there may be a time lag before it becomes effective. The drug is given intramuscularly or intravenously in four divided doses with the total daily dose being 0.25 to 0.50 mg. per kilogram of body weight. If more rapid control of brain swelling appears necessary, intravenous mannitol should be used. Mannitol in a 20 per cent solution is given in a dose of 2.0 grams per kilogram over a period of 20 minutes.

Chelating agents are used in lead poisoning to reduce the lead content of blood and tissue. Because the chelating drugs may enhance absorption of lead present in the intestinal lumen, the intestinal lead should be removed in conjunction with the beginning of therapy. Repeated small saline enemas may be used for this purpose, keeping in mind the potential danger of enemas in the presence of increased intracranial pressure. One's decision in this regard depends upon which factor he views as presenting the greatest danger.

The chelating agents utilized in therapy of lead poisoning include 2,3-dimercaptopropanol (BAL), calcium disodium edetate, and penicillamine. Penicillamine has been used less frequently than the others, and results appear less well established. Less severely ill children may be treated with calcium disodium edetate alone. During the first 48 hours of edetate therapy, there may be an exacerbation of symptoms and signs.

With more seriously ill children, a combination of edetate and BAL is recommended (Coffin et al.). An advantage of the combined agents is the much greater efficiency of BAL in removing lead from circulating red blood cells, which are the main carriers of lead in the circulation (Chisolm). Iron given orally or parenterally nullifies the beneficial effects of BAL and should not be used for anemia during chelation therapy (Chisolm, 1968). Edetate is given intravenously in a dose of 75 mg. per kilogram per day in four divided doses for five days. BAL is started simultaneously in a dose of 24 mg. per kilogram per day and is given intramuscularly every 4 hours for five days. Serial blood lead determinations are used to indicate the need for further treatment. A second course of edetate therapy is given for five days after the first is completed if the blood lead level remains elevated. Subsequent courses may be necessary, depending on the laboratory findings. Urinalysis and study of renal function should be repeated periodically when edetate is used because of its potential nephrotoxic effects.

If recovery occurs and the child returns home, efforts should be made to prevent further lead exposure. Additional laboratory examinations should be performed at periodic intervals to determine the possible need for subsequent edetate therapy. Chisolm (1968) has recommended the use of oral d-penicillamine in a dosage of 20 to 40 mg. per kilogram per day for one to six months after combined chelation therapy in children with severe lead encephalopathy.

REFERENCES

Chisolm, J. J., Jr.: Aminoaciduria as a manifestation of renal tubular injury in lead intoxication and a comparison with patterns of aminoaciduria seen in other diseases. *J. Pediat.*, **60**:1–17, 1962.

Chisolm, J. J. Jr.: Disturbances in the biosynthesis of heme in lead intoxication. *J. Pediat.*, **64**:174–186, 1964.

Chisolm, J. J. Jr.: Chronic lead intoxication in children. *Develop. Med. Child. Neurol.*, **7**:529–536, 1965.

Chisolm, J. J. Jr.: The use of chelating agents in the treatment of acute and chronic lead intoxication in childhood. *J. Pediat.*, **73**:1–38, 1968.

Chisolm, J. J. Jr., and Kaplan, E.: Lead poisoning in childhood—comprehensive management and prevention. *J. Pediat.*, **73**:942–950, 1968.

Coffin, R., Phillips, J. L., Staples, W. I., and Spector, S.:

Treatment of lead encephalopathy in children. *J. Pediat.*, **69**:198–206, 1966.

Emmerson, B. T., and Thiele, B. R.: Calcium versenate in the diagnosis of chronic lead nephropathy. *Med. J. Aust.*, **47**:243–248, 1960.

Feldman, F. Lichtman, H. C., Oransky, S., Ana, E. S., Reiser, L., and Malemud, C. J.: Serum δ-aminolevulinic acid in plumbism. *J. Pediat.*, **74**:917–923, 1969.

Freeman, R.: Reversible myocarditis due to chronic lead poisoning in childhood. *Arch. Dis. Childh.*, **40**:389–393, 1965.

Greengard, J.: Lead poisoning in childhood. *Clin. Pediat.*, **5**:269–276, 1966.

Greengard, J., Adams, B., and Berman, E.: Acute lead encephalopathy in young children. *J. Pediat.*, **66**:707–711, 1965.

Haeger-Aronsen, B.: Studies on urinary excretion of δ-aminolevulinic acid and other haem precursors in lead workers and lead-intoxicated rabbits. *Scandinav. J. Clin. Lab. Invest.*, **12**,Suppl. 47:1, 1960.

Jacobziner, H.: Lead poisoning in childhood. *Clin. Pediat.*, **5**:277–286, 1966.

Klein, M., Namer, R., Harpur, E., and Corbin, R.: Earthenware containers as a source of fatal lead poisoning. *New Eng. J. Med.*, **283**:669–672, 1970.

Kopito, L., Byers, R., and Shwachman, H.: Lead in hair of children with chronic lead poisoning. *New Eng. J. Med.*, **276**:949–953, 1967.

McFadzean, A. J. S., and Davis, L. S.: On the nature and significance of stippling in lead poisoning with reference to the effect of splenectomy. *Quart. J. Med.*, **18**:57–72, 1949.

Moore, M. T.: Human toxocara canis encephalitis with lead encephalopathy. *J. Neuropath, Exper. Neurol.*, **21**:201–218, 1962.

Morgan, J. M., Hartley, M. W., and Miller, R. E.: Nephropathy in chronic lead poisoning. *Arch. Int. Med.*, **118**:17–29, 1966.

Popoff, N., Weinberg, S., and Feigin, I.: Pathologic observations in lead encephalopathy. *Neurology*, **13**:101–112, 1963.

Sartain, P., Whitaker, J. A., and Martin, J.: The absence of lead lines in bone of children with early lead poisoning. *Amer. J. Roentgen.*, **91**:597–601, 1964.

Seto, D. S. Y., and Freeman, J. M.: Lead neuropathy in childhood. *Amer. J. Dis. Child.*, **107**:337–342, 1964.

Weissberg, J. B., Lipschutz, F., and Oski, F. A.: δ-Aminolevulinic acid dehydratase activity in circulating blood cells. A sensitive laboratory test for the detection of childhood lead poisoning. *New Eng. J. Med.*, **284**:565–569, 1971.

Whitaker, J. A., Austin, W., and Nelson, J. D.: Edathamil calcium disodium (versenate) diagnostic test for lead poisoning. *Pediatrics*, **29**:384–388, 1962.

Chapter Eleven

HEAD TRAUMA

Head injuries have become one of the leading medical causes of morbidity and death among children. With continued increase in population density, the development of new and varied forms of pleasure vehicles, such as motorcycles and sledmobiles, and ever increasing numbers of automobiles on already crowded city streets, the significance of craniocerebral trauma as a major threat to the child comes clearly into focus. Although all types of accidents have emerged as the number one cause of death in pediatric patients beyond the first few months of life, pediatric training programs in general provide insufficient experience and exposure to enable one to feel comfortable in management of the problems presented by the acutely injured child.

The prevalence of head injuries in children has been expressed statistically in many ways. Approximately one child in ten at some time experiences a head injury associated with loss of consciousness (Melchior). Accidents account for more childhood deaths than do the four most common fatal diseases of childhood combined after the age of one year. About one-fourth of these accidental deaths are due to head injuries (Mealey). It has been estimated that 200,000 children are hospitalized each year in the United States because of head injury and more than 3000 children die per year from head trauma (Mealey). It is generally agreed that boys sustain head injuries two to three times more often than girls and that the majority of childhood head injuries are mild from which complete recovery follows.

Prevention

Education of parents in the dangers of head trauma and methods of prevention could logically be incorporated into the physician's well baby care program. Such instruction could easily be provided by a nurse or other paramedical person following a relatively brief training program. The potential seriousness and long-term effects of blunt trauma to the immature brain of the infant is not appreciated by a large segment of the lay population. It is probable that many crippling injuries to small children would not occur if adults were more cognizant of the delicacy of immature central nervous system structures.

Soon after arrival home with a newborn baby, parents should be advised to survey their home or apartment to seek out possible sources of trauma, burns, or poisoning to the child as he grows and eventually becomes ambulatory. Throw rugs at the top of a flight of stairs provide an obvious hazard not only to the toddler but also to the mother carrying the infant. Unused electric outlets should be identified and plugged with inexpensive plastic safety caps. Coffee tables and other low wooden furniture with sharp, protruding corners should not be placed in an area in which the poorly coordinated 18-month-old child spends most of the time he is awake.

Stairways are danger spots for children and a frequent site of accidental falls. Although the risk cannot be entirely eliminated, it can be decreased by keeping doorways to basement steps closed, by establishing home rules preventing objects from being placed on steps, and by cushioning the wooden or cement floor at the bottom with a thick rug. Wooden gates that block the entrance to a stairway create a temporary nuisance for adults but may prevent serious brain injury to the infant and young child. Also in regard to stairways, apartment dwellers with small children should seek ground-floor accomodations whenever possible. Vacationing families use good judgment by requesting rooms at ground level in motels and resorts.

Open windows on the second story or higher represent a threat that should be eliminated by use of well installed screens in good state of repair. The dangling cord of an iron resting on a narrow ironing board presents the unknowing infant with a temptation hard to resist and can be eliminated as a source of injury only by constant preventive measures. The high chair is another device designed with little regard for the safety of the child. Although this high perch is likely to remain popular for infant feeding, mothers should be advised of the frequency with which falls occur from it.

Motor vehicle accidents resulting in childhood head injury are obviously not entirely preventable but could be significantly reduced by a more safety-minded public. An improved design of a more padded dashboard, the common site of impact of the child riding in the front seat, should be expected by the automobile-purchasing clientele. Car seats with an attached seatbelt are available for older infants and small children and would prevent many injuries if properly used. Such preventive measures are important if automobile-induced injuries are to be reduced; however, they are far exceeded by the need for operators to be constantly aware of the dangers of carelessness, unnecessary high speeds, and the effect of alcohol on one's driving ability.

Selection of toys and play objects for children is an additional consideration in which a little judgment may be a valuable factor in preventing needless injuries. A bow and arrow for the impulsive six-year-old is a questionable selection under any circumstances. Operation of a power lawnmower in the immediate vicinity of several small children likewise is an example of little safety forethought. The playground is a continual source of head injuries to youngsters, fortunately, usually mild. Playground accidents are difficult to control and perhaps are an unavoidable byproduct of this phase of a child's development. Sending an unattended three-year-old to a playground equipped with slides and swings, however, is such poor judgment that injury is to be anticipated.

Although the foregoing discussion outlines only a fraction of the seemingly endless ways by which injuries may occur, it does illustrate the importance of family education if prevention is to be attempted. The fine line between over-protection and appropriate concern is readily evident and is a matter that must be dealt with individually by every responsible parent.

Pathology

The consequences of head injury in children largely depend on the severity and location of the pathologic alterations of the brain. Fracture of the skull usually cannot be used as an index of the magnitude of the injury and is often absent, even with severe head trauma.

Cerebral concussion (commotio cerebri) refers to a head injury followed by temporary loss of consciousness and associated with a period of memory loss termed post-traumatic amnesia. Partial or total inability to recall events prior to the traumatic event is called retrograde amnesia and may cover a period of a few minutes to several hours. Post-traumatic amnesia may gradually diminish as the patient recovers from the injury, but a certain component is permanent.

The mechanism accounting for the disturbance of awareness and responsiveness (consciousness) with concussive injuries has been widely debated and remains speculative. It is generally believed that temporary alterations of the function of the reticular mechanisms in the brain stem are related to the period of loss of consciousness. Although function is briefly disturbed with concussion, structure of the brain as evident on gross observation is not altered.

Cerebral contusion and laceration are more significant lesions and are related to traumatic events in which there are grossly visible alterations of brain tissue (Fig. 11-1). Contusion may be located adjacent to the site of impact, the so-called coup lesion, or, contracoup areas of bruising may occur on the opposite side from the site of the impact. Occipital injuries frequently result in contracoup contusions of the frontal poles. Bruising of the orbital surfaces of the frontal

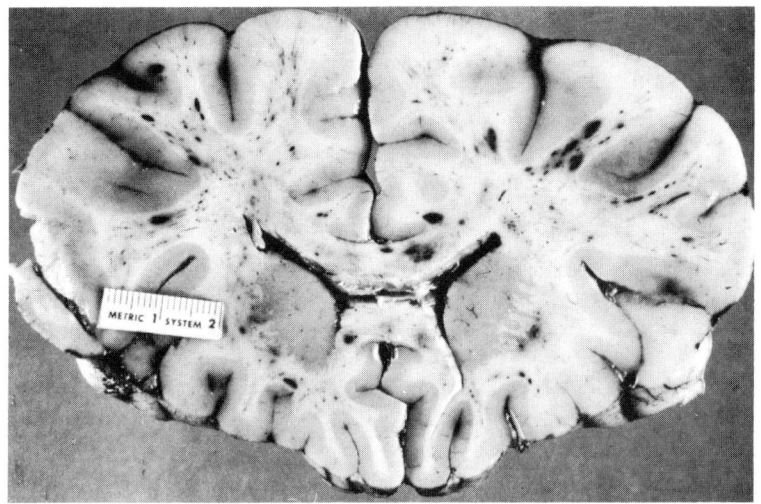

Figure 11–1. Severe, blunt trauma to the head resulting in multiple, diffuse petechial hemorrhages of various sizes. The pattern illustrated resembles that seen with cerebral fat emboli, not present in this case. Despite the severity noted on sectioning of the brain, gross observation of the external, uncut surface revealed no striking features.

lobes and tips of the temporal lobes is a common finding with diffuse head injuries (Fig. 11-2). This type of "gliding" injury occurs in areas where the cortical surface is closely approximated to the roughened skull surface. These contused areas consist of hemorrhagic lesions maximal at the gyral surface and affecting primarily the cortex with little white matter involvement. Impacts directed to the vertex of the head may produce hemorrhage and necrosis within the corpus callosum, and less commonly, frank laceration of the callosal bundles (Fig. 11-3).

Lindenberg and Freytag have emphasized the tendency for blunt trauma to the head in infancy to result in linear tissue tears within white matter. They attribute this predisposition to tearing rather than the more conventional contusion observed in older children, to the soft consistency of the poorly myelinated brain of the infant. These clefts may be either grossly visible or recognizable only on microscopic examination. Similar to other lesions resulting from blunt head trauma, they are most conspicuous on the orbital surface of the frontal lobes and in the temporal lobes.

Strich has made reference to nerve fiber shearing as a cause of permanent brain damage from head injury. She states that patients who sustain tearing of nerve fibers in the cerebral white matter typically exhibit overt and persistent neurologic signs immediately after the impact, thus excluding anoxic or vascular factors as an explanation. Subsequent examination of the brain in patients with this form of traumatic lesion reveals ventricular dilatation and retraction balls at the ends of interrupted nerve fibers but with the cerebral cortex remaining reasonably intact.

Brain stem traumatic lesions often occur in association with hemorrhagic involvement of the cerebrum or cerebellum (Fig. 11-4). Clinical evidence of morphologic compromise of the brain stem frequently suggests a fatal out-

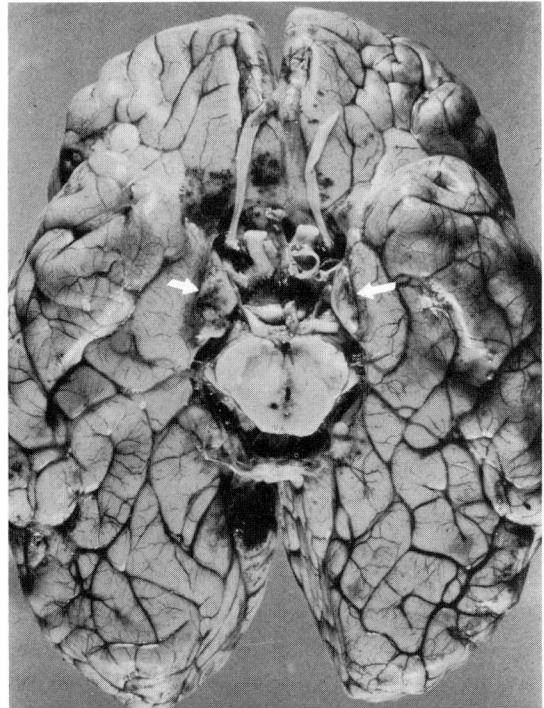

Figure 11–2. Diffuse head trauma resulting in multiple, hemorrhagic contusions of the orbital surfaces of the frontal lobes. There are bilateral uncal herniations with necrosis of the unci medial to tentorial grooves (arrows).

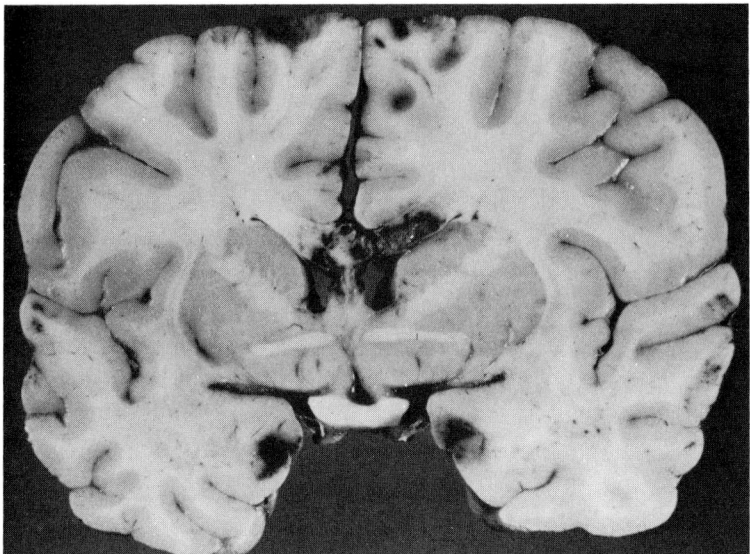

Figure 11–3. Effects of blunt trauma to the vertex of the head. There are bilateral vertex contusions beneath the site of the impact as well as uncal contusions resulting from compression of medial temporal lobe structures against the unyielding tentorium. Note the hemorrhagic necrosis of the corpus callosum.

come and almost always is associated with residual deficits if the patient survives. Primary traumatic lesions of the brain stem are usually laterally placed in the tegmentum of the midbrain or pons and are the result of impacts to the occipital region more often than elsewhere (Crompton). The cause of this type of lesion is conjectural but is believed to be the result of mechanical distortion of the brain stem with stretching or shearing forces applied to nerve fibers and vessels.

With any of the previously described traumatic insults, bleeding into the subdural, epidural, or subarachnoid spaces may coexist. Missiles penetrating the skull may lacerate brain tissue with hemorrhage. This type of injury may subsequently be complicated by meningitis or a brain abscess that can become more life-threatening than the original traumatic episode. An additional type of injury in childhood secondarily resulting in cerebral damage is trauma to the tonsillar bed by a foreign body, such as a lollipop, which can lead to carotid artery occlusion and ischemic infarction (Frantzen et al., Pitner).

Cerebral pathology with head injuries may be complicated by anoxic changes if airway obstruction occurs or by ischemic involvement if shock is part of the clinical picture. Since head trauma is frequently accompanied by skeletal fractures elsewhere, fat embolization to the brain is an additional complicating factor that may influence the neuropathologic findings.

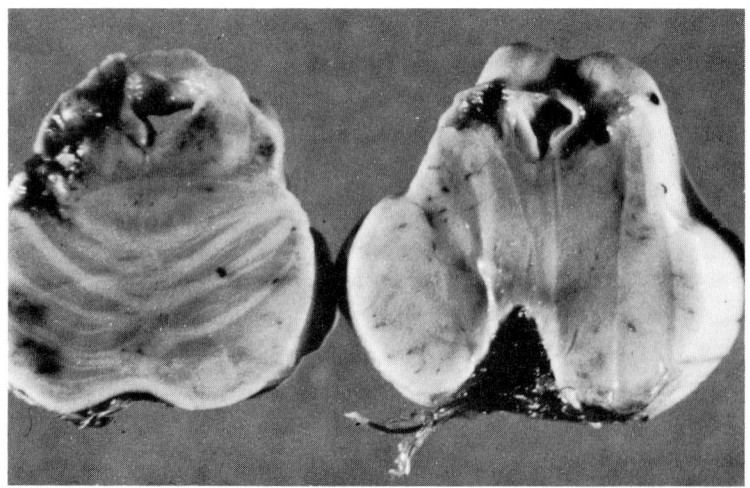

Figure 11–4. Traumatic lesions of the brain stem. The necrotic lesion involving the superior cerebellar peduncle of the pons is largely unilateral while in the midbrain, the tectum is softened bilaterally. Such lesions of the dorsal surface of the upper brain stem may result from impact of these areas against the rigid tentorium.

Clinical Aspects

Most head injuries in children are mild and are followed by prompt recovery from which no apparent sequelae remain (Hjern and Nylander). Consciousness may be briefly impaired or, more often, the child is described as being temporarily dazed or stunned, followed by a period of irrational or confused behavior. Even with such trivial impacts, children frequently vomit one or more times and a desire to sleep then ensues. For the next several hours, listlessness or tiredness may be apparent and appetite remains poor. Complete recovery usually has occurred 24 to 48 hours after the episode.

Mild head trauma of this sort is occasionally followed by ataxia, which can persist for several days. Transient complete blindness also may follow otherwise trivial head injuries in children (Griffith and Dodge). The site of impact is usually the occipital region in these cases and pupillary reactions remain intact during the period of visual loss. Recovery of vision follows within minutes to four hours, but the experience may evoke considerable anxiety for the patient and parents until visual function is restored.

Extraocular muscle weakness causing diplopia may follow either mild or severe head trauma and may be temporary or persistent. Following head trauma, sixth nerve paresis is more common than deficits of other extraocular nerves but various combinations may occur in some cases. With mild injuries, ocular muscle weakness is usually attributable to contusion of the nerve, whereas severe trauma may cause extraocular paralysis by either peripheral or central lesions. Carotid-cavernous fistula is a rare manifestation of head trauma in childhood and leads to pulsatile exophthalmos with functional deficits of cranial nerves within the cavernous sinus.

Although most children recover rapidly following concussive injuries, an occasional child continues to complain of headaches, fatigue, and dizziness, analogous to the post-concussion syndrome in adults (Dillon and Leopold). Complaints more often expressed in children subsequent to concussion include nightmares, fear of certain situations not previously present, nervousness, and renewal of bedwetting.Personality changes after traumatic episodes are frequent in children but usually diminish progressively with time.

With severe head injuries due to blunt trauma, unconsciousness is more prolonged, variable neurologic signs are evident, depending on the location of the lesions, and permanent sequelae are more common. The presence of dilated pupils that are unresponsive to light, extensor rigidity, and deep coma immediately after the impact suggest a midbrain lesion that usually proves fatal. Coma of prolonged duration may be attended by numerous complications, some of which may be a primary factor in causing death of the child. Systemic hypertension, gastrointestinal hemorrhage, and acute pulmonary edema are all recognized post-traumatic hazards.

The ultimate outcome of the child with an acute head injury is difficult to predict except in those with obvious and immediate evidence of severe brain stem pathology. It is evident from studies by Lewin on traumatized patients with prolonged unconsciousness that one must be cautious in advancing a definite prognosis too early. Of 102 injured patients unconscious for more than one month, 63 survived and 19 returned to their previous work or scholastic level. An additional 29 were able to return to some form of work or to perform household duties despite permanent neurologic deficits.

Brink et al. evaluated 46 children one to seven years after head injury with coma of at least one week duration after the traumatic episode. Independent ambulation and self-care was achieved in 87 per cent but all had significant neurologic sequelae. Twenty-six percent of the total series had seizures; in some the convulsions occurred in the first few days after injury, and in others the onset was many months later. The authors noted that improvement in these children continued for as long as three years subsequent to injury, although maximum gains occurred within the first year.

Management

Evaluation of the injured child includes a detailed historical review, although other aspects of management often take precedence, especially if consciousness is disturbed at the time of admission. The medical record should contain a detailed account of the circumstances surrounding the accident as well as a description of the child from the time of the impact until hospitalization. The presence or absence of consciousness should be documented, and if absent, its duration should be recorded.

Historical aspects frequently neglected in evaluation of the injured child include history of prior medical illnesses, especially allergies, immunizations, and whether the child has been receiving drug therapy for an established medical diagnosis before the accident. Previous diagnoses of diabetes mellitus, epilepsy, penicillin allergy, or cerebral palsy may significantly alter specific management of the traumatized patient or interpretation of signs on physical examination.

Children with mild blunt trauma to the head without loss of consciousness are frequently examined in the physician's office or hospital emergency room but can usually be allowed to return home after skull x-rays are taken. The parents should be instructed to make certain evaluations of the child at hourly intervals for four to six hours, including pulse rate, size and equality of the pupils, and the state of responsiveness.

Such children usually desire to sleep following blows to the head, and it is reasonable that they be allowed to do so. The concept that the child should be constantly stimulated to be kept awake after head trauma is untenable and creates a most unpleasant situation both for parents and child. A period of sleep is acceptable, but the child should be aroused at intervals of 60 to 90 minutes to be certain that consciousness can be restored and to check pupil size and reactions.

Sleep in children at this time is often characterized by restlessness with arousal being fairly easy, as opposed to the situation that pertains with the comatose patient. Parental anxiety is alleviated if the physician retains a degree of responsibility for decision making by requesting that the family call him at two-hour intervals for two or four hours and thereby report the status of the child. If responsiveness declines, a convulsion occurs, a pupil becomes dilated, or limb weakness becomes evident, admission to the hospital for further assessment is advised.

The child rendered unconscious by a blow to the head or with a skull fracture that traverses the groove of the middle meningeal artery or the lambdoidal suture warrants hospital admission for periodic assessment of vital and neurologic signs. The first consideration when assessing an unconscious child in the emergency or receiving area pertains to the adequacy of the airway and the presence or absence of blood loss or shock. Craniocerebral trauma alone does not usually account for profound systemic shock and when it is identified, one should consider other sites for its origin. External blood loss, rupture of the spleen or of other abdominal viscera, or massive hemothorax may cause death of the child unless recognized and treated accordingly. Head injuries in infants is an exception to this rule because acute subdural or epidural hemorrhage of large volume may sufficiently deplete the blood volume to cause shock in this age group.

Any disturbance of ventilation or airway obstruction should be circumvented by either suction of the airway with administration of oxygen, endotracheal intubation, or tracheostomy. Ventilation and the prevention of aspiration pneumonitis may also be enhanced by the passage of a nasogastric tube for the aspiration of air and gastric contents. While performing these initial procedures, it is important to keep in mind that the comatose child may also have sustained a cervical spine injury. Until fracture or dislocation of the cervical region is excluded by x-rays, head and neck motion should be kept minimized.

The performance of skull, cervical spine, and other x-rays is a necessary part of management of the child with head trauma but is best delayed until the foregoing, more emergent, needs have been met. Spinal fluid examination in the acutely injured patient rarely provides information that alters management and is best deferred to a later date, if performed at all. Certain patients require angiography to identify or exclude a surgically amenable intracranial hemorrhage but this decision is usually made after a brief period of observation subsequent to hospital admission.

The initial physical examination establishes a baseline of vital signs and neurologic findings, which must then be reassessed at intervals of 15 to 30 minutes for several hours. Tetanus prophylaxis, use of anticonvulsants, administration of antibiotics, and the need for substances to reduce brain swelling are determined by the type of injury and the findings on observation. Mild temperature elevations may be controlled by the use of salicylates or electric fans directed to the exposed body surface. In small children who have vomited several times, rehydration with intravenous fluids may suffice. More severe degrees of hyperthermia may require a cooling blanket.

Diabetes insipidus may complicate severe injuries in children and requires studies of blood and urine, including urine volume measurement, for identification. Since coma obviates the expression and satisfaction of thirst, the unconscious child with diabetes insipidus is dependent on the physician for the prevention of dehydration.

Progressive deterioration of various parameters of responsiveness, development of unilateral pupillary dilatation, or decrease of motor function on one side of the body within hours or a day or so after injury must be assumed to be evidence of an epidural or acute subdural hematoma and indicates the need for angiographic studies. Cerebral edema can also result in worsening with signs of increased intracranial pressure and often cannot be distinguished clinically from signs produced by an expanding intracranial hematoma. Occasionally, brain swelling appears to become pronounced several days after head trauma, producing lethargy, vomiting, and papilledema, and responding promptly to corticosteroid or mannitol therapy.

A major factor influencing the outcome of the comatose child with blunt head trauma is the quality and consistency of nursing care. Skin care, oral hygiene, prevention of decubitus ulcers and protection of the corneal surfaces are aspects expected to be managed by the nursing staff, in addition to the administration of medications and the performance of periodic observations. A physical therapy program should be initiated as soon as possible with the aim of preventing deficits of range of joint motion rather than correcting them, once they have developed. When improvement has occurred and consciousness is restored, many children require a prolonged program of rehabilitation requiring the skills of many discplines. Although resources for this lengthy and costly period of care are limited, it is a necessary component of management of the brain injured child if he is to achieve his greatest potential for recovery.

PERINATAL HEAD TRAUMA

Mechanical trauma to the head during birth may cause inconsequential soft tissue injuries or skull fractures, or may result in serious intracranial disease, most often due to hemorrhage. Factors during labor that predispose the infant to mechanical head injury are often those associated with hypoxia and asphyxia. Thus, multiple factors may coexist, making it difficult to distinguish which insult plays a greater role in the clinical abnormalities of the newborn. Perinatal injuries due to mechanical trauma or hypoxia are of great importance, not only because of the immediate abnormalities in the neonate, but also because of the relationship to subsequent deficits, including mental retardation, seizures, and cerebral palsy.

Cephalhematoma

Soft tissue and skull injuries in the newborn reflect evidence of trauma, but of themselves are not usually of much significance. Skull fracture, caput succadeneum, and cephalhematoma are the most common such superficial injuries and only infrequently are associated with underlying cerebral involvement. Cephalhematoma is usually considered to result from an accumulation of blood beneath the periosteum of the skull in the newborn infant (Fig. 11-5). Matson has included both subperiosteal hematomas and subgaleal hematomas in this category.

Cephalhematoma occurs in approximately 2.5 per cent of live births (Kendall and Woloshin). They are usually unilateral, most are located in the parietal region, and about 25 per cent are associated with an underlying linear skull fracture (Kendall and Woloshin).

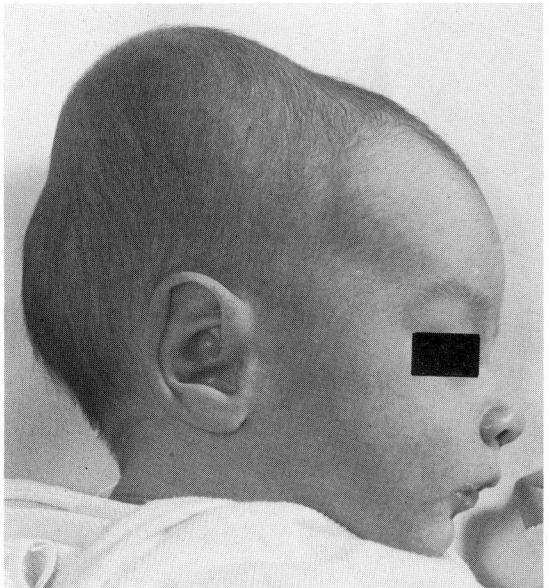

Figure 11-5. Cephalhematoma in two-week-old infant. Lesion was noted on the first day of life and resolved spontaneously by six weeks of age.

Obstetric factors predisposing to this lesion are primiparity, delivery by forceps, and large size of the infant. An occipital cephalhematoma located in the midline may be confused with an encephalocoele until it is apparent that spontaneous resolution is occurring and that no bony defect is present.

Subperiosteal hemorrhage does not extend across suture lines, being limited in its extension by the periosteal attachment at the periphery of the involved bone. Palpation of this lesion reveals a distinct, circular edge, which may give the false impression of a depressed fracture. Calcification frequently occurs within a cephalhematoma, which may be visualized as a calcified ridge at the periphery on x-ray. Subgaleal hemorrhage differs in the newborn in that it is not limited by suture lines and may extend over the entire scalp if extensive enough. In countries where vitamin K is not administered after birth, massive subgaleal bleeding secondary to hemorrhagic disease of the newborn may result in severe anemia or exsanguination and death (Robinson and Rossiter).

Cephalhematomas are generally benign lesions that resolve spontaneously within a few weeks after birth. Rarely, permanent bone deformity with hyperostosis persists. Anemia may occur with large or bilateral lesions, and hyperbilirubinemia is occasionally noted because of resorption of the hemorrhagic mass (Rausen and Diamond). A more serious complication, although rare, is localization of infection within a cephalhematoma in a septic baby (Levy et al., Burry and Hellerstein, Lee and Berg). Suppuration within a cephalhematoma may precede osteomyelitis of the skull adjacent to the abscess or even bacterial meningitis from intracranial extension through an underlying skull fracture (Cohen et al.). An infected cephalhematoma may be an indolent process, not easily recognized from the clinical signs. It is managed by incision and drainage in addition to antibiotic therapy. Most uncomplicated cephalhematomas resolve spontaneously and should not be aggressively treated. Needle drainage is not indicated because of the possibility of introducing infection.

Intracranial Hemorrhage in the Newborn

Intracranial hemorrhage is the most common serious consequence of perinatal mechanical head trauma. Intracranial bleeding does not always originate, however, from strictly mechanical forces exerted on the head during labor and delivery. The massive intraventricular hemorrhage characteristic of the low birth weight infant is believed to result from venous stasis in the deep venous drainage system. Periventricular infarction of hypoxic origin with associated damage to the delicate veins in the periventricular matrix leads to extension of hemorrhage into the lateral ventricles and subsequently throughout the subarachnoid space (Towbin).

Supratentorial subdural hemorrhage occurs mainly at term and in oversized infants. Lateral compression of the head during labor may result in molding of the cranial bones sufficient to disrupt bridging venous channels passing to the sagittal sinus. Clinical evidence of extensive bleeding into the subdural spaces in the infant at birth is not common but more often leads to signs of increased pressure recognized two to eight months after birth. The newborn with vitamin K deficiency hemorrhagic disease, severe thrombocytopenia, or consumption coagulopathy may exhibit signs of subdural hemorrhage as well as bleeding elsewhere. Defects in coagulation with subsequent subdural hemorrhage may also be the result of severe perinatal asphyxia (Chessells and Wigglesworth). Newborns with osteogenesis imperfecta may acquire large subdural hematomas during the birth process because of the fragile skull, which provides little protection to the intracranial contents (Fig. 11-6).

Severe distortion of head shape during the birth process may disrupt the tentorium or the junction of the falx cerebri and the tentorium. Lacerations of the tentorium may be associated with tears of the lateral or straight sinuses causing posterior fossa subdural hemorrhage, which rapidly becomes life threatening. Infants with this lesion may show variable signs but most become hypotonic, develop disturbances of respiratory rate and rhythm, exhibit brain stem signs including nystagmus, and have rapid head enlargement because of fourth ventricle obstruction (Gilles and Shillito, Carter and Pittman). Clinical diagnosis is difficult but requires ventriculography to demonstrate anterior and superior displacement of the fourth ventricle and aqueduct. Surgical evacuation of a neonatal posterior fossa subdural hematoma is possible, but most babies who survive have

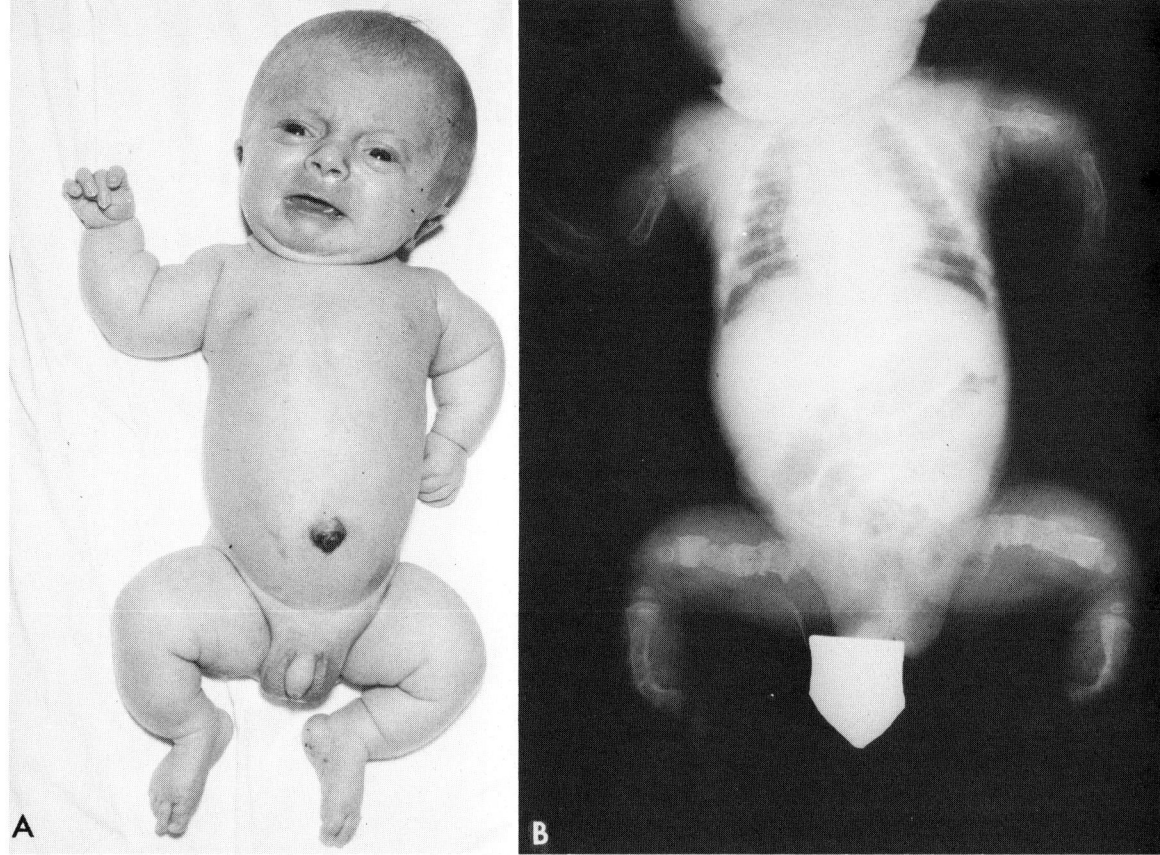

Figure 11-6. Infant with osteogenesis inperfecta with bilateral subdural hematomas present at birth. Infant was irritable and had a tense fontanel. Note the shortened and curved extremities (micromelia) characteristic of this condition. Multiple long bone fractures of various ages were found on x-ray.

residual communicating hydrocephalus (Carter and Pittman).

Other traumatic lesions associated with the stresses of labor and delivery include cerebral contusion, lacerations of the brain stem (Towbin), subarachnoid hemorrhage, and circumscribed intraventricular hematoma (Murtagh and Baird). In addition to the detrimental effects on immature brain tissue, traumatic lesions associated with subarachnoid bleeding are an important cause of communicating hydrocephalus in those who survive (Lourie and Berne).

SKULL FRACTURES

Fractures of the skull in children may be linear, depressed, or comminuted. A diastatic fracture refers to traumatic separation of the cranial bones at the site of the cranial sutures and may occur with or without other types of fractures (Fig. 11-7). Linear fractures are usually of no great significance and do not alter the principles of management of closed head injuries. A linear skull fracture does provide evidence of prior head trauma but does not necessarily indicate that the traumatic event was severe. Even mild blows to the head that are considered trivial and of no consequence may result in fractures. Fractures extending across the grooves of the middle meningeal artery are of potential significance because of the possibility of arterial disruption and epidural hemorrhage.

Fractures of greater potential significance include those that are depressed, those that involve one of the air-containing paranasal sinuses or mastoid process, or those that extend into the base of the skull. Depressed fractures carry an appreciable risk of complication by intracranial infection, hemorrhage from laceration of an adjacent venous sinus, or impingement on the brain leading to a meningocerebral scar and subsequent posttraumatic epilepsy (Miller and Jennett). De-

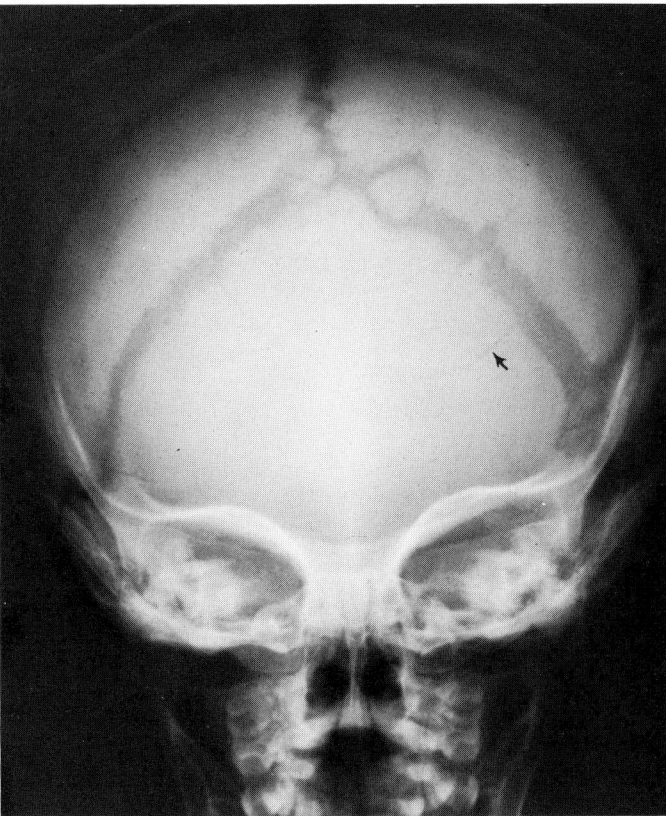

Figure 11-7. Traumatic suture diastasis. Skull film, anteroposterior view. Blunt trauma to the child's head was delivered by the fist of an adult. There is also a linear fracture extending to the lambdoidal suture (arrow).

pressed fractures of the skull require surgical elevation. Other aspects of management of the injured patient are often more important and surgical correction of the fracture is not usually considered urgent.

Basal skull fractures may be difficult to visualize roentgenographically and are the result of injuries of considerable magnitude. Fracture of the base is suspected by the presence of certain physical signs, including bleeding into the nasopharynx or middle ear, orbital and conjunctival ecchymoses, and ecchymotic lesions of the skin over the mastoid process referred to as Battle's sign. Peripheral facial paralysis or other cranial nerve deficits may also be noted. Cerebrospinal fluid leaks predisposing the child to bacterial meningitis are an additional potential complication of basal skull injuries. The pituitary stalk may be traumatized producing transient or permanent diabetes insipidus.

Skull Fractures in the Neonate

Skull fractures in the newborn may be acquired in utero before onset of labor, during labor and delivery, or in the neonatal period. Intrauterine skull fractures may occur secondary to physical trauma to the maternal abdomen or pelvis, or more commonly, because of contact of the fetal head with the promontory of the sacrum (Alexander and Davis).

Despite the pliability of the newborn's skull, fractures may also be sustained during the birth process and from forces induced by the application of forceps. Bruises of the skin, a cephalhematoma, or a palpable depression of the infant's cranium is a clue to an underlying fracture and warrants skull x-ray examination.

Neonatal skull fractures may be linear or depressed, but more often a portion of one parietal bone is buckled inward much like an indentation of a ping-pong ball. There may be no break in the bony continuity in such cases, even though these injuries are dealt with in the same manner as depressed skull fractures.

A remarkable feature of this type of non-fractured, depressed injury of the neonatal skull is the marked abnormality on the anteroposterior and posteroanterior views with

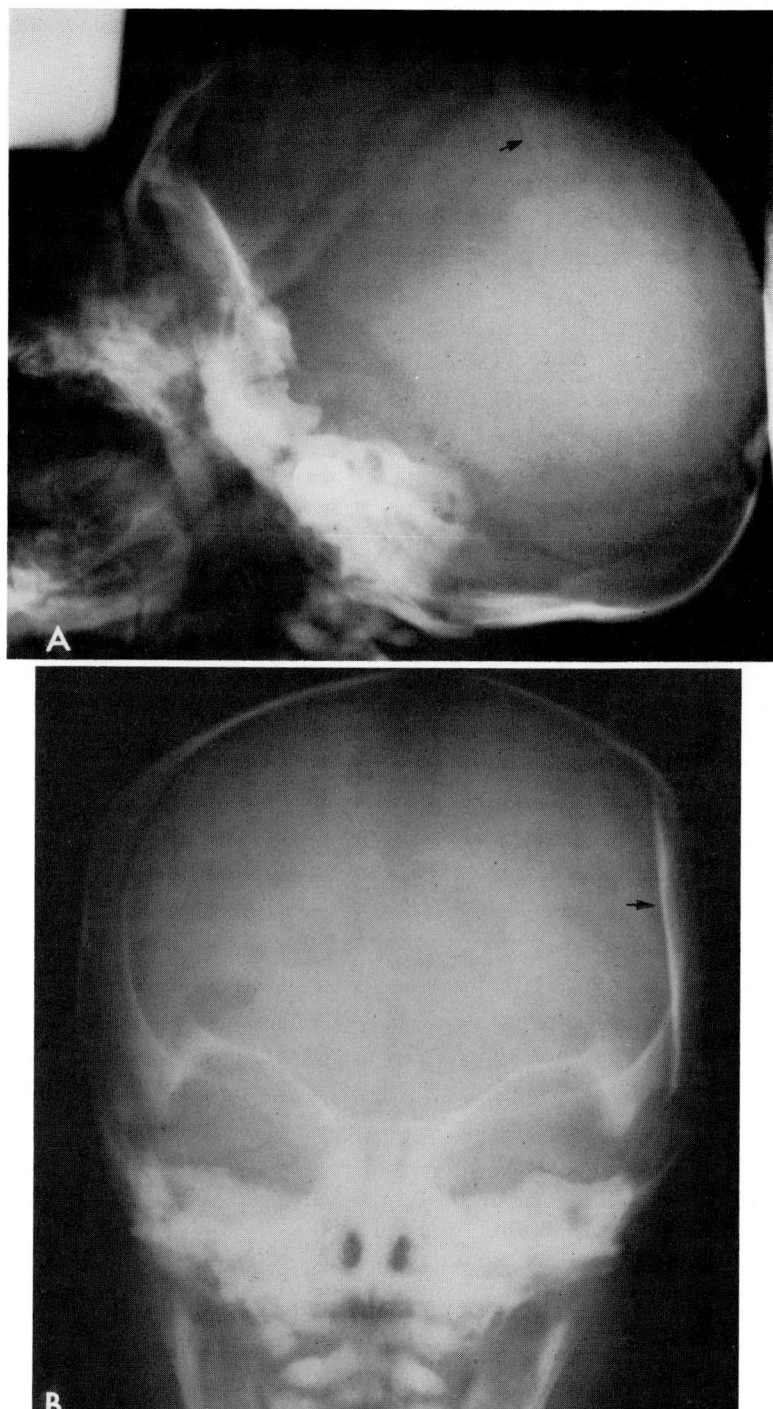

Figure 11–8. Neonatal "depressed" skull fracture. *A,* Lateral view reveals only short-segment linear fracture without evidence of depression (arrow). *B,* Posteroanterior view shows the linear density produced by buckling of the skull associated with the insignificant linear fracture in *A.*

a nearly normal appearance of the lateral view (Fig. 11-8). A distinct vertical line of increased density displaced medially from the expected site of the lateral margin of the skull is evident on the anteroposterior skull film. The lack of significant abnormalities on the lateral projections is explained by the absence of bony overlapping, which ordinarily creates the increased density observed with fractures that are depressed.

Neonatal depressed skull fractures as well as the buckling, or ping-pong ball, injury that resembles a depressed fracture should be surgically elevated to enable normal brain growth beneath. This can be safely done in the first few days of life but may be deferred if the child has other more threatening problems, such as respiratory distress, cardiac failure, or sepsis. Nonsurgical methods of elevating depressed fractures in the newborn have included the use of a breast pump (Schrager) or digital pressure (Raynor and Parsa) and deserve further consideration.

Subepicranial Hydroma

A benign complication of skull fracture in children that results in signs that may be diagnostically confusing is referred to as subepicranial hydroma (Epstein et al.). This consists of an accumulation of cerebrospinal fluid beneath the galea causing a soft, fluctuant swelling under the scalp that resembles diffuse scalp edema. The swelling gradually progresses after trauma and may eventually encompass the entire calvarium including the eyelids. The area of swelling is either not tender or only mildly so, and transilluminates when a flashlight is placed flush to the scalp.

During the stage of profound swelling of the soft tissues, the child is generally irritable and may experience recurrent vomiting. The source of the fluid is the subarachnoid space, and the fluid gains access to the epicranial soft tissues following a skull fracture that usually traverses a suture. Laceration of the dura and disruption of the arachnoid allows fluid to flow from the subarachnoid space through the fracture line and into the subgaleal space beneath the scalp.

Treatment is conservative and spontaneous absorption of the fluid usually occurs within a few weeks. Needle aspiration is not advisable because of the danger of superimposed infection. Skull x-rays should be repeated a few months after resolution of the process to be certain that a post-traumatic leptomeningeal cyst has not developed.

Pneumocephalus

Pneumocephalus is a potentially serious complication of facial or cranial fractures that involve the paranasal sinuses or mastoid process (Turner, Kahn and Daywitt). Intracranial accumulation of air subsequent to these injuries may be located in the epidural, subdural, or subarachnoid space, within the brain, or in the lateral ventricles. In some cases of traumatic pneumocephalus, air gains entrance through the fracture and the lacerated dura to more than one of these locations simultaneously. Pneumocephalus may be present immediately after the traumatic event or may develop several days later.

Luckett (1913) described air within the lateral ventricles in a patient examined after head trauma and has been credited by some as the founder of the concept of ventriculography for this observation. The pathway by which air reaches the ventricles in such cases is usually unclear but is probably from the subarachnoid space through the fourth ventricle foramina in most cases. Direct tears of the brain extending to the ventricle is another possible, but less common, route.

Meningitis creates a constant threat to the patient with traumatic pneumocephalus, analogous to the situation with rhinorrhea, which may coexist. The identification of intracranial air after trauma is sufficient evidence of bacterial contamination that intravenous antibiotics are indicated after lumbar puncture is performed for cultures. Antibiotics are continued until the air is absorbed, usually within two to three weeks. Persistence or reaccumulation of intracranial air longer than three to four weeks after fracture usually warrants surgical repair of the dural defect.

POST-TRAUMATIC LEPTOMENINGEAL CYSTS

An unusual complication of linear skull fractures in infants and young children is a pulsating leptomeningeal cyst, also known as a "growing skull fracture" (Vas and Winn, Gruber, Lende and Erickson). The injuries that result in these lesions are usually parietal or parieto-occipital. Fractures that are subsequently complicated by the development of leptomeningeal cysts are those with diastasis of 4 mm. or greater (Taveras and Ransohoff). Pulsating leptomeningeal cysts are largely restricted to infants and children who sustain the initiating fracture under three years of age.

The prerequisite for the formation of a post-traumatic leptomeningeal cyst is the occurrence of a dural tear at the time the fracture is incurred. In some children, the traumatic episode is compounded by the for-

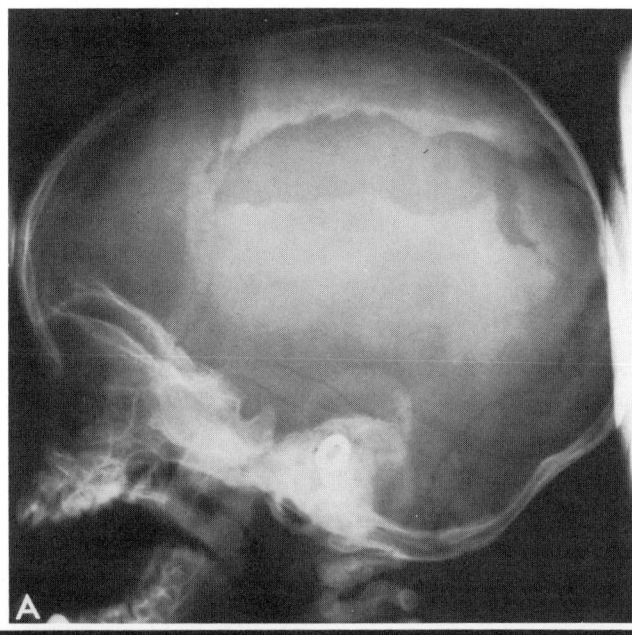

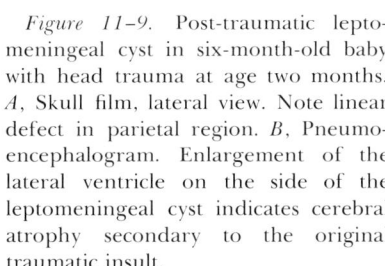

Figure 11-9. Post-traumatic leptomeningeal cyst in six-month-old baby with head trauma at age two months. *A*, Skull film, lateral view. Note linear defect in parietal region. *B*, Pneumoencephalogram. Enlargement of the lateral ventricle on the side of the leptomeningeal cyst indicates cerebral atrophy secondary to the original traumatic insult.

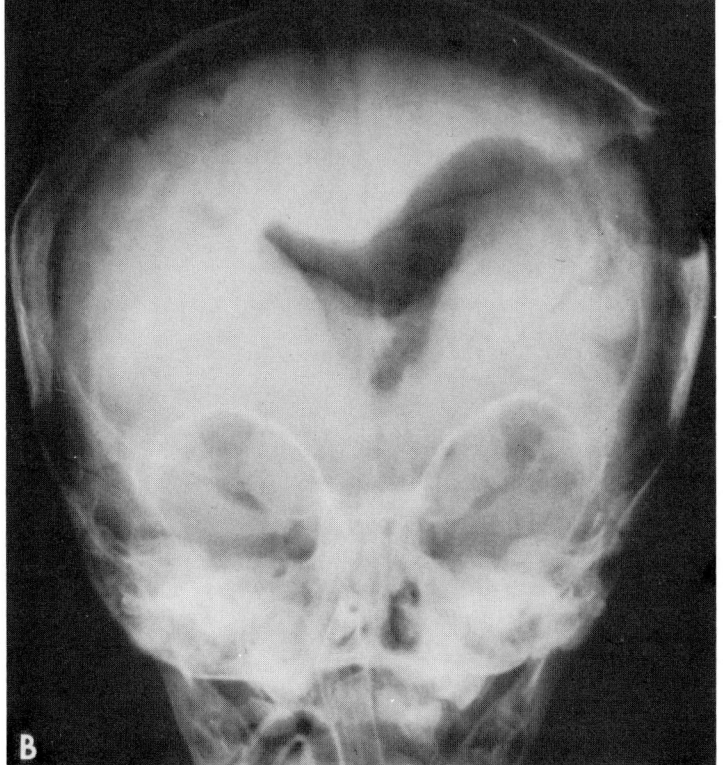

mation of a subepicranial hydroma within days after injury, with the leptomeningeal cyst becoming apparent several months later. Associated with the dural laceration beneath the fracture is arachnoidal herniation into the fracture line. Cerebral tissue may also herniate into the skull defect and eventually becomes infarcted (Tenner and Stein). Transmitted pulsations within the arachnoid produces gradual erosion of the bony margins of the fracture, resulting in eventual wide separation at the old fracture site. The pulsating, fluctuant mass can then be observed and palpated beneath the soft tissues of the scalp. These lesions may be recognized within four months after the inciting fracture or may not become apparent for several years.

The child with a post-traumatic leptomeningeal cyst may be entirely asymptomatic, and the mother discovers the lesion while washing or combing the hair. Long-standing lesions may be associated with seizures, hemiparesis, headache, or local discomfort. In addition to pulsation evident by observation and palpation, transillumination of the cyst is usually possible. Roentgenographically, a post-traumatic leptomeningeal cyst is recognized by an elongated area of lucency with scalloped and irregular margins usually located in the parietal region (Fig. 11-9). The old fracture line may still be evident at one end of the defect. The inner table of the skull is often more eroded than the outer table. Pneumoencephalography may demonstrate enlargement of that portion of the lateral ventricle beneath the cyst or a large porencephalic defect extending to the surface lesion.

Gradual, progressive enlargement is characteristic of a post-traumatic leptomeningeal cyst. For this reason, surgical correction with repair of the dural defect is indicated. Cranioplasty may be necessary for large skull lesions. The other important management principle is preventive in that children under three years of age with parietal fractures should be reexamined four to six months after the injury. Surgical correction is simplified and meningocerebral scarring diminished by early identification.

SUBDURAL HEMATOMA

Subdural hematomas and effusions were referred to in the past as pachymeningitis interna hemorrhagica (Sherwood). Subdural collections of fluid that are grossly bloody or consist of bloody fluid are called subdural hematomas and those that are xanthochromic are designated as subdural effusions. Most subdural hematomas result from preceding head trauma and most of these in the pediatric age group are identified in the first two years of life.

With dissolution of red blood cells within the clot and imbibition of fluid from adjacent compartments, a hematoma is gradually converted to an effusion, which enlarges progressively as fluid enters the mass. Subdural effusions are also well known to occur with bacterial meningitis, a complication likewise with a striking predisposition for infants.

Subdural hematomas have been divided into acute, subacute, and chronic, depending on the lapse of time from injury until identification of the lesion. Those identified within three days after injury are acute, those becoming apparent three days to three weeks after injury are subacute, and those discovered more than three weeks after trauma are classified as chronic.

Subacute or chronic subdural hematoma may occur at any time in childhood, although the peak age at which symtoms occur is two to eight months. It becomes considerably less common after the age of two years and is infrequently observed in children between 5 and 16 years of age. History of trauma is not always elicited and it is believed that trauma during birth may be the initial source of subdural bleeding in some patients.

Disruption of superficial veins entering the dural sinuses may result from excessive molding or distortion of the head during parturition, especially with precipitous deliveries or with dystocia. Accidental falls and other forms of head trauma in the infant may also be at fault. Purposefully inflicted head injury has become a widely recognized cause of subdural hematoma in the infant and should be considered in any child in whom the cause is not readily apparent.

Routine screening with chest x-ray and a long bone survey to identify unsuspected fractures of various ages is an important adjunct to other diagnostic studies. Guthkelch has suggested that bilateral subdural hematomas in physically abused children may result from violent shaking of the child, using his upper limbs as handles. The whiplash effect of this repeated acceleration-deceleration force could be sufficient to lacerate vessels passing to the dural sinus, producing subdural bleeding without fractures or other external evidence of injury. Subdural hematomas may also occur as a complication of shunting procedures in hydrocephalus (Anderson, Davidoff, and Feiring), during hemodialysis (Del Greco and Krumlovsky), subsequent to intravenous infusion of urea (Marshall and Hinman), and as a complication of pneumoencephalography (Calkins et al., Khalifeh et al.). Except for subdural hematomas that develop secondary to shunts, those mentioned have been recognized mainly in adults.

Symptoms and Signs

Symptoms and signs in the infant with chronic subdural hematomas are variable, although most patients have certain clinical findings that are at least suggestive of the diagnosis. The lesions are bilateral in 80 to 85 per cent of cases in infancy (Matson), in part accounting for the bilaterality of signs, such as hyperreflexia, or increased muscle tone. Infants with recent head trauma with bloody subdural fluid may exhibit numerous neurologic abnormalities, including convulsions, coma, or hemiparesis. These findings are often more indicative of cerebral contusion sustained at the time of injury and are not necessarily dependent upon the presence of subdural hemorrhage. Such babies may show little improvement with drainage of the acute or subacute subdural hematomas and prognosis is determined more by the degree of cerebral trauma.

The infant with chronic, bilateral subdural hematomas may slowly develop abnormal head enlargement and tenseness of the fontanel with few other abnormalities. Hydrocephalus is usually suspected in this instance until subdural taps reveal the true nature of the illness. More often, the history includes several complaints of which irritability, poor food intake, and recurrent vomiting are of cardinal importance.

Seizures, either focal or generalized, have occurred in approximately 50 per cent of patients (Matson, Till) and retardation of developmental skills is frequent in those over six months of age. Some patients exhibit papilledema, but retinal or subhyaloid hemorrhages constitute a more common finding indicative of subdural bleeding. Anemia secondary to blood loss and compounded by poor dietary intake is frequently present. Skull x-rays are not usually helpful except for the demonstration of suture spread due to increased intracranial pressure.

Diagnosis

Diagnosis of subdural hematomas in infancy is comfirmed by transfontanel or transcoronal subdural taps after the infant's head has been adequately prepared for the procedure. The hair should be shaved a distance well removed from the site of needle injection and the examination accomplished under strict aseptic conditions. A few drops or as much as 1 ml. of clear fluid with a protein content approximately twice that of normal cerebrospinal fluid may be obtained in the normal child.

Fluid in the subdural space soon after trauma may be frankly bloody. With more chronic lesions, the fluid becomes liquid but yellow or brown-tinged and has a high protein content. If abnormal fluid is obtained on the first side that is tapped, not more than 20 ml. should be removed and the opposite side then investigated. If fluid is also encountered on the other side, an equal amount is removed and the procedure terminated. Subdural fluid should be permitted to drip freely from the needle and aspiration under pressure should not be attempted.

Treatment

The initial diagnostic subdural tap, when positive, also initiates treatment, which thereafter consists of repeated taps on alternate sides on alternate days. The amount of fluid removed from each side on subsequent days is arbitrary, although many authors have expressed concern over the removal of more than 35 ml. at one time. A representative sample from each procedure should be labeled and retained for comparison with future specimens. In addition, samples of each tap should be examined for protein content and submitted for culture. In some cases, the volume of fluid obtained gradually decreases and the procedure may be discontinued after several days. The child's head circumference should be measured and recorded not less than every second day during this period.

Large subdural fluid collections are less likely to diminish with periodic taps. The source of the fluid that reaccumulates has

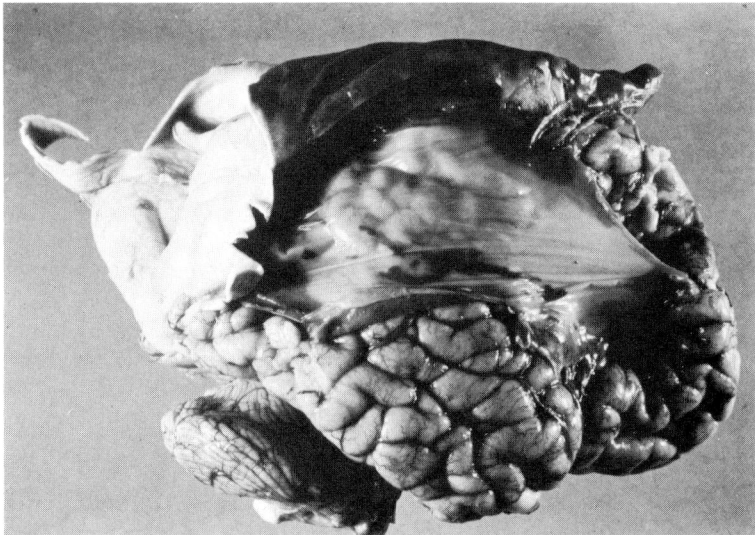

Figure 11–10. Chronic subdural hematoma. The hemorrhagic, thick outer membrane is reflected upward and the delicate, transparent inner membrane is seen on the surface of the brain. The liquid content of the hematoma between the two membranes escaped during removal of the brain. Note the indentation and atrophic changes of the brain secondary to the subdural mass.

been controversial, although studies by Rabe et al. using I^{131}-labeled albumin administered intravenously have indicated the origin of this fluid is from plasma. Persistence of significant volumes of subdural fluid after 10 to 12 subdural taps justifies consideration of more aggressive neuro-surgical therapy.

Infants with large, long-standing subdural effusions usually have inner and outer membranes of variable thickness that encapsulate the fluid collection (Fig. 11-10). The inner membrane, which lies external to the arachnoid, is usually thin and transparent, the outer membrane may be composed of a thick layer of fibrous tissue resembling the dura. In 1930, Sherwood suggested that neomembranes of this type might constrict cerebral growth and thus should be surgically excised. Matson proposed that after several subdural taps to decrease the fluid volume, a burr hole should be placed bilaterally to ascertain the presence or absence of constricting membranes. If membranes were present, a bone flap was turned and wide resection of the membranes performed. The large residual space between the atrophic brain and the dura permits reaccumulation of fluid, which usually requires further taps postoperatively until the brain has reexpanded.

Shulman and Ransohoff questioned the advisability of surgical removal of less than well developed subdural membranes and recommended subdural-pleural shunts to allow reexpansion of the brain in chronic cases. Others have preferred subdural-peritoneal shunts (Moyes et al.) or even vascular shunts in intractable situations in which fluid persists after several taps. These internal diversionary procedures eliminate the loss of protein and avoid the need for repetitive taps, which may require prolonged hospitalization. Our current level of knowledge does not allow conclusions in regard to the ideal method of treatment of patients who do not respond to repeated subdural taps. Decisions must be individualized and are largely determined by the past experience of the surgeon involved with the child's care. The general trend in recent years has been more conservative in most centers, with craniotomies being restricted to those in whom dense membranes have definitely become established.

Prognosis in infants with chronic subdural hematomas is determined by several factors, including the effect of the traumatic incident on the brain, the degree of cerebral atrophy secondary to the fluid collections, the effect of constricting membranes, and the adequacy and promptness of treatment. Yashon et al. evaluated the outcome of 92 patients at least two years after treatment and found that 21 (23 per cent) had died. Fifty-five (59 per cent) of the total series were described as doing well, seven, (8 per cent) children were in fair condition, and nine (10 per cent) were doing poorly.

Subdural Hematomas in Older Children

Chronic subdural hematomas in older infants in whom the fontanel has closed create major diagnostic problems. Vomiting and intense irritability may be the only evident clinical manifestations, with neurologic examination being necessarily restricted because of the child's lack of cooperation. Suture spread on x-ray and the lack of lateralizing signs are likely to be misinterpreted as indicative of a midline cerebellar neoplasm unless seizures or head trauma is elicited in the history. Adolescence is not entirely spared and in this age group, likewise, clinical diagnosis is difficult (Rahme and Green).

Headaches and signs of increased pressure predominate in older children with subdural hematomas. The presence of mild ataxia may tend to mislead clinical localization. The pos-

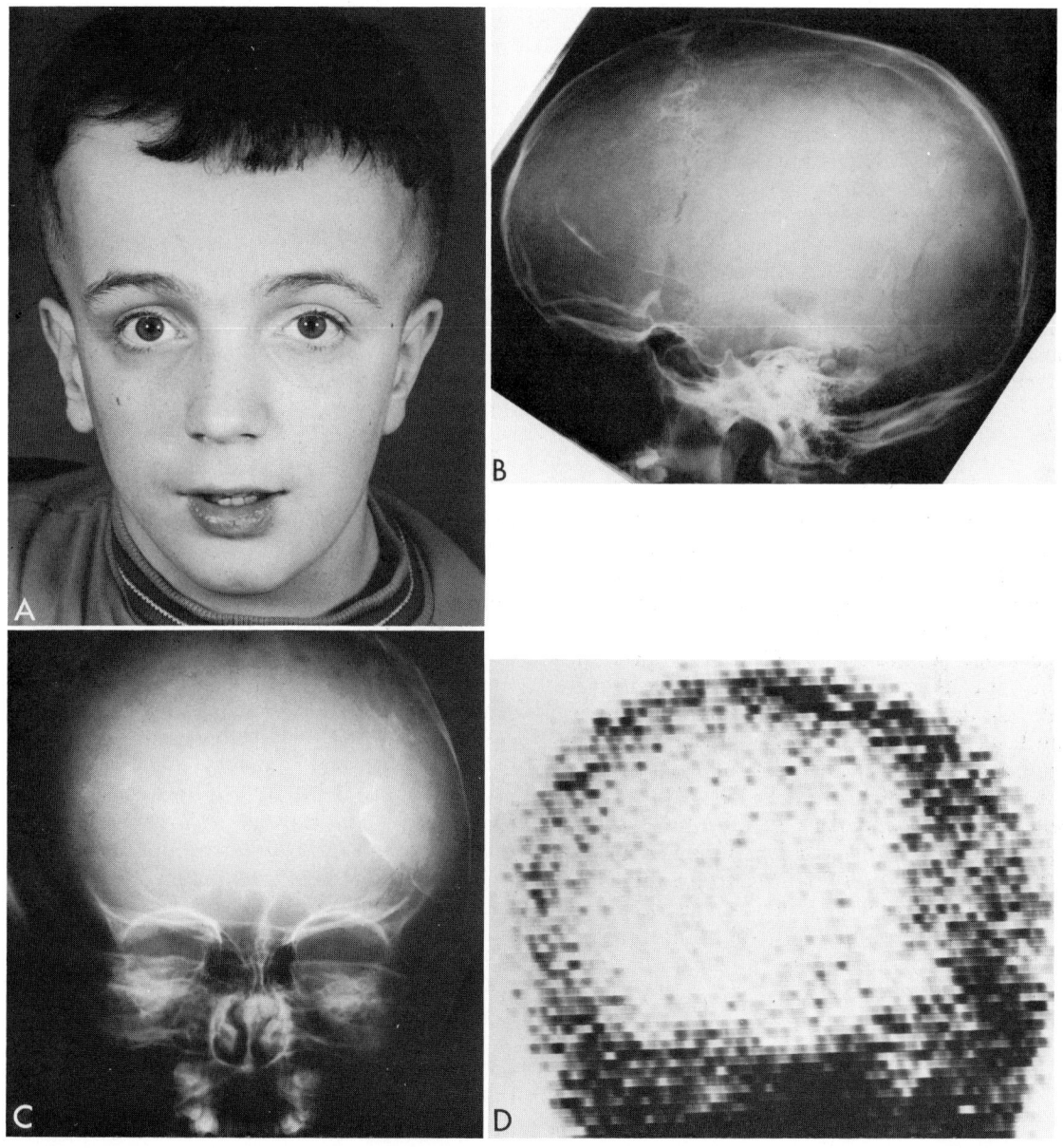

Figure 11–11. Calcified, chronic subdural hematoma. *A*, Fourteen-year-old boy with congenital communicating hydrocephalus. History of head trauma at age two years. *B*, Skull x-ray, lateral view. The head is large and mineralization is evident. *C*, Posteroanterior view. Note triangular plaque of mineralization over the convexity of the brain. *D*, Radioactive brain scan, anterior view. There is increased uptake of the radioactive material over the cerebral convexity on the side of the chronic subdural hematoma. The cause of the uptake is speculative. Abnormal brain tissue beneath the lesion may account for this finding, or dense, fibrotic membranes may be the site of accumulation of the radioactive material.

sibility of this supratentorial lesion is one reason an electroencephalogram should be performed before contrast procedures in a child suspected of having a cerebellar tumor. Although electroencephalography may be normal in patients with subdural hematomas, the finding of diffuse slow activity with marked voltage suppression over one hemisphere is strongly suggestive of this lesion. When the possibility is suspected, confirmation is best obtained by carotid angiography, which reveals the characteristic displacement of superficial vessels away from the inner table of the skull.

Chronic subdural hematomas may become densely mineralized and be identified on x-rays in older children evaluated for mental retardation, seizures, or long-standing hemiparesis (Fig. 11-11). Surgical removal of this calcified mass is not usually indicated (McLaurin and McLaurin). These lesions are not believed to progressively enlarge, although they may be associated with gradual decline of the child's intellectual skills.

EPIDURAL HEMATOMA

Hemorrhage within the epidural space is a diagnostic and therapeutic emergency unparalleled by other traumatic lesions of the nervous system, except those associated with external blood loss or airway obstruction. Although epidural hematoma is generally thought of as a lesion observed in young or middle-aged adults, it spares no age group and may even occur in the newborn (Campbell and Cohen). The lack of rarity of this traumatic lesion in infancy and childhood is evidenced by reports of 20 cases by Campbell and Cohen, 20 cases by Ingraham et al., and 16 by Hawkes and Ogle. Matson summarized 44 children under 12 years of age seen in his clinic with traumatic epidural hematomas, almost half of which occurred in patients less than two years of age.

Symptoms and Signs

The well known pattern characteristic of the adult with an acute epidural hematoma serves as a model for the findings expected in his pediatric counterpart. The child presents with certain variations from the adult picture sufficiently often that atypical features are almost considered to be the rule (Hawkes and Ogle).

The classic description in the adult includes trauma to the head with loss of consciousness from which recovery ensues within minutes. A "lucid interval" follows, during which the patient is alert with only mild complaints and without overt neurologic abnormalities. After several hours, headache becomes progressively worse in addition to recurrent vomiting, leading to drowsiness and subsequent further decline in responsiveness.

Dilatation of the pupil on the same side as the enlarging epidural clot precedes ptosis and other manifestations of an oculomotor paralysis. Rigidity, hyperreflexia, and a pathologic toe sign on the contralateral side of the body occur coincident with gradual decline in awareness and response to painful stimulation. Deep coma supervenes and decerebrate rigidity accompanies the development of bradycardia and respiratory irregularity.

Both pupils become dilated and fixed to light stimulation, and death follows within three days after onset unless the progression is interrupted by surgical intervention. Skull x-rays in such a case would reveal a linear or depressed fracture crossing the groove of the middle meningeal artery.

The events described as occurring in the older child or adult with an epidural hematoma are explained by laceration of branches of the middle meningeal artery at the time of the traumatic insult. The initial loss of consciousness is analogous to that in cerebral concussion and is not primarily related to middle meningeal artery disruption. Occasionally, contusion of the brain at the time of injury is considerable and the patient remains unconscious while the epidural clot is forming. As arterial bleeding continues, the increasing volume of blood in the epidural space results in increasing intracranial pressure and shift of the brain from the lesion, correlating with worsening of headache and decline of consciousness.

Transtentorial herniation of medial temporal lobe structures on the side of the mass compresses the third nerve, producing pupillary dilatation. Further herniation compromises brain stem function, with pressure on the cerebral peduncle causing spastic signs on the opposite side of the body. Continued brain stem distortion and subsequent midbrain and pontine hemorrhage lead to bilateral long tract signs signaling the irreversibility of the process.

The infant or child with an epidural hematoma may not sustain immediate loss of consciousness with the traumatic event and thus not exhibit the "lucid interval" characteristic of the adult. Roentgenographic evidence of skull fracture is less common in children and the rate of progression of neurologic signs may be considerably slower.

Onset of symptoms after trauma may be as short as 15 minutes or as long as seven days (Ingraham et al.). Once symptoms and neurologic signs do appear, progression may be extremely rapid or several days may pass before the child shows evidence of brain stem compression. The more gradual evolution of the process in children is seen in those in whom the source of epidural bleeding is ruptured dural veins rather than the more common lacerated meningeal artery.

Papilledema is infrequent in adults with epidural hematoma because of the rapid course. Children with more gradual progression may develop papilledema and may also show retinal hemorrhages. In addition to the foregoing variations, the infant with 100 to 400 ml. of blood within the epidural space has lost a significant percentage of his blood volume and may develop systemic shock therefrom.

Epidural hematomas are almost always unilateral and only rarely have been described as occurring in the posterior fossa (Gage). As in most types of head injuries in children, males are affected more often than females. Most have been identified in previously normal children but hemophilia and other coagulation disorders may predispose one to this and other forms of intracranial hemorrhage (Silverstein). Accidental falls are the usual form of injury leading to an epidural hemorrhage. Any type of head trauma may be at fault, including athletic injuries, motor vehicle accidents, and blows purposefully inflicted to the child's head.

Diagnosis

Diagnosis of this condition rests largely on awareness of the possibility following even relatively mild head trauma, and evidence of progressive stupor plus the characteristic neurologic signs. It should be suspected in any child with a skull fracture that traverses the path of the middle meningeal artery or who has traumatic diastasis of the lambdoidal suture. Normal skull x-rays however, do not eliminate the possibility of an epidural hematoma.

In certain instances, the seriousness of the child's condition warrants immediate transport to the operating room even before skull films are obtained. The necessity for prompt diagnosis and emergency surgical treatment usually precludes the performance of other diagnostic studies. A reasonable probability of an acute epidural hematoma is a contraindication to lumbar puncture because of the danger of the procedure with impending tentorial herniation. Furthermore, it is unlikely that any useful information can be obtained from spinal fluid analysis that will alter management of the child.

Carotid angiography is neither desirable or needed in most cases and unnecessarily delays specific surgical management. In the unusual situation in which the clinical picture varies markedly from the expected pattern and when the child's condition is not in jeopardy, angiography may be indicated to establish the diagnosis and exclude other possible considerations.

One cannot depend on transfontanel or suture needle taps in the infant to exclude an epidural hemorrhage because partially clotted arterial blood may not escape, even through a large bore needle. Epidural clots in the subtemporal region or those in the posterior parietal area would not be accessible by this approach. In addition, even if needle drainage could be accomplished, it would not be adequate therapy because the source of continued bleeding would probably still exist.

Treatment

An acute epidural hematoma is surgically removed as rapidly as possible after diagnosis is made. It is imperative to present children with this lesion to the neurosurgeon before a state of coma or decerebration has been reached if death or permanent sequelae are to be avoided. When transportation over many miles is necessary for definitive surgical care, air travel should be considered. Mannitol and other hypertonic agents are best avoided preoperatively because of the potential ability to enhance bleeding. Acute blood loss in a child with an epidural hemorrhage may result in severe anemia or even shock and usually requires administration of blood, preferably begun before the induction of anesthesia. Diagnosis of an epidural hematoma is confirmed by placement of burr holes and the lesion is evacuated completely by craniotomy. Bleeding vessels must then be identified and ligated.

Complete recovery is expected if the epidural hematoma is removed before coma had developed or signs of brain stem compression have become severe. The mortality rate increases precipitously when these signs have developed before the surgical procedure is accomplished. In some children, residual deficits may include a hemiparesis, behavioral abnormalities, or seizures. Patients with cerebral contusion or laceration from the trauma responsible for the epidural hemorrhage are more likely to have lasting neurologic defects.

"BATTERED CHILD SYNDROME"

In 1962, Kempe et al. introduced the term "battered child syndrome" in reference to infants and children who sustain physical injury from purposeful abuse by others in their environment. With the passage of time and the accumulation of further observations, the term has been expanded to include children abused not only by physical attack, but also those willfully deprived nutritionally and emotionally (Kempe). The incidence of significant physical trauma wantonly inflicted upon small children is unknown. Kempe has estimated that approximately 25 per cent of all fractures in children under two years of age originate in this fashion.

In any series of physically abused children, varying degrees of craniocerebral trauma are a prominent feature. Skull fractures may occur because of blows to the child's head without apparent cerebral injury, or severe contusion or laceration of the brain may lead to death or permanent sequelae (Fig. 11-12). Subarachnoid hemorrhage, subdural hematomas, or vertebral and spinal cord injuries (Swischuk) may follow impulsive or premeditated violence, at times inflicted by astonishing methods.

The "battered child syndrome" should be considered in any child with subdural hematomas or other evidence of head trauma in whom the cause is not reasonably well established. Fresh retinal or subhyaloid hemorrhages are not specific for this form of injury, but in infancy can be accepted as strong presumptive evidence of recently acquired

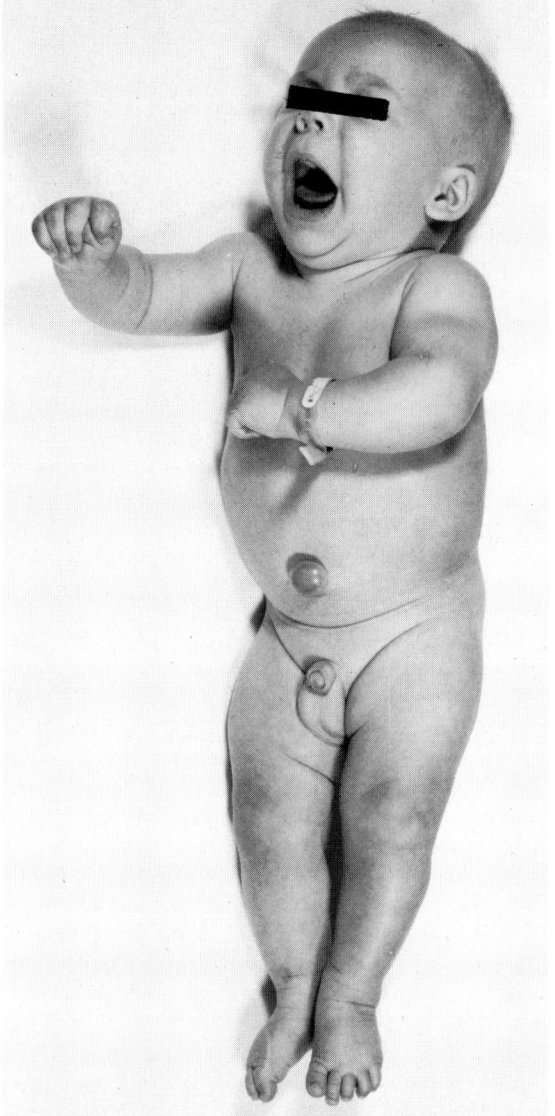

Figure 11-12. "Battered child syndrome." Three-month-old infant "suddenly became limp" two weeks before hospital admission. The patient was seen by a local physician who noted facial bruises. Child was then described as well until the morning of admission when he again "suddenly became limp." On examination, he was unresponsive and had recurrent convulsions. Skull x-rays revealed that sutures were spread and the cerebrospinal fluid was uniformly bloody. Fresh blood was present in subdural spaces bilaterally. Illustration shows child six weeks after admission. All four limbs are markedly spastic and developmental retardation is profound. Sequelae of traumatic encephalopathy is undoubtedly severe and permanent.

head trauma. Cutaneous lesions on other parts of the body may also be present, serving either as clues to or proof of needless but purposeful physical abuse (Fig. 11-13). Mul-

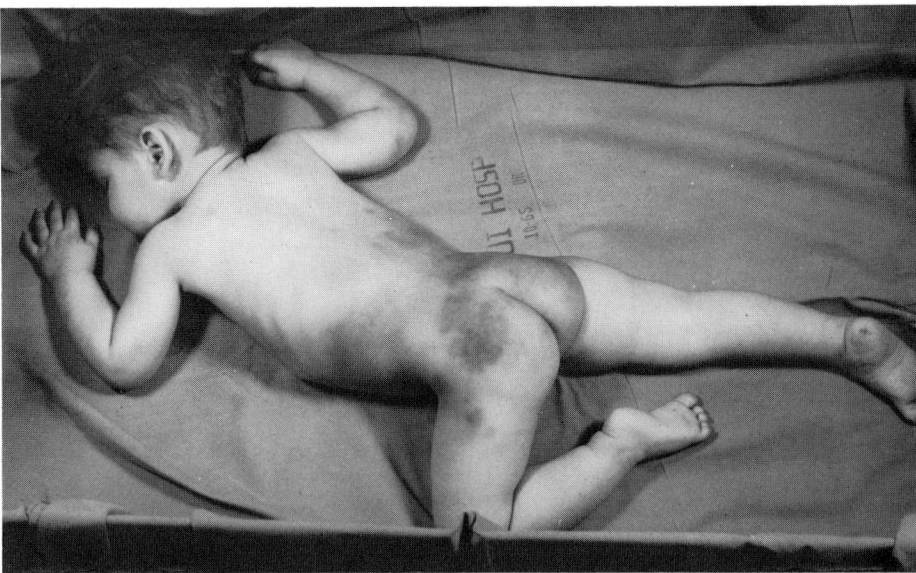

Figure 11–13. "Battered child syndrome." Fifteen-month-old child who cried and then initiated a breath-holding episode. As a reprimand for this behavior, he was "spanked vigorously." Soon thereafter, he allegedly fell while in a walker. On hospital admission, he was unresponsive to painful stimuli and exhibited a left hemiparesis in addition to retinal hemorrhages. The cerebrospinal fluid was grossly bloody. The child died two days after admission; cerebral contusions and edema were present at necropsy.

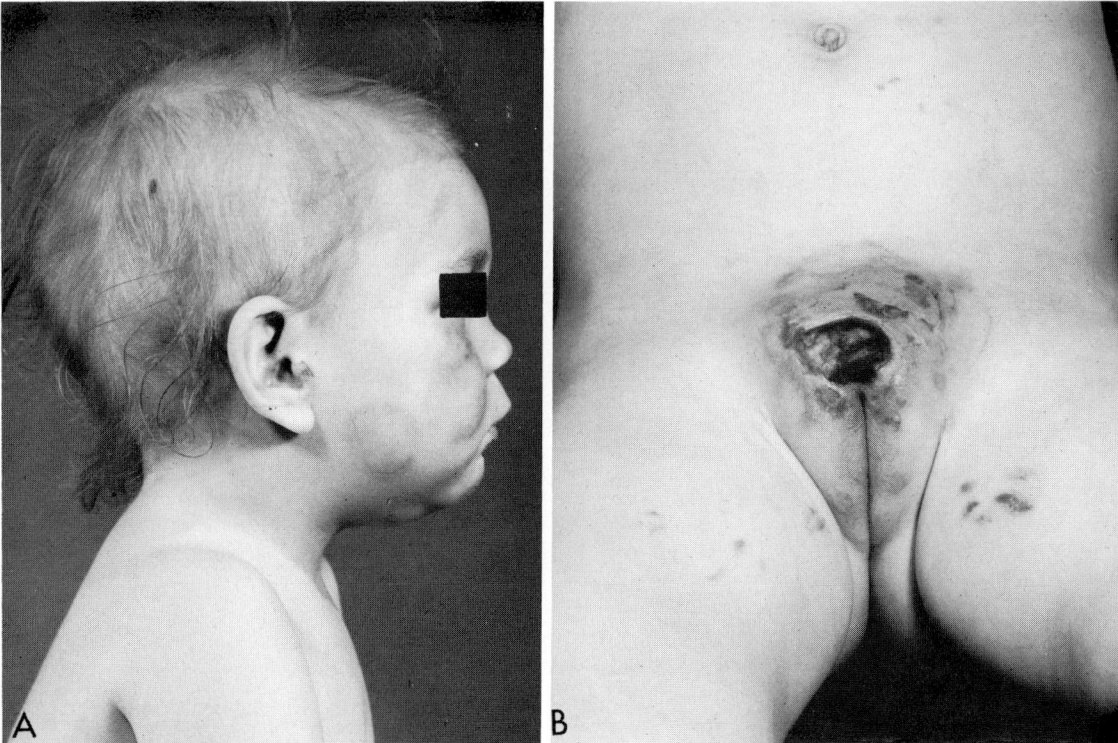

Figure 11–14. Physically abused child with variety of cutaneous lesions. *A*, Circular lesion over the angle of the mandible was inflicted by the bite of an adult attacker. *B*, Cause of denudation of the area shown did not become evident.

tiple bruises of different ages, bite marks on the skin, cigarette burns, or whip marks produced by a belt or rope may be observed (Fig. 11-14).

Discrepancies and inconsistencies in the explanation of the events surrounding the head injury must also be viewed as possible evidence of the "battered child syndrome." Bilateral subdural hematomas and bruises on the buttocks of a six-month-old child attributed to a fall from a bed to a carpeted floor should be viewed suspiciously. Severe head injury with retinal hemorrhages allegedly resulting from blows from a 15-month-old sibling, himself barely able to walk, is an obvious improbability. The denial of trauma in the infant, previously well, who suddenly became "limp" and unresponsive and who has skull fractures and subarachnoid bleeding is an additional implausible situation. Significant delay in seeking medical advice after head injury to an infant who is undoubtedly ill is also suggestive of physical abuse.

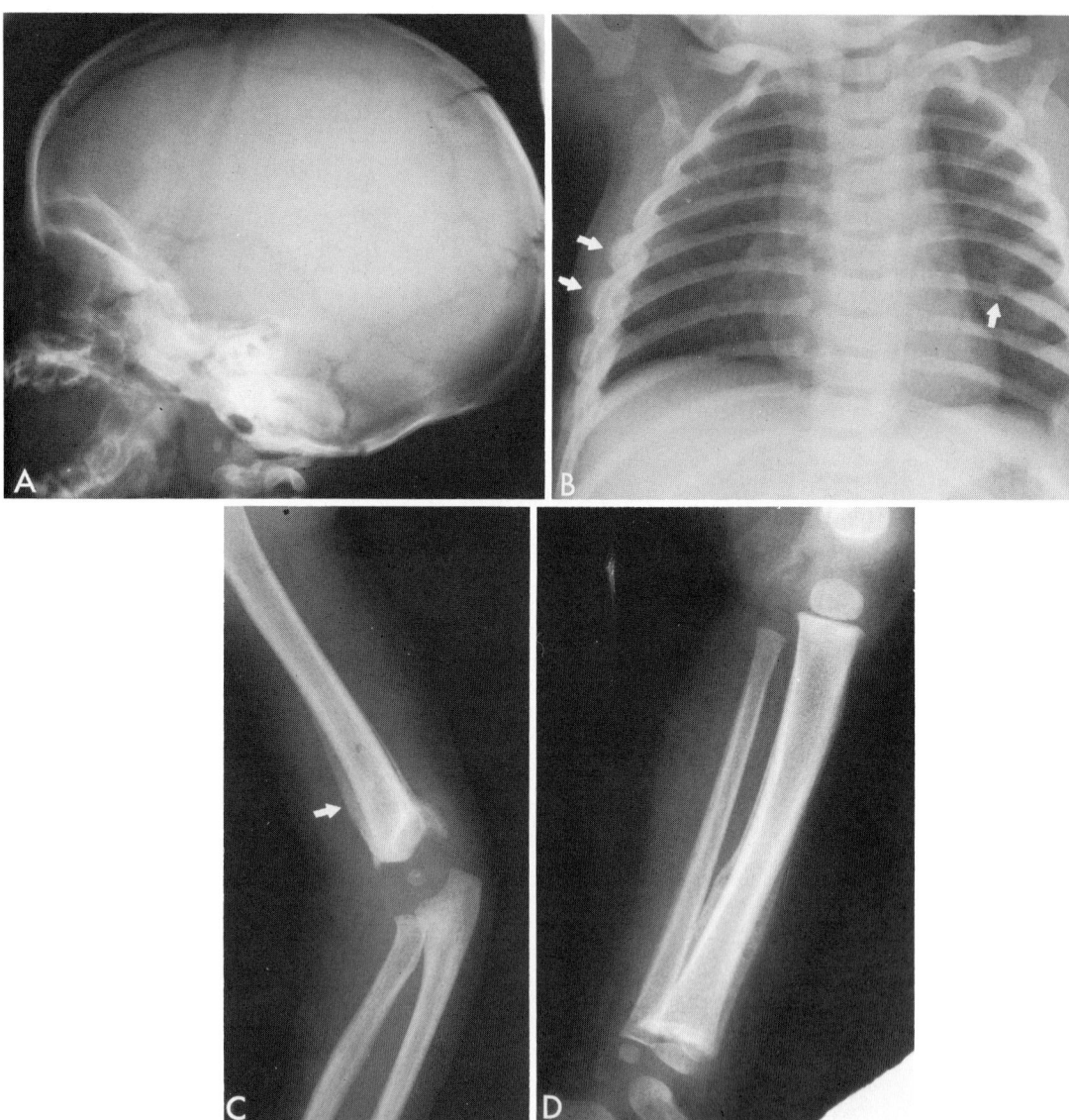

Figure 11-15. The x-ray findings in four children purposefully physically abused. *A*, Skull film, lateral view, showing multiple fractures. *B*, Chest x-ray, revealing rib fractures of various ages. Fracture on patient's left side (arrow) is recent, whereas those on the right side are older as indicated by the callous formation. *C*, Torsion injury with old fracture of metaphysis of the humerus. Note calcium deposition in subperiosteal hemorrhage cloaking the distal humerus (arrow). *D*, New-bone formation surrounding the distal tibia, indicative of an old metaphyseal fracture with subperiosteal bleeding.

Roentgenographic examination plays an important role in the identification of battered children in that it provides a means of recognition of injuries that otherwise remain silent (Fig. 11-15). The radiologic hallmark of this syndrome is the presence of multiple, traumatic skeletal lesions of different ages. Rib fractures are particularly common and may be recent with no evidence of healing or may be virtually healed but dated because of marked callous formation. Long bone fractures may be of any type and may be single or multiple. The most characteristic evidence of limb trauma on x-ray is the metaphyseal injury associated with subperiosteal hemorrhage, causing periosteal elevation and followed by newbone formation. Such injuries are usually produced by a torsion force on the child's extremity with the attacker clenching the child's wrist or forearm and twisting it forceably.

Physical attacks on small children may occur from a variety of persons, although the most common include the parents, step-parents, babysitters, a separated mother's boyfriend, and older siblings. Only one child among several siblings may be selectively subjected to abuse, or the history may include unexplained or allegedly explained traumatic deaths in siblings during the infant period.

Certain types of children seem predisposed to battering, including the step-child, the child who is the result of an undesired or illegitimate pregnancy, the low birth weight infant, and the hyperkinetic and destructive child. Not uncommonly, the mother who batters her child was herself the recipient of similar insults in her childhood years. No particular personality types are consistently involved and no socioeconomic group is excluded. On interviewing battering parents one is often impressed by their genuine concern for their injured child's welfare and their sense of responsibility in community activities.

After the immediate medical needs of the battered child have been met, the physician's primary obligations are to recognize this syndrome and to report to the appropriately designated authorities. Laws have been established in all states (Helfer and Kempe), that facilitate such reports and also provide protection for the reporting physician. Recognition and reporting are the prerequisites for the prevention of further injury, or perhaps death, of the involved child as well as other siblings. It is also the stepping stone to the initiation of appropriate treatment of the person or persons responsible for the child's injuries.

REFERENCES

Alexander, E., Jr., and Davis, C. H., Jr.,: Intra-uterine fracture of the infant's skull. *J. Neurosurg.*, **30**:446–454, 1969.

Anderson, F. M.: Subdural hematoma, a complication of operation for hydrocephalus. *Pediatrics.*, **10**:11–18, 1952.

Brink, J. D., Garrett, A. L. Hale, W., Woo-Sam, J., and Nickel, V. L.: Recovery of motor and intellectual function in children sustaining severe head injuries. *Develop. Med. Child Neurol.*, **12**:565–571, 1970.

Burry, V. F., and Hellerstein, S.: Septicemia and sub-periosteal cephalhematomas. *J. Pediat.*, **69**:1122–1135, 1966.

Calkins, R. A., Van Allen, M. W., and Sahs, A. L.: Subdural hematoma following pneumoencephalography. *J. Neurosurg.*, **27**:56–59, 1967.

Campbell, J. B., and Cohen, J.: Epidural hemorrhage and the skull of children. *Surg. Gynec. Obstet.*, **92**:257–280, 1951.

Carter, L. P., and Pittman, H. W.: Posterior fossa subdural hematoma of the newborn. *J. Neurosurg.*, **34**:423–426, 1971.

Chessells, J. M., and Wigglesworth, J. S.: Coagulation studies in severe birth asphyxia. *Arch. Dis. Childh.*, **46**:253–256, 1971.

Cohen, S. M., Miller, B. W., and Orris, H. W.: Meningitis complicating cephalhematoma. *J. Pediat.*, **30**:327–329, 1947.

Crompton, M. R.: Brain stem lesions due to closed head injuries. *Lancet*, **1**:669–673, 1971.

Davidoff, L. M., and Feiring, E. H.: Subdural hematoma occurring in surgically treated hydrocephalic children. With a note on a method of handling persistent accumulations. *J. Neurosurg.*, **10**:557–563, 1953.

Del Greco, F., and Krumlovsky, F.: Subdural hematoma in the course of hemodialysis. *Lancet*, **2**:1009–1010, 1969.

Dillon, H., and Leopold, R. L.: Children and the post-concussion syndrome. *J.A.M.A.*, **175**:86–92, 1961.

Epstein, J. A., Epstein, B. S., and Small, M.: Subepicranial hydroma. A complication of head injuries in infants and children. *J. Pediat.*, **59**:562–566, 1961.

Frantzen, E., Jacobsen, H. H., and Therkelsen, J.: Cerebral artery occlusions in children due to trauma to the head and neck. *Neurology*, **11**:695–700, 1961.

Gage, E. L.: Recurrent extradural cerebellar hematoma. *Amer. J. Dis. Child.*, **84**:82–83, 1952.

Gilles, F. H., and Shillito, J., Jr.: Infantile hydrocephalus: Retrocerebellar subdural hematoma. *J. Pediat.*, **76**:529–537, 1970.

Griffith, J. F., and Dodge, P. R.: Transient blindness following head injury in children. *New. Eng. J. Med.*, **278**:648–651, 1968.

Gruber, F. H.: Post-traumatic leptomeningeal cysts. *Amer. J. Roentgen.*, **105**:305–307, 1969.

Guthkelch, A. N.: Infantile subdural haematoma and its relationship to whiplash injuries. *Brit. Med. J.*, **2**:430–431, 1971.

Hawkes, C. D., and Ogle, W. S.: Atypical features of epidural hematoma in infants, children, and adolescents. J. Neurosurg., **19**:971–980, 1962.

Helfer, R. W., and Kempe, C. H.: *The Battered Child.* Chicago, The University of Chicago Press, 1968.

Hjern, B., and Nylander T.: Acute head injuries in children. *Acta Pediat.*, Suppl., **152**:5–37, 1964.

Ingraham, F. C., Campbell, J. B., and Cohen, J.: Extradural hematoma in infancy and childhood. *J.A.M.A.*, **140**:1010–1013, 1949.

Kahn, R. J., and Daywitt, A. L.: Traumatic pneumocephalus. *Amer. J. Roentgen.*, **90**:1171–1175, 1963.

Kempe, C. H.: Pediatric implications of the battered baby syndrome. *Arch. Dis. Childh.*, **46**:28–37, 1971.

Kempe, C. H., Silverman, F. N., Steele, B. F., Droegemueller, W., and Silver, H. K.: The battered child syndrome. *J.A.M.A.*, **181**:17–24, 1962.

Kendall, N., and Woloshin, H.: Cephalhematoma associated with fracture of the skull. *J. Pediat.*, **41**:125–132, 1952.

Khalifeh, R. R., Van Allen, M. W., and Sahs, A. L.: Subdural hematoma following pneumoencephalography in an adult. *Neurology*, **14**:77–80, 1964.

Lee, Y., and Berg, R. B.: Cephalhematoma infected with *Bacteroides. Amer. J. Dis. Child.*, **121**:77–78, 1971.

Lende, R. A., and Erickson, T. C.: Growing skull fractures of childhood. *J. Neurosurg.*, **18**:479–489, 1961.

Levy, H. L., O'Conner, J. F., and Ingall, D.: Bacteremia, infected cephalhematoma, and osteomyelitis of the skull in the newborn. *Amer. J. Dis. Child.*, **114**:649–651, 1967.

Lewin, W.: Severe head injuries. *Proc. Roy. Soc. Med.*, **60**:1208–1212, 1967.

Lindenberg, R., and Freytag, E.: Morphology of brain lesions from blunt trauma in early infancy. *Arch. Path.*, **87**:298–305, 1969.

Lourie, H., and Berne, A. S.: A contribution on the etiology and pathogenesis of congenital communicating hydrocephalus. *Neurology*, **15**:815–822, 1965.

Luckett, W. H.: Air in ventricles of brain, following fracture of skull. *Surg. Gynec. Obstet.*, **17**:237–240, 1913.

Marshall, S., and Hinman, F., Jr.: Subdural hematoma following administration of urea for diagnosis of hydrocephalus. *J.A.M.A.*, **182**:813–814, 1962.

Matson, D. D.: *Neurosurgery of Infancy and Childhood.* Springfield, Ill., Charles C Thomas, 1969.

McLaurin, R. L., and McLaurin, K. S.: Calcified subdural hematomas in childhood. *J. Neurosurg.*, **24**:648–655, 1966.

Mealey, J., Jr.: *Pediatric Head Injuries.* Springfield, Ill., Charles C Thomas, 1968.

Melchior, J.: The incidence of head injuries in children. *Acta Pediat.*, **50**:47–50, 1961.

Miller, J. D., and Jennett, W. B.: Complications of depressed skull fracture. *Lancet*, **2**: 991–995, 1968.

Moyes, P. D., Thompson, G. B., and Cluff, J. W.: Subdural peritoneal shunts in the treatment of subdural effusions in infants. *J. Neurosurg.*, **23**:584–587, 1965.

Murtagh, F., and Baird, R. M.: Circumscribed intraventricular hematoma in infants. *J. Pediat.*, **59**:351–355, 1961.

Pitner, S. E.: Carotid thrombosis due to intraoral trauma. *New Eng. J. Med.*, **274**:764–767, 1966.

Rabe, E. F.: Subdural effusions in infants. *Ped. Clin. N. Amer.*, **14**:831–850, 1967.

Rabe, E. F., Flynn, R. E., and Dodge, P. R.: Subdural collections of fluid in infants and children. *Neurology*, **18**:559–570, 1968.

Rahme, E. S., and Green, D.: Chronic subdural hematoma in adolescence and early adulthood. *J.A.M.A.*, **176**:424–426, 1961.

Rausen, A. R., and Diamond, L. K.: Enclosed hemorrhage and neonatal jaundice. *Amer. J. Dis. Child.*, **101**:164–169, 1961.

Raynor, R., and Parsa, M.: Nonsurgical elevation of depressed skull fracture in an infant. *J. Pediat.*, **72**:262–264, 1968.

Robinson, R. J., and Rossiter, M. A.: Massive subaponeurotic hemorrhage in babies of African origin. *Arch. Dis. Childh.*, **43**:684–687, 1968.

Schrager, G. O.: Elevation of depressed skull fracture with a breast pump. *J. Pediat.*, **77**:300–301, 1970.

Sherwood, D.: Chronic subdural hematoma in infants. *Amer. J. Dis. Child.*, **39**:980–1021, 1930.

Shulman, K., and Ransohoff, J.: Subdural hematoma in children. The fate of retained membranes. *J. Neurosurg.*, **18**:175–181, 1961.

Silverstein, A.: Intracranial bleeding in hemophilia. *Arch. Neurol.*, **3**:141–157, 1960.

Strich, S. J.: Shearing of nerve fibres as a cause of brain damage due to head injury. *Lancet*, **2**:443–448, 1961.

Swischuk, L. E.: Spine and spinal cord trauma in the battered child syndrome. *Radiology*, **92**:733–738, 1969.

Taveras, J. M., and Ransohoff, J.: Leptomeningeal cyst of brain following trauma with erosion of skull. *J. Neurosurg.*, **10**:233–241, 1953.

Tenner, M. S., and Stein, B. M.: Cerebral herniation in the growing fracture of the skull. *Radiology*, **94**:351–355, 1970.

Till, K.: Subdural haematoma and effusion in infancy. *Brit. Med. J.*, **3**:400–402, 1968.

Towbin, A.: Central nervous system damage in the human fetus and newborn infant. *Amer. J. Dis. Child.*, **119**:529–542, 1970.

Turner, J. S.: Pneumocephalus with facial fractures. *Laryngoscope*, **78**:713–727, 1968.

Vas, C. J., and Winn, J. M.: Growing skull fractures. *Develop. Med. Child. Neurol.*, **8**:735–740, 1966.

Yashon, D., Jane, J. A., White, R. J., and Sugar, O.: Traumatic subdural hematoma in infancy. *Arch. Neurol.*, **18**:370–377, 1968.

Chapter Twelve

BRAIN ABSCESS

Abscess formation within the parenchyma of the brain may be solitary or multiple and may not be associated with an extracranial suppurative focus. Brain abscesses are less often identified during infancy than in older children. In the infant, the lesion may become enormous before it is recognized, more often results from gram-negative bacilli, and is frequently followed by hydrocephalus in those who survive (Hoffman et al.). In older children, conditions that predispose to the development of brain abscess include chronic otitis or mastoiditis, suppurative sinusitis, pulmonary infection, and cyanotic congenital heart disease. Suppurative skin lesions and dental extractions are other potential sources of sepsis that may lead to the formation of a brain abscess. Cerebellar abscess may develop secondary to infection within a dermoid cyst at the termination of a congenital dermal sinus in the posterior fossa.

In a significant percentage of cases, an unsuspected brain abscess is identified at surgery in a child believed to have a neoplasm without an obvious antecedent suppurative illness. Penetrating cranial trauma also may be the source of entry of bacteria leading to abscess within the brain. Such injuries in children may be deceptively subtle with evidence of penetration of the skull by a foreign body not being initially apparent. Small missiles, such as fragments of wire, may be propelled by power machinery, or an accidental fall on a sharpened pencil may result in transmission of foreign material into the brain leading to abscess formation (Horner et al.). Symptoms of intracranial suppuration may not appear for months or years after the injury.

Congenital Heart Disease and Brain Abscess

Congenital heart disease, especially of the cyanotic type, has become one of the most important factors predisposing the child to the development of cerebral abscess (Matson and Salam, Raimondi et al. Calkins and Bell (Fig. 12-1) In children under two years of age with congenital heart disease, acquired neurologic dysfunction is more often due to vascular occlusive disease; in those over two years of age, abscess must be considered in any cyanotic child who develops headaches, seizures, or other focal neurologic signs.

Tetralogy of Fallot is the most common associated cardiac lesion, although brain abscess may develop in any condition with a right to left intracardiac shunt or with a pulmonary arteriovenous fistula (Stern and Naffziger). Venous to arterial shunts within the heart allow recirculation of poorly oxygenated venous blood through the systemic circulation, bypassing the filtering effects of the lungs. This exposes the brain to bacteria ordinarily present in the circulation only briefly, as in transient bacteremia. Polycythemia secondary to arterial desaturation increases blood viscosity, leading to a reduction in the rate of cerebral blood flow. These factors are important in the pathogenesis of brain abscess formation in children with cyanotic heart disease, although previous tissue damage from hypoxia may also be necessary.

Groff's experiments in animals revealed that bacteremia does not result in the formation of an abscess unless preceding brain infarction has occurred. In view of the disturbed hemodynamics and alterations in

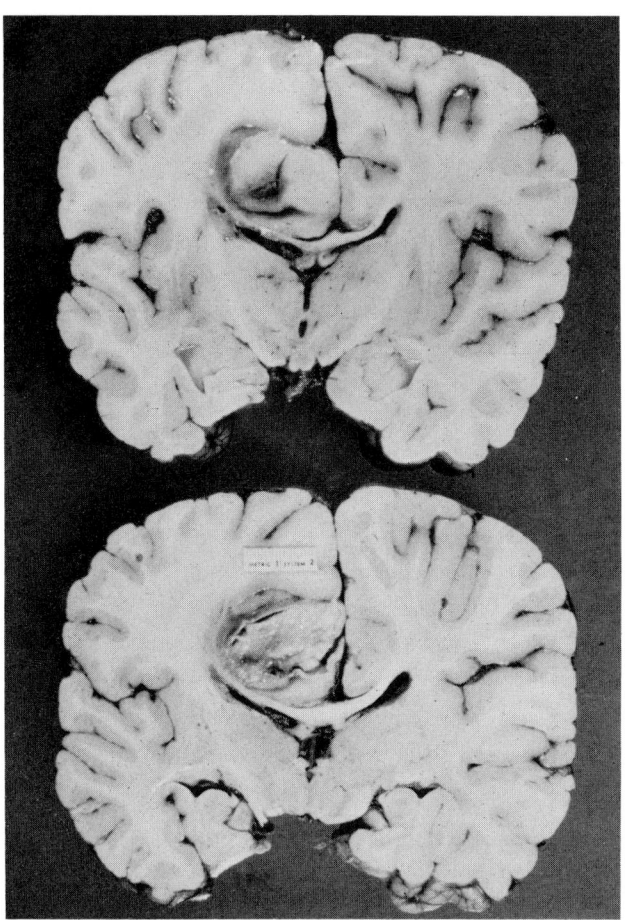

Figure 12-1. Parietal lobe (left) abscess in a nine-year-old boy with cyanotic congenital heart disease. His first symptoms of the cerebral abscess occurred two days before hospital admission and consisted of recurrent focal motor seizures involving his right leg and were followed by flaccid weakness of the same extremity. Severe, generalized headache developed in addition to repeated episodes of vomiting.

The child was afebrile when admitted to the hospital. White blood cell count and erythrocyte sedimentation rate were normal. On the fourth day of hospitalization, he became lethargic and soon thereafter developed a decerebrate posture and respiratory arrest. Postmortem examination revealed that the abscess in the cingulate gyrus had ruptured through the corpus callosum into the adjacent lateral ventricle.

blood flow in children with cyanotic heart disease, ample opportunities exist for hypoxic or ischemic cerebral insults to occur. Bacterial endocarditis is usually not present in those found to have brain abscesses; preceding infections, including otherwise insignificant bacteremia, are frequently not identified. Surgical procedures, including the Potts and Blalock anastomoses, do not eliminate the possibility of the subsequent development of a brain abscess (Wishingrad et al., Clark and Clarke). These shunt procedures increase pulmonary blood flow, but persistence of the ventricular defect permits venous contamination of systemic blood.

Pathological Considerations

Abscesses may be located in various positions within the cerebrum or cerebellum. Those associated with cyanotic heart disease are usually solitary and are generally in the frontal, temporal or parietal lobe. Chronic suppurative otitis or mastoiditis results in either temporal lobe or cerebellar hemisphere suppuration; abscess secondary to sinusitis is more commonly frontal.

Tarkkanen reported 99 cases of otogenic brain abscesses, 78 per cent of which were secondary to chronic otitis and 22 per cent resulted from acute otitis media. Children were much less often affected with this complication than adults, and males comprised 71 per cent of cases. Cerebral abscess occurred in 54 of the 99 cases, almost all being within the temporal lobe. In 42 patients, the abscess was within the cerebellum, and three patients harbored both cerebral and cerebellar lesions. The mortality rate in this series was 66 per cent; however, it included cases seen as early as 1930.

Abscesses within the brain stem or basal nuclei and thalamus are rare. Brain abscesses in infants with staphylococcal sepsis or with infected meningomyelocoeles and secondary ventriculitis are more often multiple than solitary.

Streptococci, staphylococci, and pneumococci are the organisms most frequently recovered from cerebral abscesses (Raimondi et al., Wright and Ballantine, Tarkkanen). Many types of anaerobic bacteria have been identified in brain abscesses, indicating the need for both aerobic and anaerobic cultures of all abscess material (Heineman and Braude). Gram-negative bacilli are more often found in infants with brain abscess and, with all age groups, a significant percentage result in no bacterial growth on culture. Multiple cerebral microabscesses may occur with fungal infections including those due to Candida (Roessman and Friede) and Aspergillus (Hughes).

Nocardia asteroides is a rare but widely recognized cause of brain abscess, especially in patients who are debilitated or taking corticosteroids or cytotoxic agents (Rankin and Javid, Shuster et al.). The portal of entry of this organism is the lung in most cases, with hematogenous dissemination resulting in potential abscess formation in multiple organs, including the brain. Nocardial brain abscesses may be either solitary or multiple (Fig. 12-2). Lack of encapsulation is a characteristic feature of cerebral abscess due to this organism.

The earliest stage of development of a cerebral abscess consists of a poorly demarcated area of septic cerebritis with softening, hyperemia, and infiltration of inflammatory cells. Necrotic changes occur centrally, followed by liquifaction and the subsequent formation of purulent material comprising the abscess (Fig. 12-3). Fibroblastic activity at the circumference of the abscess, in addition to gliosis, eventually results in encapsulation of the lesion. In most instances, profound edema of white matter is present in the region of a brain abscess and may extend several centimeters from its periphery. Schurr has stated that a minimum of four weeks is required for encapsulation following the initial state of cerebritis.

Symptoms and Signs

Symptoms and signs produced by a brain abscess depend on several factors, including the age of the child, the location and size of the lesion, whether it is single or multiple, and the degree of associated brain swelling. During the cerebritis stage, headache, fever, lethargy, or seizures may occur, but more often, no clinical evidence of illness is present until the process manifests itself as a mass lesion. During infancy, abnormal head enlargement, vomiting, and seizures are usual manifestations of a brain abscess and may readily be confused with other space-occupying lesions, including subdural effusions and neoplasm.

The older child with a cerebral abscess usually exhibits a progressively worsening clinical course with symptoms and signs being those of focal neurologic dysfunction in conjunction with manifestations of increased intracranial pressure. Headaches, vomiting, and drowsiness are often accompanied by a hemiparesis and a homonymous hemianopsia if the optic radiations are involved. Papilledema is present in most cases and abducens weakness with diplopia frequently develops as a false localizing sign.

Posterior frontal or anterior parietal lobe abscesses often cause focal motor or sensory seizures on the opposite side, but generalized convulsions may also be described. An abscess within the cerebellar hemisphere results in papilledema and other signs of increased pressure in addition to coordination disturb-

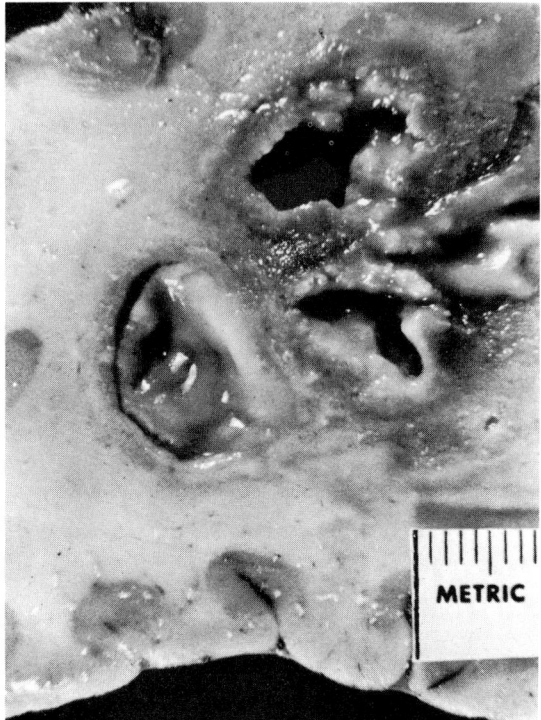

Figure 12-2. Frontal lobe abscess due to *Nocardia asteroides*. The abscess is multiloculated and poorly encapsulated. Granulomatous changes of brain tissue surrounding the cavitary lesions are evident.

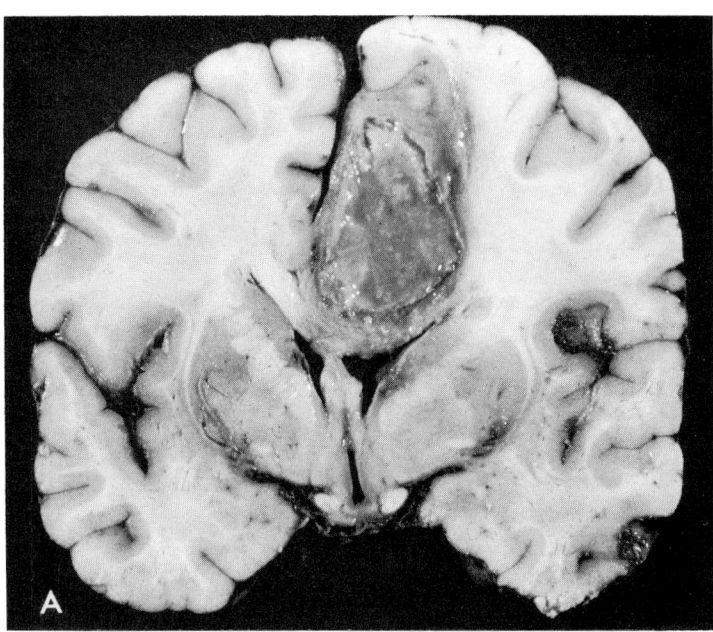
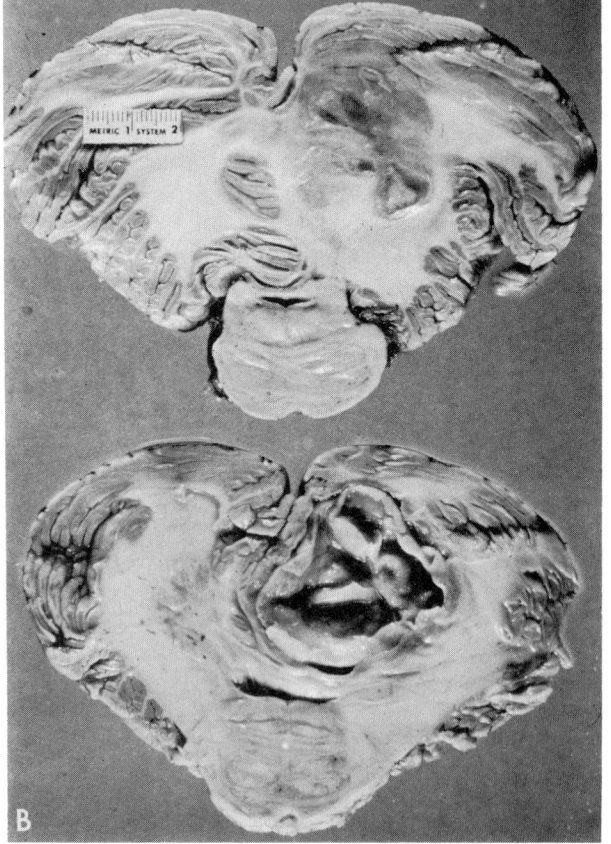

Figure 12-3. A, Cerebral abscess. The lesion is located in the parasagittal region of the frontal lobe and has caused inflammatory softening of the corpus callosum. Purulent material is surrounded by a poorly developed fibrotic capsule. B, Cerebellar abscess. The section at the top shows softening and necrotic changes while that at the bottom reveals multilocular cavities containing purulent material and surrounded by a poorly formed capsule.

ances. The gait is usually ataxic and dysmetria is present in the limbs on the homolateral side. Horizontal nystagmus, more marked on gaze to the same side as the lesion, is further evidence of posterior fossa localization.

Sudden deterioration of the clinical status of patients with cerebral or cerebellar abscesses generally indicates either internal herniation of the medial temporal lobe or cerebellar tonsils, or spontaneous rupture of the abscess with extension of pus into the ventricular system. Although not invariably fatal, these complications markedly worsen the outlook for the child and indicate the desirability of prompt diagnosis and treatment before such catastrophes have occurred.

Another event that may prove fatal in the patient with a cerebral abscess is massive hemorrhage into the lesion. This may occur spontaneously or in the child with thrombocytopenia or other bleeding disorders. It has also been described as a complication of inappropriate anticoagulation therapy for presumed cerebrovascular occlusive disease (Abbott and Stern).

Laboratory and Ancillary Studies

Fever and blood leukocytosis are suggestive of an infectious process when present; however, absence of these factors in no way excludes the possibility of a brain abscess. Of 19 patients reported by Raimondi et al., only six had temperature elevation exceeding 101° F. The white blood cell count, likewise, is variable and cannot be considered a consistently reliable indicator of a suppurative lesion in the brain. Marked elevation of the total white count with an increased number of immature forms is more often seen when meningitis is present in conjunction with an abscess.

The cerebrospinal fluid is usually clear, colorless, and without organisms unless rupture of the lesion has produced meningitis. The spinal fluid pressure is almost always elevated and the protein content is modestly elevated. The cell count may be normal, although 10 to 100 cells per cubic millimeter is more characteristic. The cellular response may be either primarily lymphocytic or a combination of lymphocytes and polymorphonuclear leukocytes. As a generalization, a more chronic and encapsulated abscess is associated with a lymphocytic pleocytosis, whereas more acute lesions exhibit a higher percentage of polymorphonuclear cells in the spinal fluid.

Among 23 patients with intracranial abscesses described by Wright and Ballatine, three had completely normal findings on lumbar puncture. A spinal fluid examination may be of diagnostic assistance; however, when an abscess is strongly suspected and meningitis can be excluded with reasonable certainty from the clinical signs, spinal tap is best avoided because of the potential hazard. Such patients are in urgent need of contrast procedures and the results of the lumbar puncture rarely alter the method of further investigation.

Roentgenograms of the skull in children with brain abscesses are of little definitive help except for evidence of increased pressure manifested by suture spread. An unusual finding on skull x-ray in children with cerebral abscesses is the presence of gas within the abscess cavity (Norrell and Howieson). Most such cases have followed penetrating head wounds with the abscess due to a gas-forming bacillus. Differentiation of a gas-containing abscess from traumatic pneumocephalus may be difficult although the clinical findings of the two lesions are usually dissimilar. Sinus and mastoid films may reveal a potential source of infection and views of the petrous apices are useful to exclude the possibility of osteomyelitis in this region secondary to chronic middle ear disease.

Electroencephalography provides a valuable tool for localization of the cerebral hemisphere abscess. The abnormality is in the form of a high voltage, delta slow focus originating from the region of the suppurative lesion. In certain cases in which findings are equivocal but an abscess is believed to be developing, repeated electroencephalograms at intervals of several days may add much needed information by showing the presence and progression of a focal, slow abnormality.

Radioactive brain scan, like the electroencephalogram, is an additional procedure that can be safely performed and that may localize the site of the lesion with great precision. The available literature does not allow conclusions regarding the percentage of cerebral abscesses identified by scanning techniques. At least some may be outlined by this method, and the possibility warrants its performance when abscess is suspected, assuming that it can be done without undue delay.

Confirmation of the localization of an in-

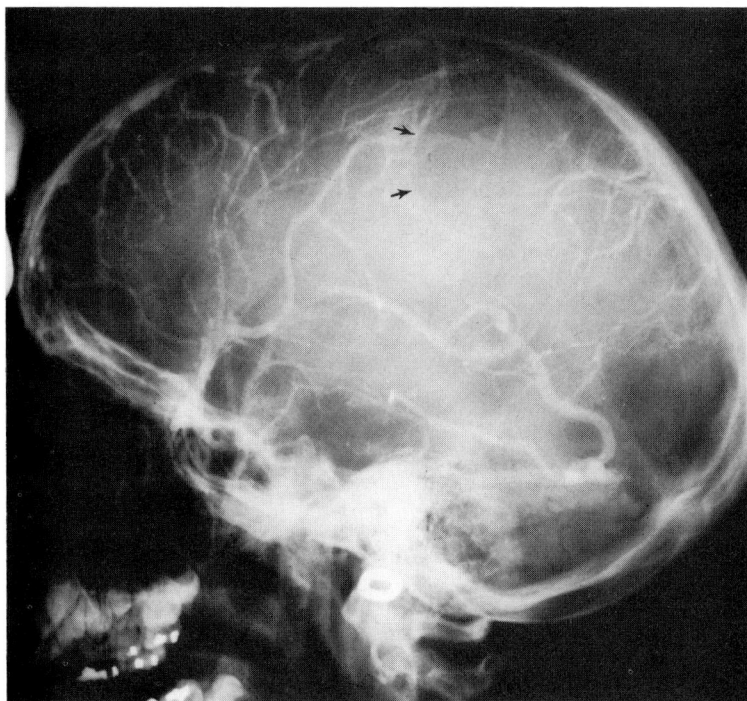

Figure 12-4. Parietal lobe abscess in a nine-year-old girl with cyanotic congenital heart disease. Carotid angiogram, venous phase, demonstrates an avascular mass surrounded by a faint halo of increased vascularity.

tracranial abscess requires contrast procedures before formulating a surgical attack of the lesion. Abscesses involving the cerebral hemispheres are most safely and accurately localized by carotid angiography which also may provide an estimate of the size of the mass (Fig. 12-4). Even in patients with cyanotic heart disease with polycythemia and reduced cerebral blood flow, the risk of angiography appears less than the hazard of cannulation of the congested brain required for air ventriculography. Cerebellar abscess is best localized by ventriculography. In most instances, the lateral ventricles are dilated because of fourth ventricle obstruction and thus are readily entered by the ventricular cannula.

Treatment

Treatment of a brain abscess includes the intravenous administration of antibiotics, attempts to reduce brain swelling, and surgical removal or evacuation of the lesion. Anti-convulsant therapy should be initiated preoperatively in a child suspected of harboring a brain abscess, even though seizures may not yet have occurred.

Infusion of antibiotics should also be started before surgery in any case in which an abscess is a reasonable consideration. Selection of the antibiotic regimen is never concise in this situation since the organism is yet unknown. The prominence of the staphylococcus as a cause of brain abscess is well established, and for this reason, either methicillin or oxacillin should be included in the regimen. Until the agent is isolated, methicillin in a dosage of 300 mg. per kilogram of body weight intravenously and kanamycin in a dosage of 10 mg. per kilogram intramuscularly per day would be a logical combination. In the rare case in which Nocardia is suspected or identified, sulfadiazine would be the drug of choice.

If signs of increased pressure are marked and include high-grade papilledema, lethargy, and bradycardia, dexamethasone, intravenously at 0.25 to 0.5 mg. per kg. per day, or mannitol, 2 grams per kilogram intravenously over 30 minutes, would be advisable. Mannitol should be avoided, however, in the child with heart disease if cardiac failure is present or impending. The sudden increase in intravascular volume resulting from use of this preparation may overload the heart, leading to pulmonary edema.

Surgical management of an intracranial abscess has been a controversial subject for many years. Some have favored aspiration of the contents or drainage by marsupialization, while others have recommended total excision whenever possible. It would appear that no one form of surgical management would be suitable for all cases and that individualization on the basis of size and location of the lesion plus condition of the child would be necessary.

The old concept of delaying surgery to permit the abscess to become encapsulated should be abandoned because this only invites disaster in the form of spontaneous rupture or internal herniation (Wright and Ballantine). Most believe that the clinical diagnosis of an intracranial abscess supported by the demonstration of an avascular mass on angiography or a cerebellar mass on ventriculography should be followed by operation without delay.

Large lesions that are poorly encapsulated are usually best managed by cannula drainage at craniotomy. The same is true of deeply located abscesses that involve the internal capsule or basal ganglia. Wright and Ballantine advocate complete excision of cerebral abscesses and claimed their results were more favorable with this approach than with simple aspiration or drainage. The condition of the child at the time of surgery is an additional factor that must be considered. A lengthy operative procedure may be poorly tolerated by the patient who is in a precarious state before operation.

REFERENCES

Abbott, M., and Stern, W. E.: Intracerebral hemorrhage associated with brain abscess. A complication of inappropriate anticoagulation. *J.A.M.A.*, **207**:1111–1114, 1969.

Calkins, R. A., and Bell, W. E.: Cerebral abscess and cyantoic congenital heart disease. *J. Lancet*, **87**:403–410, 1967.

Clark, D. B., and Clarke, E. S.: Brain abscess as complication of congenital cardiac malformation. *Tr. Am. Neurol. Assoc.*, **77**:73–76, 1952.

Groff, R. A.: Experimental production of abscess of the brain of cats. *Arch. Neurol. Psychiat.*, **31**:199–204, 1934.

Heineman, H. S., and Braude, A. I.: Anaerobic infection of the brain. *Amer. J. Med.*, **35**:682–697, 1963.

Hoffman, H. J., Hendrick, E. B., and Hiscox, J. L.: Cerebral abscesses in early infancy. *J. Neurosurg.*, **33**:172–177, 1970.

Horner, F. A., Berry, R. G., and Frantz, M.: Broken pencil points as a cause of brain abscess. *New Eng. J. Med.*, **271**:342–345, 1964.

Hughes, W. T.: Generalized aspergillosis. *Amer. J. Dis. Child.*, **112**:262–265, 1966.

Matson, D. D., and Salam, M.: Brain abscess in congenital heart disease. *Pediatrics*, **27**:772–789, 1961.

Norrell, H., and Howieson, J.: Gas.containing brain abscesses. *Amer. J. Roentgen.*, **109**:273–276, 1970.

Raimondi, A. J., Matsumoto, S., and Miller, R. A.: Brain abscess in children with congenital heart disease. I. *J. Neurosurg.*, **23**:588–595, 1965.

Rankin, J., and Javid, M.: Nocardiosis of the central nervous system. *Neurology*, **5**:815–820, 1955.

Roessman, U., and Friede, R. L.: Candidal infection of the brain. *Arch. Path.*, **84**:495–498, 1967.

Schurr, P.: Brain abscess in childhood. *Develop. Med. Child. Neurol.*, **7**:433–435, 1965.

Shuster, M., Klein, M. M., Pribor, H. C., and Kozub, W.: Brain abscess due to Nocardia. *Arch. Intern. Med.*, **120**:610–614, 1967.

Stern, W. E., and Naffziger, H. C.: Brain abscess associated with pulmonary angiomatous malformation. *Ann. Surg.*, **138**:521–531, 1953.

Tarkkanen, J. V.: Otogenic brain abscesses. A study of 99 cases including 24 follow-up examined. *Acta. Otolaryng.*, Suppl. 185, 1963.

Wishingrad, L., Rosenthal, I. M., and Cascino, J. P.: Brain abscess seven years after a Potts anastomosis in case of tetralogy of Fallot. *J.A.M.A.*, **164**:1465–1466, 1957.

Wright, R. L., and Ballantine, H. T., Jr.: Management of brain abscesses in children and adolescents. *Amer. J. Dis. Child.*, **114**:113–122, 1967.

PART
III

Intracranial Tumors In Childhood

Chapter Thirteen

GENERAL COMMENTS

It is generally stated that primary intracranial neoplasms comprise the second most common type of neoplastic disease in childhood, exceeded only by the leukemias. Intracranial tumors may occur in a variety of locations, thereby producing variable clinical manifestations depending on the structures involved and the presence or absence of increased intracranial pressure. Any age in childhood may be affected, although the peak incidence is in the second half of the first decade.

A number of differences are apparent when one compares intracranial tumors in children with those in adults. Meningiomas, pituitary adenomas, and acoustic neurinomas are reasonably common in adults but are rarely seen in childhood. Conversely, medulloblastomas, cystic astrocytomas of the cerebellum, optic gliomas, pontine gliomas and diencephalic gliomas are generally considered more characteristic of the pediatric years. The infrequent occurrence of pituitary, meningeal, and nerve sheath tumors in children, plus the predominance of diencephalic, brain stem, and cerebellar astrocytomas explains the higher percentage of gliomas in children than in adults.

The predominant location of brain tumors also tends to be different in children and in adults. Approximately 70 per cent of primary brain tumors in adults occur above the tentorium, whereas in children, tumors below the tentorium have been more common in most reported series. In their classic monograph on intracranial tumors in childhood, Bailey et al. noted that 67 per cent of 103 tumors occurred below the tentorium. Keith et al. found that 66 per cent of 427 intracranial tumors in children were infratentorial, whereas Ingraham and Matson found 60 per cent of 313 intracranial neoplasms in children under 12 years of age to be infratentorial.

Of tumors in the series of Ingraham and Matson, 80 per cent were gliomas, whereas Bailey et al. found that 76 per cent of intracranial tumors in childhood were gliomas, and Walker and Hopple noted that 78 per cent were glial in origin. In the large series reported by Keith et al., 84 per cent were gliomas. This high incidence of glial tumors in childhood is in contrast to the much lower incidence of gliomas in adults. In Cushing's 1932 series of 2023 intracranial tumors in all age groups, 42.6 per cent were gliomas. Among 2326 patients of all ages with brain tumors, Grant found gliomas to comprise 50.2 per cent. Courville reviewed 3010 intracranial tumors, including all age groups, and found 41.5 per cent of the total number were gliomas. In summary, 60 to 70 per cent of all intracranial tumors in children occur below the tentorium and 70 to 80 per cent of all intracranial tumors are gliomas.

The frequency of different intracranial masses in childhood has appeared to change considerably over the years. In 1889, Starr found that 50.6 per cent of 300 intracranial masses in children were tuberculomas. In 1937, a subsequent review of intracranial masses in the childhood years revealed only a 6 per cent incidence of tuberculous lesions (Stern). Tuberculomas of significant size are now uncommon in the United States, but this is not true in other parts of the world where granulomatous lesions continue to account for a large percentage of intracranial mass

Table 13-1. Types of Intracranial Tumors in Childhood. Compiled from Seven Reported Series* (Total of 1518 Cases).

	Series Included	Number	Percentage
Astrocytoma (site unspecified)	1–7	409 of 1518	26.9
Ependymoma (site unspecified)	1–7	135 of 1518	8.8
Glioblastoma (site unspecified)	1–7	99 of 1518	6.5
Medulloblastoma	1–7	307 of 1518	20.2
Craniopharyngioma	1–7	104 of 1518	6.8
Pontine glioma	2,4,5	72 of 819	8.7
Optic nerve glioma	4,5,6	33 of 802	4.0
Pineal tumors	2,4,5,6,7	14 of 1004	1.3
Meningioma	2,3,4,5,6,7	21 of 1091	1.9
Other			14.9

*Series 1: Keith, McK.Craig, and Kernohan, 1949 (427 cases). Series 2: Walker and Hopple, 1949 (100 cases). Series 3: Smith and Fincher, 1942 (87 cases). Series 4: Cushing, 1927 (154 cases). Series 5: Matson, 1964 (565 cases). Series 6: Cuneo and Rand, 1952 (83 cases). Series 7: Bailey, Buchanan, and Bucy, 1939 (102 cases).

lesions in children. Thus, Dastur has stated that 48.5 per cent of all brain tumors in children in India are tuberculomas.

In an attempt to arrive at a reasonable approximation of the incidence of various types of brain neoplasms in childhood, seven large reported series were combined (Table 13-1). Although the various reports were not always comparable, the total number of cases in the seven series was 1518. Astrocytoma, including those in the optic system and brain stem, was the most common childhood tumor (39.6 per cent); however, this figure has limited meaning, because most reports did not distinguish cerebral from cerebellar astrocytomas. Medulloblastomas accounted for 20.2 per cent and craniopharyngiomas for 6.8 per cent of all intracranial tumors in children.

Interpretation of the results of several different series such as this may be misleading in some areas. In certain reports, diagnosis of a particular type of tumor was dependent upon surgical or autopsy verification. Because brain stem or pineal tumors are rarely operated upon, these lesions would often not be included in such statistics. Therefore, the frequency of these lesions in children is most likely greater than is apparent from Table 13-1.

The relative occurrence of different types of gliomas in the cerebellum is difficult to ascertain from the literature. Walker and Hopple (1949) described 25 medulloblastomas and 15 astrocytomas in their series of cerebellar tumors in childhood. Of 115 posterior fossa tumors in children, Matson (1956) found that 34 were cerebellar astrocytomas and 36 were medulloblastomas. In the older literature, however, a different tendency is noted; Bailey et al. (1939) found 24 cerebellar astrocytomas and only 13 medulloblastomas. Cushing's material (1931) showed 76 cerebellar astrocytomas and 62 medulloblastomas.

The incidence of different histologic types of tumors occurring in the cerebral hemispheres in children has been reviewed by Low et al. These authors described 123 cases of cerebral tumors in childhood of which 115 were examined histologically. The findings in this series support the generally recognized concept that cerebral hemisphere tumors are apt to be morphologically bizarre. Solid astrocytomas were present in 29 per cent of the 115 cases and cystic astrocytomas in 17 per cent. However, several of these were mixed tumors, including astroglial elements plus other neoplastic components. Of the remaining tumors approximately 12 per cent were glioblastomas, 12 per cent were oligodendrogliomas, and 8 per cent were ependymomas. Several other histologic types, including sarcomas, gangliogliomas, teratomas, and neuroblastomas, occurred in the hemispheres in lesser numbers.

CLASSIFICATION AND PATHOLOGIC ASPECTS OF INTRACRANIAL TUMORS

Cell types found in normal brain tissue include microglia, astrocytes, ependymal cells, oligodendroglia, and neurons. Variations of these cell types are found in various areas, such as the Bergmann cells and granule cells of the cerebellum and pituicytes of the posterior pituitary gland. The astrocyte is the cell type most commonly involved in brain tumors, followed by ependymal cells and less often the oligodendroglia and microglia. Nerve cells only rarely become neoplastic in the brain.

Numerous classifications of brain tumors have been developed. The area of greatest debate regarding nomenclature has concerned the glioma group of intracranial neoplasms. Perhaps the most widely recognized classification of the gliomas to gain favor in the first half of this century was that developed by Bailey and Cushing in 1926 (Table 13-2). These authors based their classification on a histogenic concept, indicating that cells observed in the various gliomas resembled embryonic cells present in the developing nervous system. Thus, they proposed that the astroblastoma, for example, developed from cellular elements consisting of the primitive astroblast present during embryonic development.

The term spongioblastoma multiforme had been used earlier by Globus and Strauss (1925) and was used by Bailey and Cushing to refer to a more rapidly growing type of glial tumor. In 1927, Bailey suggested that the term glioblastoma multiforme replace the previously proposed spongioblastoma multiforme. Glioblastoma multiforme has become firmly entrenched in neurologic nomenclature and refers to a rapidly growing, invasive glial tumor with characteristic microscopic features. The term has continued to distress morphologists, however, because it is difficult to reconcile with the histogenetic concept of glial tumors. Many have argued that there is no embryonic counterpart in the

Table 13-2. Bailey and Cushing (1926) Classification of the Gliomas

1. Medulloepithelioma
2. Medulloblastoma
3. Pineoblastoma
4. Pinealoma
5. Ependymoblastoma
6. Ependymoma
7. Neuroepithelioma
8. Spongioblastoma
   A. multiforme
   B. unipolare
9. Astroblastoma
10. Astrocytoma
11. Oligodendroglioma
12. Neuroblastoma
13. Ganglioneuroma
14. Papilloma choroideum

Table 13-3. Comparison of Previous Classifications with that Proposed by Kernohan et al. (1949)

Previous Classifications	Kernohan et al. (1949)
Astrocytoma	Astrocytoma, grade 1
Astroblastoma	Astrocytoma, grade 2
Glioblastoma multiforme	Astrocytoma, grade 3, 4
Ependymoma	Ependymoma, grade 1
Ependymoblastoma	Ependymoma, grades 2 to 4
Medulloepithelioma	Ependymoma, grade 4
Oligodendroglioma	Oligodendroglioma, grade 1
Oligodendroblastoma	Oligodendroblastoma, grades 2 to 4
Medulloblastoma	Medulloblastoma
Neurocytoma	
Ganglioneuroma	Neuroastrocytoma, grade 1
Gangliocytoma	
Ganglioglioma	
Neuroblastoma	
Spongioneuroblastoma	Neuroastrocytoma, grades 2 to 4
Glioneuroblastoma	

brain that might be referred to as a glioblast. This type of reasoning resulted in a growing belief that the more malignant intracranial gliomas resulted from anaplastic change or dedifferentiation of more mature glial cells.

In 1949, Kernohan et al., proposed a simplification of the classification of intracranial gliomas based on the degree of anaplasia present on microscopic examination. Tumors were graded from one through four on the basis of the gradual transition from most mature to most malignant (Table 13-3). Thus, astrocytoma, grade 1, corresponds to the astrocytoma of the older classification. Astrocytoma, grade 2, replaces the previous term astroblastoma. Grade 3 and 4 astrocytomas were substituted for the term glioblastoma multiforme.

The classification described by the Mayo Clinic group has the advantage of being consistent with the concept of change of the degree of malignancy within a single tumor with the passage of time. It has the disadvantage of excluding certain descriptive terms, such as spongioblastoma polare, that connote meaning regarding histologic appearance and even environment of the tumor. An additional problem with any classification of brain tumors concerns the variable degree of anaplasia within different parts of a single tumor. Tissue obtained by surgical biopsy

Table 13-4. Classification of Intracranial Tumors (Summarized from Russell and Rubinstein)

1. Congenital tumors
    A. Teratoma
    B. Dermoid and epidermoid cysts
    C. Craniopharyngioma
    D. Lipoma
    E. Ectopias and hamartoma
    F. Dysgenetic syndromes with tumor formation
        (1) Lindau's syndrome
        (2) Tuberous sclerosis
        (3) Neurofibromatosis
2. Tumors of the meninges
    A. Benign meningiomas
    B. Malignant meningiomas
    C. Primary sarcoma of the meninges
3. Tumors of reticular tissue
    A. Leukemia
    B. Lymphoma
        (1) Hodgkin's disease
        (2) Follicular lymphoma
        (3) Microgliomatosis and reticulum cell sarcoma
        (4) Lymphosarcoma
    C. Plasmacytoma and multiple myelomatosis
4. Tumors and hamartomas of blood vessels
    A. Hemangioblastoma
    B. Blood vessel hamartoma
        (1) Capillary telangiectases
        (2) Cavernous angioma
        (3) Venous and arteriovenous malformations
5. Primary tumors of neuroectodermal origin
    A. Tumors of glial series
        (1) Astrocytic group
            (a) Astrocytoma
                protoplasmic
                fibrillary
                pilocytic
                gemistocytic
                anaplastic
            (b) Astroblastoma
            (c) Polar spongioblastoma
        (2) Oligodendroglioma
        (3) Ependyma and homologues
            (a) Ependymoma
            (b) Subependymal glomerate astrocytoma
            (c) Papilloma of the choroid plexus
            (d) Colloid cyst of the third ventricle
        (4) Glioblastoma multiforme
    B. Pineal neoplasms
        (1) Teratomas
        (2) Pinealomas
        (3) Glial tumors
        (4) Cysts
    C. Retinoblastoma
    D. Tumors of neuron series
        (1) Medulloblastoma
        (b) Medulloepithelioma
        (3) Neuroblastoma
        (4) Ganglioneuroma
        (5) Ganglioglioma
6. Secondary neoplasms of the nervous system
    A. By direct extension
        (1) Pituitary tumor
        (2) Glomus jugulare tumor
        (3) Osteoma-osteochondroma
        (4) Chordoma
        (5) Bone sarcoma
        (6) Rhabdomyosarcoma
        (7) Carcinoma
    B. Hematogenous metastasis

from the margin of a tumor may reveal only mature glial tissue. Deeper parts of the lesion may contain highly anaplastic tissue consistent with a malignant glioma but not evident from the material obtained on the biopsy.

A currently widely used text on the pathology of tumors of the nervous system approaches the subdivision as outlined in Table 13-4 (Russell and Rubinstein), and is the classification most commonly used by authorities. Classic terminology is adhered to with the inclusion of categories such as astroblastoma, glioblastoma multiforme, and medulloepithelioma.

PATHOLOGY

Pathologic characteristics of certain intracranial tumors are described here that are not discussed in the section on specific tumors.

Astrocytoma

Astrocytomas have been divided into several types on the basis of the histologic characteristics of the lesion. Russell and Rubinstein recognize protoplasmic, fibrillary, pilocytic, gemistocytic, and anaplastic astrocytomas. These tumors may occur in various areas of the nervous system and produce clinical symptoms and signs more dependent on the location than the histology of the lesion (Fig. 13-1).

Protoplasmic astrocytomas are infrequent and occur primarily within the gray matter of the cerebral hemispheres. The cellular elements of this tumor contain swollen cytoplasm with few astrocytic processes being evident. Microcystic degeneration, evident by small, vacuolar spaces on microscopic examination, is often present. Protoplasmic astrocytomas of the cerebrum are frequently located superficially and lack sharply defined

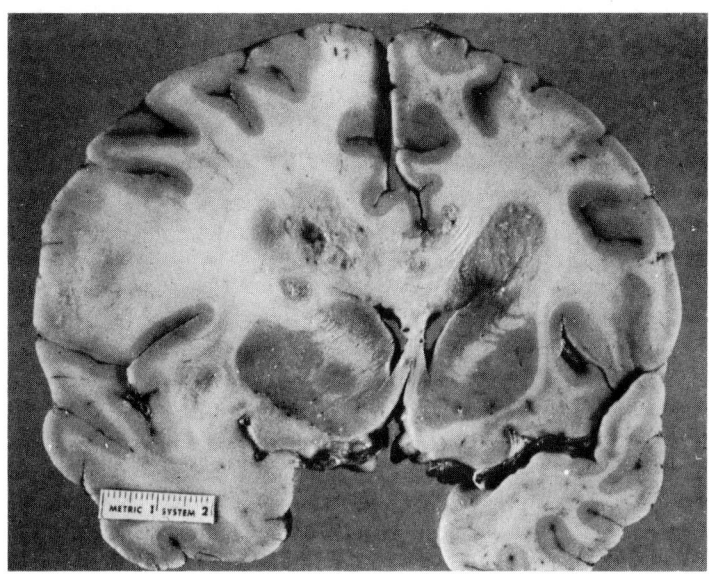

Figure 13-1. Frontal lobe infiltrative astrocytoma. Neoplasm is deep-seated, invasive, and involves both frontal lobes and the corpus callosum. There is considerable white matter edema adjacent to the tumor, resulting in flattening of the surface gyri and narrowing of the sulci. Note that delineation of the ventricular system by pneumoencephalography in this case would not completely localize the extent of tumor involvement.

margins. A gelatinous or spongy consistency may be noted on palpation.

Fibrillary astrocytomas are slow-growing neoplasms, which in children, may occur in several different areas, including the cerebrum, cerebellum, hypothalamus, and brain stem. The fibrillary astrocytoma tends to be gray to white in appearance, firm on palpation, and usually without definite demarcation from the surrounding brain. In the cerebrum, fibrillary astrocytomas are commonly solid; in the cerebellum, cysts are often present. Microscopically, the cells of the fibrillary astrocytoma vary in size and shape and are dispersed unevenly. The nuclei of the neoplastic cells approximate those of normal astrocytes, although they may be larger. Well defined glial fibrils form the stroma of the neoplasm and are nicely demonstrated by the phosphotungstic acid–hematoxylin stain. In the low-grade astrocytoma, mitotic divisions, areas of necrosis, palisading, rosette-formation, and proliferation of vascular endothelium are not observed.

The pilocytic astrocytoma is characterized by parallel arrangement of fibrils within the tumor. In certain areas of the brain, the explanation for the pilocytic arrangement of the cellular components is not evident. In other regions, the elongated bipolar cells with fibrils in parallel rows appear to represent an adaptation to the local environment. This tendency is noted when the tumor develops in the region of nerve tracts, such as in the corpus callosum or pons.

Gemistocytic astrocytoma is an unusual histologic type of tumor that occurs within the cerebral hemispheres. This tumor is composed of large cells closely packed together with small and eccentric nuclei. The cytoplasm is abundant, causing the cells to assume a globoid appearance with an eosinophilic quality. Russell and Rubinstein suggest that some gemistocytic astrocytomas may undergo further anaplastic change, resulting in the histologic pattern of a glioblastoma multiforme.

The subependymal glomerate astrocytoma is rarely symptomatic and has been identified predominately in adults. The tumor is characteristically discrete, lobulated, and grows into the adjacent ventricle with only minor compression of the underlying tissue. These lesions seem particularly apt to occur in the region of the floor of the fourth ventricle where they may be multiple (Fig. 13-2). Those projecting into the lateral ventricle may arise from the septum pellucidum. The bulk of the tumor tends to be intraventricular with only superficial penetration of the parenchyma at the site of attachment.

Histologically, the subependymal glomerate astrocytoma consists of clusters of ependymal tumor cells embedded in a thick mass of astroglial fibers. Because of the location and the combination of cellular elements present, this tumor has been classified among the ependymomas by some and with the astrocytomas by others. Scheinker (1945) was the first to recognize this lesion as a distinct histologic entity and referred to it as subependymoma. Boykin et al. (1954) stressed the

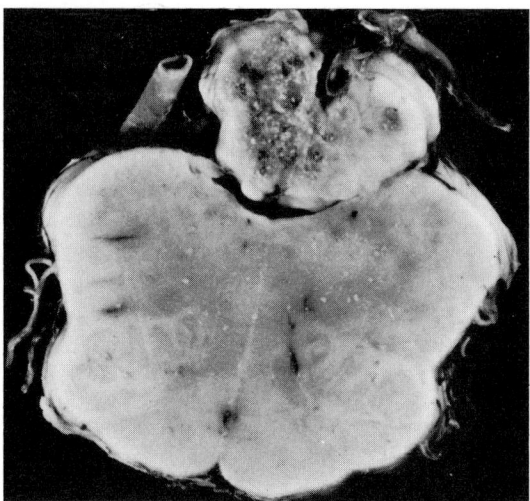

Figure 13-2. Subependymal glomerate astrocytoma. The tumor is located within the fourth ventricle with no obvious infiltration or compression of the adjacent medulla.

intraventricular location of these neoplasms and suggested the term subependymal glomerate astrocytoma. Chason emphasized the combination of neoplastic ependymal and astrocytic cells in this tumor and suggested the term subependymal mixed glioma, to avoid confusion.

Astroblastoma

The astroblastoma is a rare neuroectodermal neoplasm, which corresponds to one type of the astrocytoma, grade 2, of Kernohan et al. It is a very unusual tumor in childhood and occurs more often in the cerebrum in young adults. The tendency for infiltration, hemorrhage, and degeneration within the tumor resembles that seen in the glioblastoma multiforme. However, the lesser degree of malignancy is indicated by the longer period of survival of patients with astroblastomas as compared to those with glioblastomas (Courville, 1967). The most outstanding histologic feature of the astroblastoma is the tendency of the neoplastic cells to be arranged radially around vessels, referred to as pseudorosette formation.

Glioblastoma

The term glioblastoma multiforme refers to a malignant glioma that corresponds to the grade 3 and 4 astrocytomas as classified by Kernohan et al. Glioblastomas are far more common among adults and occur most often in the frontal or temporal lobes. More than one lobe of the brain frequently is involved. The neoplasm also may develop in the region of the corpus callosum and infiltrate bilaterally to involve both cerebral hemispheres. The tumor may originate in one hemisphere, infiltrate the corpus callosum, and gain access to the opposite side of the brain by this route.

In addition to being one of the most malignant types of glioma, the glioblastoma is the most common when all age groups are considered. In Courville's series (1967), which included 1259 gliomas, 52 per cent were judged to be glioblastoma multiforme.

The gross appearance of the cut surface of a glioblastoma reveals a variable pattern in different areas of the tumor (Fig. 13-3). Hemorrhagic areas are often noted and small cysts containing clear xanthochromic fluid may be present. Necrosis within the tumor may cause a gray or yellowish discoloration. The borders of the neoplasm may be fairly well delineated grossly, giving the false impression of lack of infiltration or even encapsulation. However, encapsulation does not occur with glioblastomas; microscopic examination will show tumor cells invading adjacent brain tissue. Considerable edema may surround the lesion.

The microscopic features of this tumor are marked by variability from field to field and heterogenicity of the cellular appearance. The cell population is mixed, containing astrocytes, spongioblasts, astroblasts, and a multiplicity of anaplastic cells with hyperchromatic or multiple nuclei. Multinucleated giant cells are present and contain abundant eosinophilic cytoplasm. Mitotic figures may be numerous and may appear in bizarre forms. Palisading is a prominent aspect of this tumor and refers to the arrangement of neoplastic cells in parallel rows pointing toward a zone of necrosis (Fig. 13-4). When the patch of necrosis is small or circular, the radial arrangement of tumor cells at its periphery may be misinterpreted as rosette or pseudorosette formation, as seen in other tumors.

A striking feature within the substance of the glioblastoma is a variable degree of endothelial hyperplasia of the contained blood vessels (Fig. 13-5). This hyperplastic change is most marked in capillaries but may occur in other vessels as well. Thickening of the vessel wall causes the lumen to become more and more narrow.

The hyperplastic endothelial cells within a glioblastoma may assume neoplastic proper-

General Comments

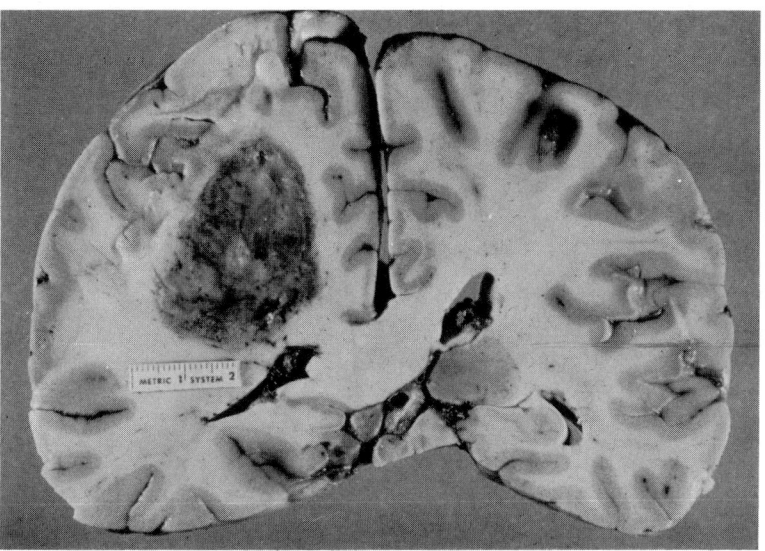

Figure 13-3. Glioblastoma multiforme. The gross appearance of the neoplasm suggests well defined margins, although microscopic examination demonstrates invasive and infiltrative tendencies. The tumor is one of variable patterns including small areas of necrosis, of hemorrhage, and of cystic degeneration with cysts of different sizes. The entire hemisphere containing the tumor is larger than the opposite hemisphere and the homolateral ventricle is markedly depressed.

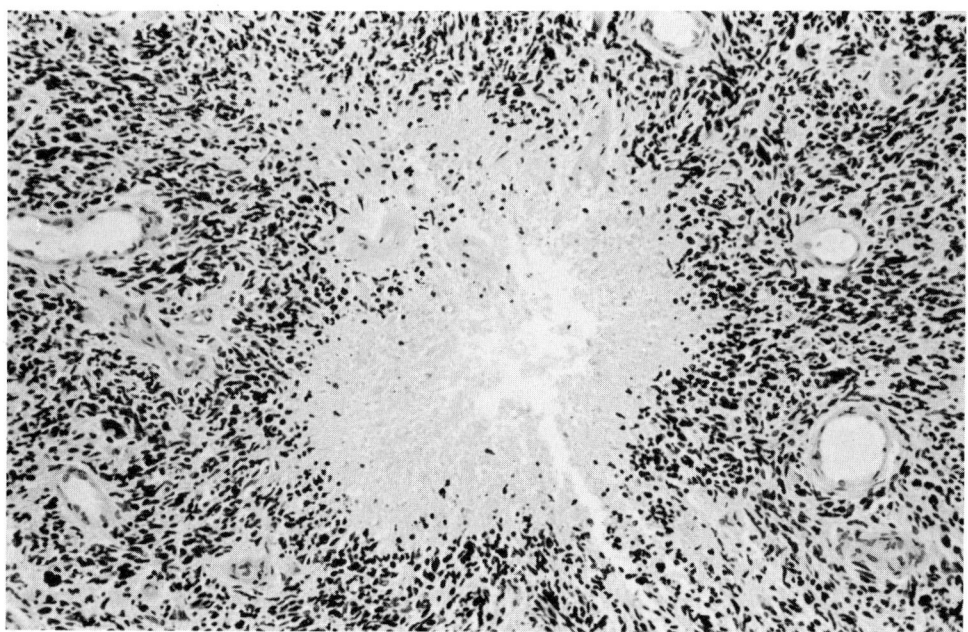

Figure 13-4. Glioblastoma multiforme. Neoplastic cells with hyperchromatic nuclei are arranged around a zone of central necrosis. This pattern is referred to as palisading and is one of the main histologic patterns characteristic of the glioblastoma multiforme.

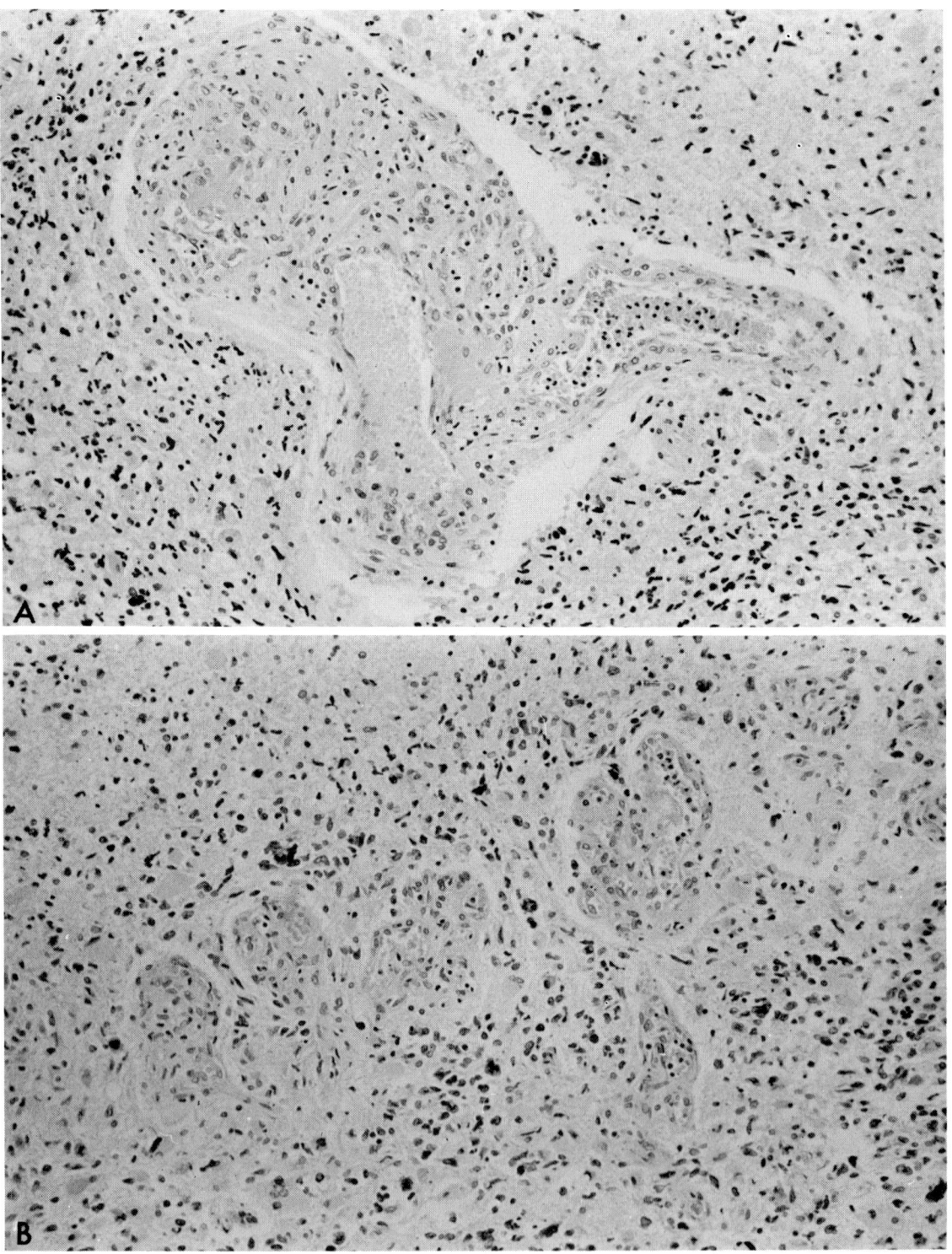

Figure 13-5. Glioblastoma multiforme. A, Marked endothelial proliferation within the tumor. The neoplastic cell population surrounding the abnormal vessel is mixed with cells of various sizes, most with hyperchromatic nuclei and some with multiple nuclei. B, The clusters of perivascular endothelial proliferation are referred to as "glomeruloids," a feature often observed within a glioblastoma. Tumor giant cells and multinucleated cells are also observed within the neoplasm.

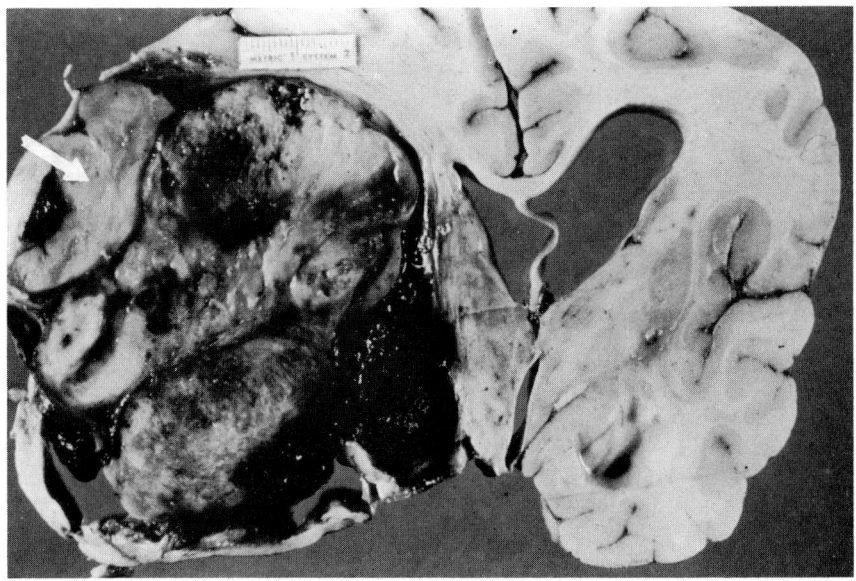

Figure 13-6. Glioblastoma of one cerebral hemisphere is located adjacent to a sarcomatous tumor (arrow). Sarcomatous change within a malignant glioma is believed to originate from hyperplastic endothelial cells within the primary neoplasm.

ties, producing sarcomatous changes within the substance of the intracranial glial tumor (Feigin et al.) (Fig. 13-6). When this occurs, one finds two malignant tissues, one being glioblastoma, the other, a spindle-cell sarcoma, within a large neoplastic lesion. In rare instances, glioblastomas with sarcomatous degeneration may spread extracranially to the lungs (Ehrenreich and Devlin) or to cervical lymph nodes (Garret). Both neoplastic components have been observed within the metastatic lesions. In other instances, extracranial spread to the lungs has occurred from a glioblastoma without associated sarcomatous changes (Giok and Schoot).

Extracranial spread of glioblastoma appears to be unusual; however, Smith and colleagues described visceral metastases in 23 adult cases. Prior neurosurgical intervention and prolonged postoperative survival were the most important factors associated with the development of extracranial metastasis in these cases. Infiltration and distortion of surrounding brain tissue is usual; in some instances, leptomeningeal dissemination may occur (Towbin and Bell).

Oligodendroglioma

The separation of oligodendroglia from other forms of neuroglia was accomplished by del Rio Hortega in 1921. Seven years later, the same author proposed that oligodendroglia are related to myelin formation in the central nervous system as Schwann cells are in the peripheral nervous system. In 1926, Bailey and Cushing identified intracranial tumors of the oligodendroglial series and chose the name oligodendroglioma. This tumor occurs primarily in adults and predominantly in the cerebral hemispheres. It is usually regarded as a slowly growing neoplasm, which may reach considerable size before definitive symptoms or signs are observed. This is variable, however, because some appear to proceed at a rapid rate.

Calcification is often present in the oligodendroglioma and may be sufficiently dense to be evident on roentgenographic examination. The tumor is composed of small cells that are densely packed with little stroma between cell bodies. The cell nuclei are round to oval, deeply stained, and appear to be floating in cytoplasm that is faintly visible. Tumors in which the nuclei contain less chromatin with frequent mitotic figures are referred to by some as oligodendroblastomas.

Certain tumors of the oligodendroglial type contain spongioblastic, astroblastic, or astrocytic cell forms in variable proportions. Occasionally, a single tumor is clearly oligodendroglial in one area and astrocytic in another. Ravens et al. described oligodendrogliomas with transition of the cellular components to astroglial cell types. Although the oligodendroglioma is generally regarded as a slowly growing tumor, arachnoidal dissemination may occur. In rare instances, arachnoidal dissemination can provoke a fibrotic response from the leptomeningeal cells, disturbing cerebrospinal fluid absorption and producing increased intracranial pressure (Korein et al.).

Ependymoma

The ependymomas are an important group of intracranial tumors in childhood, although they are considerably less common than tumors of the astroglial series. They may occur either above or below the tentorium, corresponding to the sites of ependymal tissue. In the posterior fossa, the ependymoma often originates from the floor of the fourth ventricle, projecting into the ventricular lumen and resulting in obstructive hydrocephalus.

Microscopic features commonly observed in ependymomas include true rosettes in which neoplastic ependymal cells are arranged in a halo, forming a tubular structure. Pseudorosettes are also seen in which the radially arranged ependymal cells encircle a blood vessel. Blepharoplasts are occasionally noted and refer to lightly stained, rodlike structures near the nucleus of the cell. The blepharoplasts are best visualized with the phosphotungstic acid—hematoxylin stain.

Various cellular patterns occur in the ependymomas in addition to different degrees of malignant change. Tumors with more marked pleomorphism, including giant forms, hyperchromatic nuclei, and frequent mitoses have been referred to as ependymoblastomas. These lesions are characteristically quite vascular and may contain considerable endothelial hyperplasia, as in other gliomas.

Papillary ependymoma describes an ependymal tumor composed of cuboidal cells lined in papillary fashion and covering a central core of connective tissue. Myxomatous degeneration of this central stroma may occur and has led to the term "myxopapillary type of ependymoma." The cellular type of ependymoma consists of a less orderly arrangement of neoplastic ependymal cells, although pseudorosettes may still be present. Cells of oligodendroglial origin may be intermixed within the cellular ependymoma.

Arachnoidal dissemination of neoplastic cells of the ependymoma may occur with secondary implantation occurring at sites remote from the primary lesion.

Medulloepithelioma

Classification of the medulloepithelioma has remained controversial with some authorities denying its existence. Others have placed it among the poorly differentiated ependymomas. The medulloepithelioma is described by Russell and Rubinstein as a neuroectodermal tumor of extremely primitive character with cell elements that resemble primitive medullary epithelium. Columnar cells without blepharoplasts are arranged in a palisade fashion, abutting on a limiting membrane. Thus, the cellular components of the medulloepithelioma appear to recapitulate embryonic neural tube formation in a haphazard fashion, distinguishing it from the ependymoma group. The nuclei of the columnar cells may be elongated, and numerous mitoses may be present.

Treip described a medulloepithelioma developing in the midbrain of an eight-month-old infant. Van Epps et al. reported a five-year-old child with this type of tumor in the temporal lobe from which extracranial metastasis occurred to posterior cervical lymph nodes. Diffuse leptomeningeal invasion also occurred in this patient. Support for the concept that the medulloepithelioma is a tumor of embryonic origin is provided by the case described by Deck in which maturation along ependymal and ganglionic cell lines occurred.

Ganglioglioma

Ganglioglioma is a mixed type of tumor containing neoplastic ganglionic and glial cells. The presence of neoplastic glial elements separates this tumor from the ganglioneuroma in which ganglion cells comprise the neoplastic component embedded in a non-neoplastic glial stroma. The relative amounts of ganglion and glial elements in a ganglioglioma are variable; either may predominate. These tumors have been described more often in children and young adults. The location may be the cerebral hemisphere, the floor of the third ventricle, or the hypothalamus. Gangliogliomas occurring in the pituitary region may result in diabetes insipidus, hypopituitarism, or visual deficits. Those located in the posterior hypothalamus may cause isosexual precocious puberty.

On gross examination, this tumor is usually firm with well defined margins. Microscopic examination of the ganglioglioma reveals cells of neuronal origin, some well differentiated and others bizarre in form. Giant or multinucleated cells of the neuron series may be present. The glial component of this tumor includes evidence of neoplastic proliferation as seen in a pleomorphic astrocytoma. The neoplastic glial cells may be spongioblastic or gemistocytic in variable proportions. In rare instances, cerebral ganglioglioma has been associated with tuberous sclerosis (Davis and Nelson).

Microglioma

Microglioma refers to a neoplasm derived from microglial cells or the primitive reticulum cell precursors. In 1919, del Rio Hortega distinguished the microglia from other small cells of the nervous system. These cells of mesoblastic origin respond promptly to various stimuli and become actively phagocytic. Tumors of microglial origin are rare and occur primarily in the cerebrum.

The outstanding gross characteristic of the microglioma is the strikingly granular appearance to the cut surface of the lesion (Fig. 13-7). Histologically, the neoplasm tends to be densely cellular. The cells are large with prominent nuclei of various shapes within cytoplasm that is less distinct. Mitoses are usually readily evident. These neoplasms have been described under numerous titles, including perivascular sarcoma, reticuloendothelioma, Hodgkin's sarcoma, reticulum cell sarcoma, and microglioma. They may occur at any age, including infancy and childhood, but are most often seen in middle-aged adults (Burstein et al.). Mention has been made of the onset with intestinal or encephalitic type of symptoms in some cases which, in association with rapid clinical progression, may create considerable diagnostic confusion (Adams and Jackson).

REFERENCES

Adams, J. H., and Jackson, J. M.: Intracerebral tumors of reticular tissue: The problem of microgliomatosis and reticulo-endothelial sarcomas of the brain. *J. Path. Bact.*, **91**:369–381, 1966.

Bailey, P.: Further remarks concerning tumors of the glioma groups. *Johns Hopk. Hosp. Rep.*, **40**:354–389, 1927.

Bailey, P., and Cushing, H.: *A Classification of Tumors of the Glioma Group on a Histogenic Basis with a Correlated Study of Prognosis.* Philadelphia, J. B. Lippincott Co., 1926.

Bailey, P., Buchanan, D. N., and Bucy, P.: *Intracranial Tumors of Infancy and Childhood.* Chicago, University of Chicago Press, 1939.

Boykin, F. C., Cowen, D., Iannucci, C, A. J., and Wolf, A.: Subependymal glomerate astrocytoma. *J. Neuropath. and Exper. Neurol.*, **13**:30–49, 1954.

Burstein, S. D., Kernohan, J. W., and Uhlein, A.: Neoplasms of the reticuloendothelial system of the brain. *Cancer*, **16**:289–305, 1963.

Chason, J. L.: Subependymal mixed gliomas. *J. Neuropath. and Exper. Neurol.*, **15**:461–470, 1956.

Courville, C. B.: Intracranial tumors. Notes upon a series of three thousand verified cases with some current observations pertaining to their mortality. *Bull. Los. Ang. Neurol. Soc.*, **32**:Suppl. 2:1–80, 1967.

Cuneo, H. M., and Rand, C. W.: *Brain Tumors in Childhood.* Springfield, Ill., Charles C Thomas, 1952.

Cushing, H.: The intracranial tumors of preadolescence. *Amer. J. Dis. Child.*, **33**:551–584, 1927.

Cushing, H.: Experiences with cerebellar astrocytomas. *Surg. Gynec. and Obst.*, **52**:129–204, 1931.

Cushing, H.: *Intracranial Tumors. Notes upon a Series of Two Thousand Verified Cases with Surgical-Mortality Percentages Pertaining Thereto.* Springfield, Ill., Charles C Thomas, 1932.

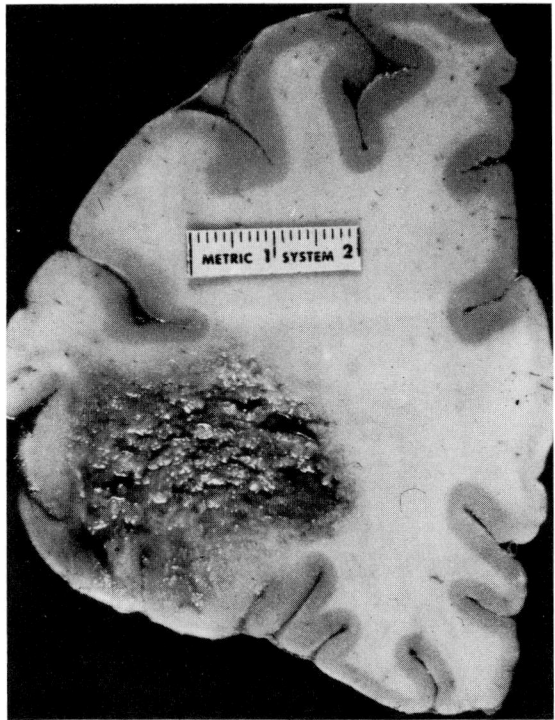

Figure 13-7. Microglioma of the frontal lobe. Granular appearance with infiltrative features is a characteristic gross finding in this tumor.

Dastur, D. K., and Udani, P. M.: The pathology and pathogenesis of tuberculous encephalopathy. *Acta. Neuropath.*, **6**:311–326, 1966.

Davis, R. L., and Nelson, E.: Unilateral ganglioglioma in a tuberosclerotic brain. *J, Neuropath and Exper. Neurol.*, **20**:571–581, 1961.

Deck, J. H. N.: Cerebral medulloepithelioma with maturation into ependymal cells and ganglion cells. *J. Neuropath. and Exper. Neurol.*, **28**:442–454, 1969.

Ehrenreich, T., and Devlin, J. F.: A complex of glioblastoma and spindle-cell sarcoma with pulmonary metastasis. *Arch. Path.*, **66**:536–549, 1958.

Feigin, I., Allen, L. B., Lipkin, L., and Gross, S. W.: The endothelial hyperplasia of the cerebral blood vessels with brain tumors and its sarcomatous transformation. *Cancer*, **11**:264–277, 1958.

Garret, R.: Glioblastoma and fibrosarcoma of the brain with extracranial metastases. *Cancer*, **11**:888–894, 1958.

Giok, S. P., and Schoot, H. C. M.: Metastasizing primary cerebral tumor. *J. Neuropath. and Exper. Neurol.*, **18**:575–579, 1959.

Globus, J. H., and Strauss, I.: Spongioblastoma multiforme: A primary malignant form of brain neoplasm: its clinical and anatomical features. *Arch. Neurol. and Psychiat.*, **14**:139–191, 1925.

Grant, F. C.: A study of the results of surgical treatment in 2,326 consecutive patients with brain tumor. *J. Neurosurg.*, **13**:479–488, 1956.

Ingraham, F. D., and Matson, D. D.: *Neurosurgery of Infancy and Childhood.* Springfield, Ill., Charles C Thomas, 1961.

Keith, H. M., McCraig, W. M., and Kernohan, J. W.: Brain tumors in children. *Pediatrics,* **3**:839–844, 1949.

Kernohan, J. W., Mabon, R. F., Svien, H. J., and Adson, A. W.: A simplified classification of the gliomas. *Proc. Mayo Clin.*, **24**:71–75, 1949.

Korein, J., Feigin, I., and Shapiro, M. F.: Oligodendrogliomatosis with intracranial hypertension. *Neurology*, **7**:589–594, 1957.

Low, N. L., Correll, J. W., and Hammill, J. F.: Tumors of the cerebral hemispheres in children. *Arch. Neurol.*, **13**:547–554, 1965.

Matson, D. D.: Cerebellar astrocytoma in childhood. *Pediatrics*, **18**:150–158, 1956.

Matson, D. D.: Intracranial tumors. *In* Farmer: *Pediatric Neurology*, New York, Hoeber, 1964.

Ravens, J. R., Adamkiewicz, L. L., and Groff, R.: Cytology and cellular pathology of the oligodendrogliomas of the brain. *J. Neuropath. and Exper. Neurol.*, **14**:142–184, 1955.

Rio Hortega, P. Del.: El tercer elemento de los centros nerviosos, I. La microglia en estado normal. II. Intravencion de la microglia en los procesos patologicos. III. Naturaleza probable de la microglia. *Bol. de la Soc. Esp. de Biol.*, **9**:69, 1919.

Russell, D. S., and Rubinstein, L. J.: *Pathology of Tumors of the Nervous System.* London, Edward Arnold, 1959.

Scheinker, I. M.: Subependymoma: A newly recognized tumor of subependymal derivation. *J. Neurosurg.*, **2**:232–240, 1945.

Smith, D. R., Hardman, J. M., and Earle, K. M.: Metastasizing neuroectodermal tumors of the central nervous system. *J. Neurosurg.*, **31**:50–58, 1969.

Smith, W. A., and Fincher, E. F.: Intracranial tumors in children: preliminary study of 100 cases. *South. Med. J.*, **35**:547–554, 1942.

Starr, M. A.: Tumors of the brain in childhood. *Med. News*, **54**:29–37, 1889.

Stern, R. O.: Cerebral tumors in children. A pathologic report. *Arch. Dis. Childh.*, **12**:291–304, 1937.

Towbin, A., and Bell, G.: Spontaneous arachnoidal dissemination of spongioblastoma multiforme. *J. Neuropath. and Exper. Neurol.*, **14**:263–275, 1955.

Treip, C. S.: A congenital medulloepithelioma of the midbrain. *J. Path. Bact.*, **74**:357–363, 1957.

Van Epps, R. R., Samuelson, D. R., and McCormick, W. F.: Cerebral medulloepithelioma. *J. Neurosurg.*, **27**:568–573, 1967.

Walker, A. E., and Hopple, T. L.: Brain tumors in children. *J. Pediat.*, **35**:671–687, 1949.

Chapter Fourteen

CLINICAL SIGNS AND DIAGNOSTIC ASSESSMENT

SYMPTOMS AND SIGNS

The symptoms and signs of intracranial tumors in childhood depend on several factors, including the age of the child, the location of the lesions, and the presence or absence of increased intracranial pressure. In some, the manifestations of increased pressure predominate or even account for all the findings observed. In others, there may be no evidence of increased pressure and only signs due to focal neurologic dysfunction. Still others show variable combinations of both types of deficits. As mentioned before, the size of the lesion and its location largely determine which factor is most important from the symptomatic standpoint.

In order to identify intracranial tumors in the early stages, one must recognize certain combinations of abnormalities that provide a strong suspicion of the presence of such a lesion. The identification of papilledema automatically raises the possibility of an intracranial tumor, regardless of the nature of the child's symptoms. The combination of visual loss, especially if progressive, and primary optic atrophy is strong suggestive evidence of a suprasellar tumor in childhood. Gliomas of the optic chiasm or nerve are especially prone to present in this fashion with few other findings. The suspicion is even greater if these deficits are noted in a child with multiple café-au-lait spots or other evidence of neurofibromatosis (Fig. 14-1). The child with acquired diabetes insipidus, visual acuity or field defects, or headaches should also be considered a candidate for a mass lesion in the region of the pituitary or anterior hypothalamus. Isosexual precocious puberty, especially in males, in combination with symptoms of increased pressure or focal neurologic signs must be considered sufficient evidence of a posterior hypothalamic tumor to warrant air contrast studies. The

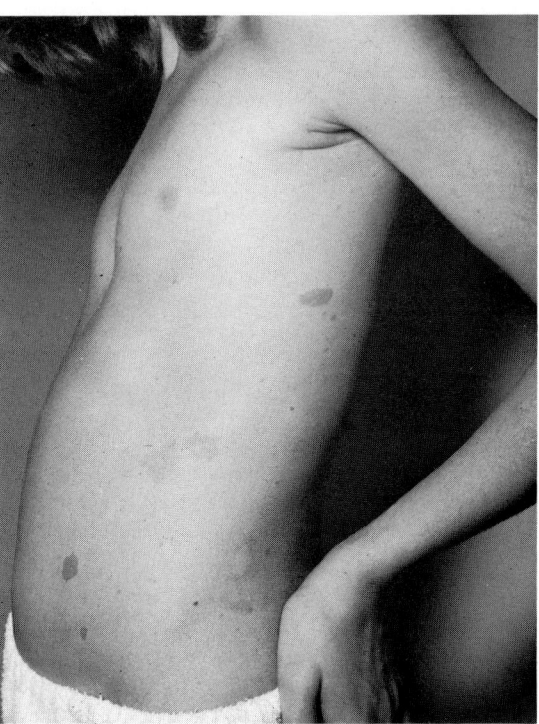

Figure 14-1. Multiple café-au-lait spots in a child with neurofibromatosis. Primary optic atrophy and visual loss in children with this disorder suggests the possibility of a glioma of the optic chiasm or nerve.

possibility of craniopharyngioma should be entertained in a child with growth failure, visual defects, or fundus changes, including either optic atrophy or papilledema.

With any of the lesions already described in or around the sella, skull x-rays are of considerable help, because distinctive abnormalities are often present. However, normal x-rays do not completely exclude the possibility, and if clinical suspicion is great enough, further studies are in order.

Cerebral hemisphere tumors may be difficult to recognize clinically, because the symptoms may mimic those of several other disorders. The previously normal young child who develops a major motor or akinetic type of convulsive disorder that shows little response to appropriate anticonvulsants must be watched closely in this regard.

A number of progressive neurologic disorders may cause intractable seizures of this type; however, hemisphere tumors must be included in the differential diagnostic consideration. The possibility becomes more overt if the electroencephalogram reveals a focal, slow abnormality. The lack of control with anticonvulsants after a reasonable trial and the focal electroencephalographic abnormality may be considered sufficient evidence for additional studies, including pneumoencephalography and angiography.

While seizures are relatively common in the childhood age group, one must be cautious about the combination of seizures in a previously normal child and a persistently focal electroencephalogram with localized slow activity. This is true for grand mal seizures, but even more so if the convulsive activity is of the focal motor type or is followed by a transient, postictal paresis. Psychomotor seizures also must be considered to be focal and if associated with a localized electroencephalographic abnormality, should raise the possibility of a temporal lobe tumor.

Other deficits of hemisphere function that point to the possibility of tumor include the combination of headaches and progressive spastic weakness of the limbs on one side of the body. These findings, often with sensory defects on the weak side, suggest a deep-seated lesion as may occur in the white matter extending into the thalamus or basal ganglia.

Tumors in the region of the posterior portion of the third ventricle usually result in signs of increased pressure early because of the proximity of the Sylvian aqueduct. Thus, a history of headaches and vomiting, plus paresis of vertical conjugate gaze, dilated pupils, and ataxia, add support to the probability of a mass lesion in the upper part of the brain stem or in the pineal region. Equally suggestive of a pineal tumor is the combination of recently acquired headaches and mineralization of the pineal gland in a child under 10 years of age. This structure is rarely visible on x-ray in this age group and must be assumed to be abnormal until proved otherwise.

The development of progressive cranial nerve palsies, incoordination of gait, and long tract signs is a clinical syndrome in childhood rarely produced by disease other than a brain stem glioma. The cranial nerve deficits may be unilateral or bilateral and most often include diplopia, strabismus, and asymmetry of facial movement. Disturbance of function of the long descending pathways within the brain stem is evidenced by hyperreflexia, ankle clonus, and extensor plantar responses. Because the fourth ventricle is not usually obstructed with tumors within the substance of the brain stem, signs of increased pressure may not occur until late in the clinical course, if at all.

Neoplasms within certain parts of the ventricular system are capable of causing obstructive symptoms and signs with little evidence of involvement of the surrounding brain tissue. Thus, cysts of the third ventricle in the region of the foramen of Monro or ependymomas of the fourth ventricle may be characterized by intermittent episodes of obstructive hydrocephalus. Severe headache of abrupt onset, precipitous bouts of vomiting, and transient periods of diplopia may occur and then terminate as promptly as the symptoms had appeared. Recurrent attacks of vomiting may be the outstanding complaint with such midline tumors, erroneously leading the examiner to consider the upper gastrointestinal tract as the probable site of disease.

Cerebellar tumors in childhood usually result in a combination of manifestations of increased pressure and signs of focal cerebellar dysfunction. Recurrent early morning headaches and vomiting are common early symptoms followed by staggering gait and other signs of an ataxic nature. The child with a medulloblastoma usually has a more abbreviated history, often with considerable weight loss at the time of admission. The ataxic abnormalities are often truncal, because this tumor has a tendency to occur in midline cerebellar structures. The child with a cystic cerebellar astrocytoma is apt to have a longer history, also with recurrent vomiting and headache as the initial complaints. If the tumor is in or near the vermis, truncal ataxia results. Cystic astrocytomas often occur in one cerebellar hemisphere, in which case the ataxic deficits are predominately unilateral, and horizontal nystagmus is marked.

Symptoms and Signs in Infancy

Recognition of intracranial tumors in infancy may be difficult because of the lack of symptoms available from the patient and the problems with identification of discreet signs on examination. In addition, it often is difficult to be certain whether neurologic abnormalities observed in the infant are due to a stable lesion, present from birth, or to a progressive disorder, as with an intracranial tumor. There are certain situations, however, in which one must suspect an intracranial neoplasm in the infant and proceed with the proper studies to include or exclude the possibility.

A rare instance is the child with failure to thrive for which no other explanation is evident. The development of nystagmus, optic atrophy, vomiting, and suture spread on x-ray indicate a progressive neurologic disease. This clinical pattern is consistent with the so-called "diencephalic syndrome of infancy" due to a glioma in the hypothalamic region.

Papilloma of the choroid plexus in the small baby may create considerable diagnostic problems, because the outstanding abnormality is abnormal head enlargement. Other forms of infantile hydrocephalus are far more common, allowing one to overlook the possibility of an intraventricular tumor. Awareness of the possibility and ventriculography may be the only means of diagnosis unless one is keenly aware of the possibility and the peculiar symptoms that may result therefrom. Irritability is usually marked and vomiting often recurs. Resistance to antiflexion of the head may be observed.

Young children with lesions in the posterior fossa may regress developmentally. Ataxia in this age group may be clinically evident by tremulousness of the limbs or of the head. Tremor and dysmetria of the upper extremities and refusal to walk suggest an ataxic disorder in the previously ambulatory infant.

It is not unusual that parents of infants with posterior fossa mass lesions suddenly notice abnormalities of function in the child. Thus, the onset of symptoms, as interpreted by the observers, may have been abrupt and perhaps only first noticed a few days before medical evaluation is requested.

The frequency of insignificant infections and bumps to the head at this age is also a pitfall, because parents are likely to attribute the neurologic deficits, irritability, or vomiting to such an event. Recurrent vomiting episodes in the infant may render him sufficiently dehydrated that intermittent fever may occur, further confusing the diagnostic logic. In the infant, therefore, one must abandon many of the generally useful guidelines that ordinarily provide suspicion of the existence of a brain tumor. An illness described as abrupt in onset, only days in duration, associated with fever, noticed after head trauma, and characterized by gastrointestinal features, may be due to an intracranial tumor in the infant.

DIAGNOSTIC ASSESSMENT

The points made in the discussion of symptoms and signs indicate the importance of a detailed history and thorough physical examination to suggest the possibility of an intracranial tumor in childhood. Having accomplished this part of the evaluation, one often feels that a tumor is reasonably possible or perhaps even likely. Further diagnostic studies will be required both to exclude other possible alternative disorders and to confirm the presence and location of the neoplasm.

Under these circumstances, it is ordinarily advisable to suggest to the parents before proceeding that an intracranial tumor is under consideration as an explanation for the child's symptoms. Suggesting the possibility in this manner has two advantages. It provides a reason why the extensive diagnostic assessment is mandatory. It allows them to accept diagnostic procedures that carry a certain degree of hazard, especially in the presence of increased intracranial pressure. In addition, awareness of the possibility of tumor permits the family to adjust emotionally during the few days that the more specific studies are being accomplished. If a tumor is identified, the family receives the news better if previously advised of the possibility.

Beyond the blood count and urinalysis, further laboratory tests depend on the nature of the symptoms, the general condition of the child, and the concern about other diagnostic possibilities. For example, if the child is dehydrated from vomiting, determinations of serum electrolytes and blood urea nitrogen are in order. If generalized seizures have occurred, blood sugar and calcium determinations should be made.

As noted elsewhere, rare causes of papilledema in childhood include conditions such as adrenal insufficiency, hypoparathyroidism, and iron-deficiency anemia. These diseases are rapidly and easily excluded by the appropriate laboatory studies. If a hypothalamic or pituitary lesion is suspected, a 24-hour urine collection should be initiated for 17-hydroxycorticosteroid determination and for gonadotropins in postpubertal patients. Consideration of a neuroblastoma with dural metastases warrants a similar urine specimen for estimation of catecholamines and their urinary metabolites.

Spinal Tap

The decision to perform a lumbar puncture as part of the diagnostic evaluation is based on comparison of the probability of useful information obtained and the potential hazard of the procedure. If the diagnosis of a posterior fossa tumor is virtually certain from the available information, the procedure should be avoided. When the evidence points to a cerebral hemisphere tumor or a suprasellar mass, it is often apparent early in the evaluation that pneumoencephalography will be required for diagnostic purposes. Here again, it is wiser to delay lumbar puncture and to obtain fluid specimens for analysis at the time of the air study. The greatest value of lumbar puncture in this regard is when the illness is brief and when one cannot be completely certain that the child does not have an infectious illness. The possibility of cryptococcosis or tuberculous meningitis requires a diagnostic lumbar puncture, even if papilledema is present.

If a lumbar puncture is done during the diagnostic evaluation, an effort should be made to obtain an accurate opening pressure. The Queckenstedt test should *not* be done. If a tumor is a reasonable possibility, a specimen of fluid should be obtained and sent to the pathologist for cytologic examination. Certain tumors may shed cells into the cerebrospinal fluid that can be identified by microscopic examination.

If this study is to be performed, the pathologist should be forewarned that the specimen is being sent. It should be delivered immediately after it is collected because neoplastic cells may be very short-lived and promptly disappear unless properly handled. This technique is also valuable if one suspects recurrence of an intracranial tumor at some point following surgical therapy.

The cerebrospinal fluid protein content may be elevated in patients with intracranial tumors. Completely normal findings on lumbar puncture in no way exclude the possibility of a brain tumor. After the procedure is accomplished, it is important to record the results of the study with complete clarity in the medical record.

Skull X-Rays

Skull x-rays should be obtained whenever there is the possibility of an intracranial tumor. Abnormalities that may be observed include signs of increased intracranial pressure, of which suture spread is the most common in childhood (Fig. 14-2). Certain tumors often exhibit calcification on x-ray. In children, this may be noted in or above the sella in the craniopharyngioma, in the region of the cerebral hemispheres with astrocytomas or oligodendrogliomas, or rarely, in the posterior fossa with ependymomas or other glial tumors.

Shift of a mineralized pineal gland is rarely observed in cerebral hemisphere tumors in childhood, because the pineal gland does not usually show mineralization on x-ray before the age of 16 years. Distinct mineralization of the pineal gland under 10 years of age must be assumed to be abnormal and suggests the presence of a tumor in this region.

Other distinctive abnormalities that may be identified on skull x-ray include the characteristic multiple, osteolytic lesions of histiocytosis X and the diffuse, destructive changes in the bony tables with marked suture spread due to metastatic neuroblastoma.

In the child with visual loss and primary optic atrophy, views of the optic foramina should be obtained in addition to skull films. The normal optic foramen is generally regarded to be less than 6 mm. in diameter and the foramina on the two sides should not

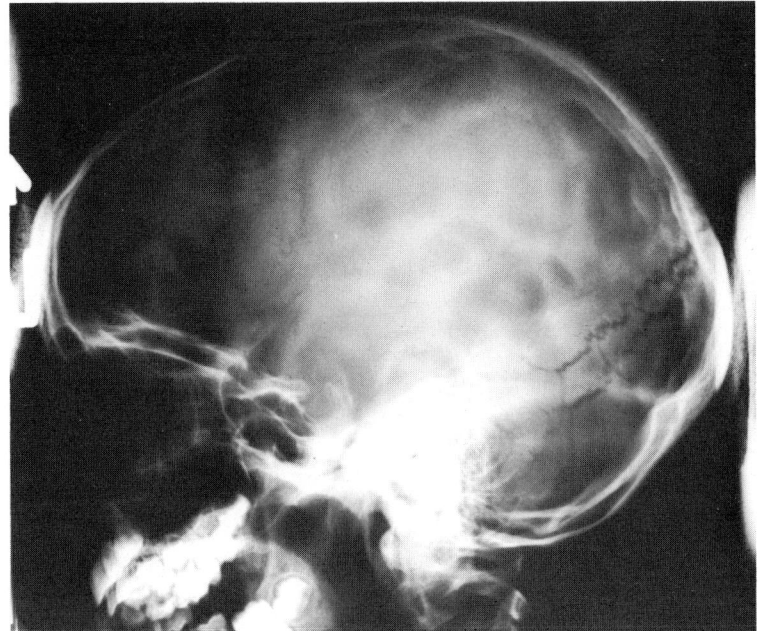

Figure 14-2. Lateral skull x-ray of a five-year-old girl with a cerebellar astrocytoma. Coronal and lambdoidal sutures are widely separated secondary to increased pressure from obstruction within the posterior fossa.

differ more than 1 mm. Abnormalities suggest a glioma of the optic nerve. Although abnormalities on skull x-rays are common in children with intracranial tumors, it must be stressed that normal skull films are not incompatible with this diagnosis. If the clinical data suggests hypopituitarism secondary to a suprasellar or intrasellar tumor, appropriate bone films should be obtained to ascertain the bone age.

Electroencephalography

Electroencephalography should be performed during the diagnostic assessment of any child who is considered to have an intracranial tumor. Although limitations of the procedure undoubtedly exist, it remains a valuable tool in conjunction with other studies in the establishment of a clinical diagnosis. Hans Berger described abnormal slow waves in the electroencephalogram in persons with cerebral neoplasms as early as 1931. Focal slow activity has remained the electroencephalographic hallmark of cerebral tumors, although it is not restricted to neoplastic lesions.

Because most cerebral tumors are glial in origin, general opinion is that abnormalities seen on the electroencephalogram do not result primarily from the tumor parenchyma directly but from functional disturbances of neuronal groups adjacent to the mass. Such involvement may result from edema surrounding the tumor, from vascular compromise, or from direct compression by the lesion.

Clinical suspicion of a cerebellar tumor warrants electroencephalographic investigation despite the nonspecific electrical abnormalities found with tumors in this area. Certain lesions of the cerebral hemispheres may cause symptoms that closely resemble those of a cerebellar tumor. A frontal lobe glioma may be manifested only by signs of increased pressure and incoordination. Rarely, a chronic subdural hematoma in childhood may result in similar signs, deluding the physician into an erroneous diagnosis of a posterior fossa mass. Although examples such as this are not common, identification of persistent focal delta activity originating from one cerebral hemisphere may provide the clue that results in correct localization of the lesion.

Electroencephalography has greater localizing value with cerebral tumors than with infratentorial neoplasms. In addition, reasonable localization is more likely with superficially located tumors than with more deeply seated neoplasms. In analysis of the electroencephalographic interpretation, one must remember that, in addition to effects of the tumor, the recording is influenced by associated increased intracranial pressure, by the effects of certain drugs that may have been administered, and by preexistent cerebral insults. A normal electroencephalogram, while not common, is not inconsistent with the existence of a cerebral tumor. Even paroxysmal bilaterally synchronous spike-wave abnormalities characteristic of idiopathic epilepsy may rarely be found in children with cerebral tumors (Madsen and Bray).

Electroencephalographic findings with posterior fossa tumors vary according to the location of the lesion and the degree of increased intracranial pressure. For example, tumors originating within the substance of the brain stem are often associated with normal electroencephalograms. Abnormalities that do occur are usually in the form of bilateral rhythmic slow activity, which may develop in various areas over the hemispheres but which often is more marked in the occipital regions.

Cerebellar or fourth ventricular tumors may produce a variety of electrical abnormalities resulting from neuronal disturbances well removed from the site of the lesion. Abnormalities often described with such tumors include rhythmic posterior delta activity, arrhythmic posterior delta slow, or generalized bursts or rhythmic slow discharges originating from both cerebral hemispheres. These abnormalities must be considered nonspecific but, when found in conjunction with other clinical symptoms and signs, add consistency to the diagnosis of a posterior fossa tumor.

The explanation for the tendency in childhood for projected slow activity to appear in the occipital regions with posterior fossa tumors remains unclear. The posterior rhythmic delta found in children with infratentorial tumors has been said to result from increased intraventricular pressure with distention of the walls of the third ventricle and distortion of the adjacent thalamic nuclei. Projected abnormalities via the thalamocortical connections are thus identified on the electroencephalogram.

Martinius et al. have suggested that the posterior arrhythmic delta activity often seen with posterior fossa tumors may result from regional disturbances, including interference with the posterior circulation or effects directly on the occipital lobes by upward pressure from the tumor. In a series of 124 children with cerebellar or fourth ventricular

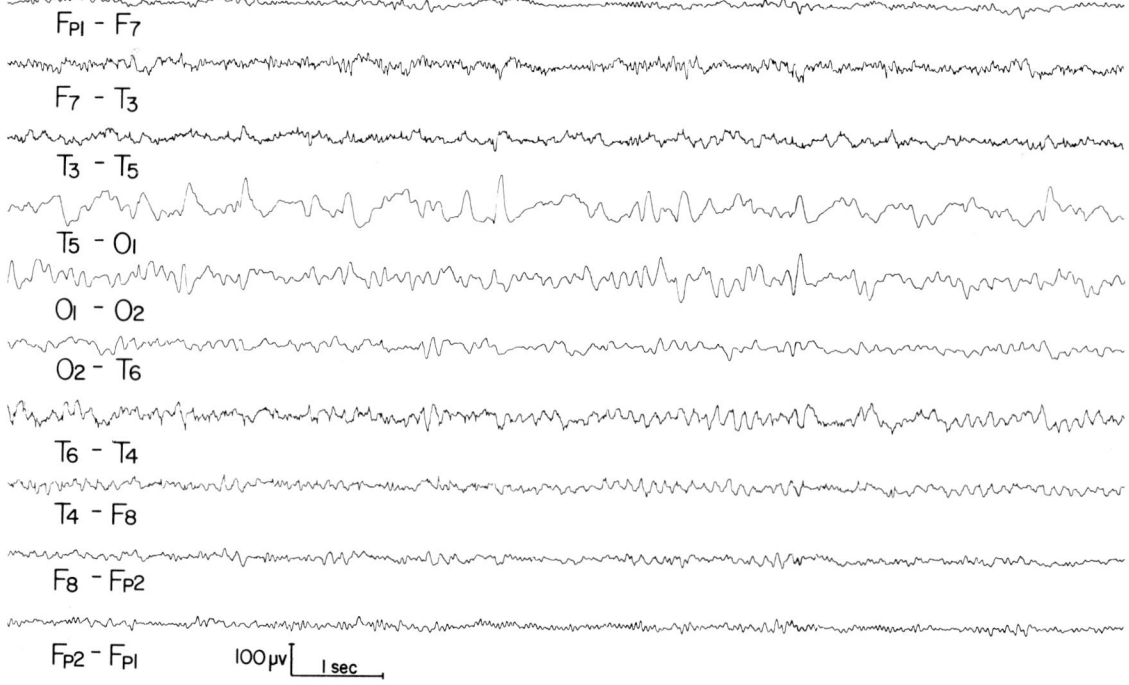

Figure 14–3. Electroencephalogram of a 15-year-old boy. There is high voltage delta slow and sharp activity in the left posterior temporal region. This type of abnormality is consistent with focal, structural cerebral disease, including neoplasm. (Courtesy of Dr. John Knott, Iowa City, Iowa.)

neoplasms, 81 per cent had abnormal electroencephalograms (Martinius et al.).

Cerebral hemisphere tumors in children usually result in electroencephalographic abnormalities, consisting primarily of focal slow disturbances (Fig. 14-3). Identification of the precise site and boundaries of the lesion cannot be anticipated from electroencephalographic analysis and depends on the clinical findings plus other ancillary procedures.

A slow focus resulting from a cerebral tumor is often displaced away from the anatomic location of the mass. Focal delta activity from a temporal lobe tumor is frequently projected forward into the anterior temporal region. Frontal and parietal lobe neoplasms may displace the focal delta discharges into the temporal region. The focal slow activity with cerebral hemisphere tumors may be continuous or episodic. The amplitude of the slow discharges is often markedly increased.

Both the slow activity and the increased amplitude may be accentuated by hyperventilation. During sleep, the slow wave focus with superficially located cerebral tumors is apt to persist and sleep spindles may be suppressed in the involved area. With more deeply placed hemisphere tumors, the focal slow abnormality may diminish or disappear in sleep. Sharp or even spike-wave activity may accompany the slow-wave focus originating from a cerebral tumor. Sharp or spike discharges are more often seen with temporal or frontotemporal lobe tumors than those located elsewhere. A localized, high-voltage spike focus with normal background activity and with accentuation during sleep is a rare abnormality with cerebral tumors and is more suggestive of a static, atrophic cortical lesion.

Deep-seated midline supratentorial tumors that impinge upon the third ventricle may produce high-voltage, bifrontal slow activity, either continuous or paroxysmal. The frontal slowing may be asymmetrical and may be associated with a diminution or disappearance of the alpha pattern when awake.

Thalamic tumors result in variable electroencephalgraphic abnormalities depending on the degree on extension of the lesion into the adjacent white matter and the presence or absence of third ventricular obstruction. Irregular slow delta activity may be present over the entire ipsilateral hemisphere in the tracing made when the patient is awake. Focal slow activity found in the tracing during wakefulness may be less well identified during sleep. The alpha rhythm on the same side as the tumor may become disorganized or may be absent.

A recently developed electrical diagnostic procedure for evaluation of brain stem integrity utilizes the electromyogram and is referred to as the pontogram. The procedure shows promise as a tool to assist the recognition of pontine gliomas, but further experience is necessary. The study takes advantage of the reflex blink of the orbicularis oculi muscle in response to electrical stimulation of the supraorbital nerve. Two components of the orbicularis response include an early ipsilateral and a later bilateral response. The bilateral response appears to be transmitted through multisynaptic reflex arcs within the brain stem. Comparison of the ipsilateral and bilateral reflex responses may indicate transmission abnormalities within the substance of the brain stem as opposed to peripheral seventh nerve involvement.

Visual Fields

Informative data from visual field testing is less often obtained in children with intracranial tumors than in adults. This is true not only because of the limitations of examination because of age but also because of the higher percentage of posterior fossa tumors in childhood.

The visual fields with posterior fossa neoplasms ordinarily reveal either no abnormalities or only enlarged blind spots secondary to papilledema. In rare instances, a bitemporal hemianopsia results from compression of the chiasm by distention of the third ventricle secondary to obstruction in the posterior fossa.

Formal visual fields by perimetric or tangent screen examination may be obtained on certain cooperative children by five years of age and on many by the age of six years. In younger children, testing for peripheral vision by confrontation is of general help but identifies only gross deficits.

A variety of techniques and instruments have been devised for visual field examination (Harrington). The particular type of instrument and method used are less important than the skill and patience of the examiner and the sustained cooperation of the patient. The patient being tested should be at ease and should understand the procedure. Visual field testing is a refined method of evaluation of one sensory modality and therefore is subject to the recognized pitfalls of subjective examination. Tangent screen testing provides excellent delineation of the central field and abnormalities therein. As a single testing device, perimetric examination is generally a more adequate and more reliable method. Certain centers perform both tangent screen and perimetric tests on each patient, with one supplementing the other.

Examination of the visual fields may be of considerable value as a screening procedure in instances in which a cerebral tumor is judged to be a remote possibility on the basis of the clinical findings. At times, one is surprised to find field abnormalities indicative of disruption of the visual pathways, thus clarifying the need for further diagnostic procedures. For example, a child with psychomotor seizures with no abnormal neurologic signs may have an electroencephalographic abnormality that does not clearly lateralize the primary site of the disorder. The identification of a left homonymous superior quadrant field defect might add enough suggestive evidence of a right temporal lobe lesion to justify right carotid angiography.

In a child with recurrent headaches of questionable etiology, the identification of spiral fields or markedly constricted fields would add support to a possible psychogenic explanation of the basic disorder, if the acuity is normal. Another example of the clinical value of visual field testing is the child with acquired diabetes insipidus in whom the cause has not become apparent. Serial visual field testing at periodic intervals in addition to careful fundus examinations is warranted in such cases. The development of a field cut or of optic atrophy would provide strong presumptive evidence of a compressive lesions in the region of the optic chiasm.

Visual field examination in children with intracranial tumors has its greatest benefits when lesions are located in or around the sella turcica. Tumors in this region often produce field defects of great localizing value. In addition, repeating the visual field examinations at intervals in the postoperative period or following irradiation therapy is helpful as an indicator of stability or rate of growth of the lesion. The most characterisitic field defect from tumors in this region is the symmetrical bitemporal hemianopsia seen with pituitary adenomas. Because pressure is initially exerted on the inferior surface of the chiasm by these lesions, the earliest field defect is often a bitemporal superior quadrantanopsia. As growth of the tumors continues, a more complete bitemporal hemianopsia eventually develops. Pituitary adenomas are exceedingly rare in childhood: however, other neoplasms in this region that cause field defects include the craniopharyngioma, glioma of the hypothalamus, glioma of the optic nerve or chiasm, and ectopic pinealoma.

A symmetrical bitemporal hemianopsia may be found in patients with craniopharyngioma, but it is more common to find an asymmetrical defect depending on the site of compression of the optic nerves or chiasm. Amaurosis on one side and temporal hemianopsia on the other indicates asymmetrical involvement with compression of the optic nerve on the blind side plus chiasmal involvement. Posterior extension of a craniopharyngioma may result in pressure on one optic tract causing an incongruous homonymous hemianopsia. Compression of the posterior rim of the chiasm containing macular fibers may result in bilateral central scotomas. This type of central field defect with craniopharyngiomas was emphasized by Wagener and Love and may lead to an erroneous impression of retrobulbar neuritis.

A cerebral hemisphere tumor results in a homonymous visual field defect if the lesion involves the optic radiations from the lateral geniculate body extending to the calcarine portion of the occipital lobe. As a generalization, more anterior lesions of the geniculocalcarine fibers cause incongruous, or asymmetrical, homonymous field defects. Lesions more posteriorly placed, in or approaching the occipital lobe, produce homonymous field abnormalities that are more congruous. A temporal lobe lesion interrupting the inferior surface of the optic radiations may produce a superior homonymous quadrant defect.

Involvement of the superior portion of the optic radiations by a parietal lobe lesion is more apt to be manifested by an inferior homonymous quadrantopsia on the side opposite to the lesion. Because of the lack of proximity to the visual system, frontal lobe tumors are less likely to be associated with localizing visual field abnormalities. Tumors at the orbital surface of the frontal lobe may be associated with unilateral optic atrophy with a central scotoma plus contralateral papilledema.

Radioactive Brain Scan

The radioactive brain scan has become a valuable ancillary tool for the identification and localization of intracranial tumors. As with other neurologic diagnostic studies, the degree of reliability of the procedure is dependent on the skill and experience of those responsible for its performance. When the procedure is properly done and interpreted, false positive scans are infrequent and the accuracy of detection of intracranial tumors in childhood is 75 to 80 per cent (Maynard and Kelsey, Mealy). Abnormalities

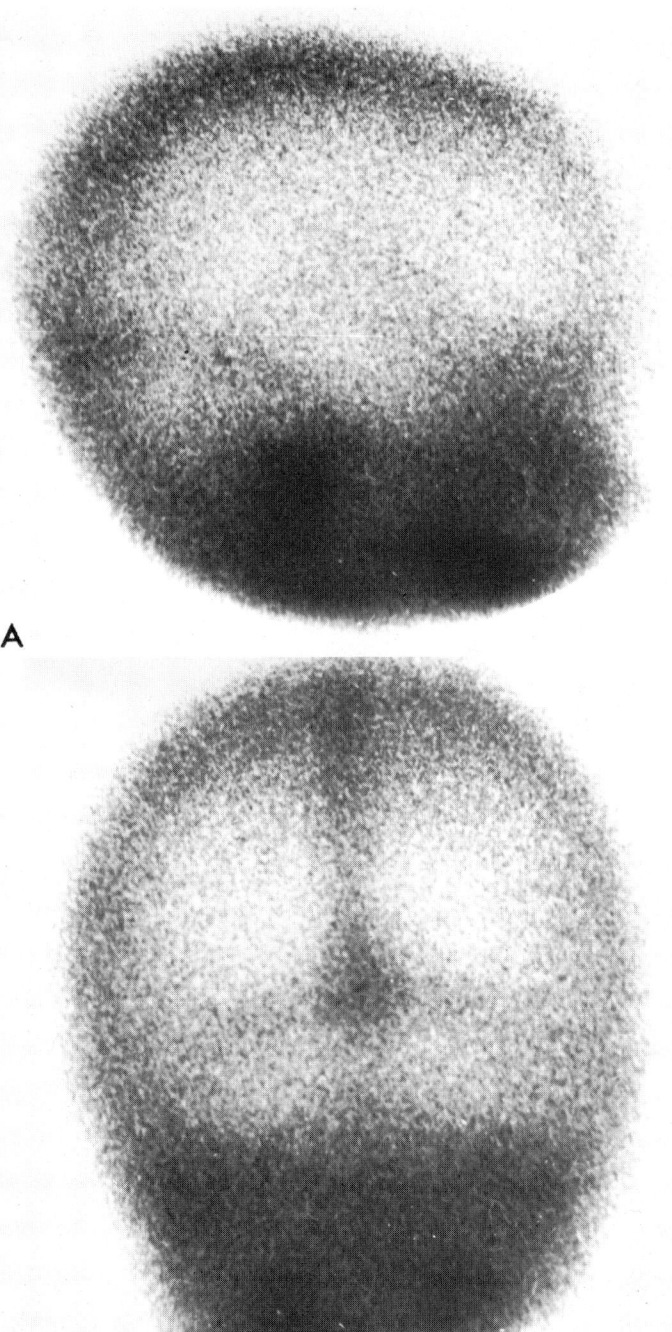

Figure 14–4. Normal radioactive brain scan, technetium-99m pertechnetate. A, Lateral view. B, Posterior view. Note uptake of radioactive material in superior sagittal and transverse sinuses. The torcula is well delineated on both projections.

identified by this procedure are not entirely specific for neoplastic disease. Positive brain scans may also occur with brain abscess, vascular malformation, intracerebral hematoma, cerebral infarction, cerebral contusion, and subdural fluid collection (Overton et al.).

A number of isotope compounds have been used as scanning agents, including chlormerodrin containing mercury 203 and 197 and more recently technetium-99m pertechnetate. The latter material is the agent of choice in most laboratories because its short half-life of six hours has considerably reduced radiation exposure to the patient. The optimal time for scanning for detection of brain tumors appears to be three to four hours after injection of this agent (Gates et al.). Uptake simulating that within a tumor is occasionally seen within the choroid plexus; however, this may be blocked by the prior administration of potassium perchlorate. Uptake of the radioactive material is also normally seen in the paranasal sinuses, the mastoid process, and major venous channels, including the the superior sagittal sinus, the transverse sinuses, and the torcula (Fig. 14-4). The latter may be erroneously considered as evidence of a posterior fossa lesion unless recognized as a normal vascular structure.

Precisely what factors contribute to the isotope uptake noted with intracranial neoplasms remains speculative. It is generally stated that more malignant tumors are more readily demonstrated by scanning techniques than benign ones and that those in the cerebral hemispheres are better identified than those in the posterior fossa (Tefft et. al.) (Fig. 14-5). The development of "angled" posterior views has facilitated the recognition of cerebellar neoplasms (Maynard and Kelsey), but tumors within the brain stem remain elusive by this diagnostic method.

Contrast Studies

Pneumoencephalography, ventriculography, and carotid angiography are the most extensively used contrast procedures for localization of intracranial tumors. Choice of procedure is determined by the probable degree of safety related to the anticipated location of the lesion and the presence or absence of increased intracranial pressure. In addition, the choice is made on the basis of the type of information one hopes to obtain judged from the clinical localization of the tumor.

In past years, many authors felt that

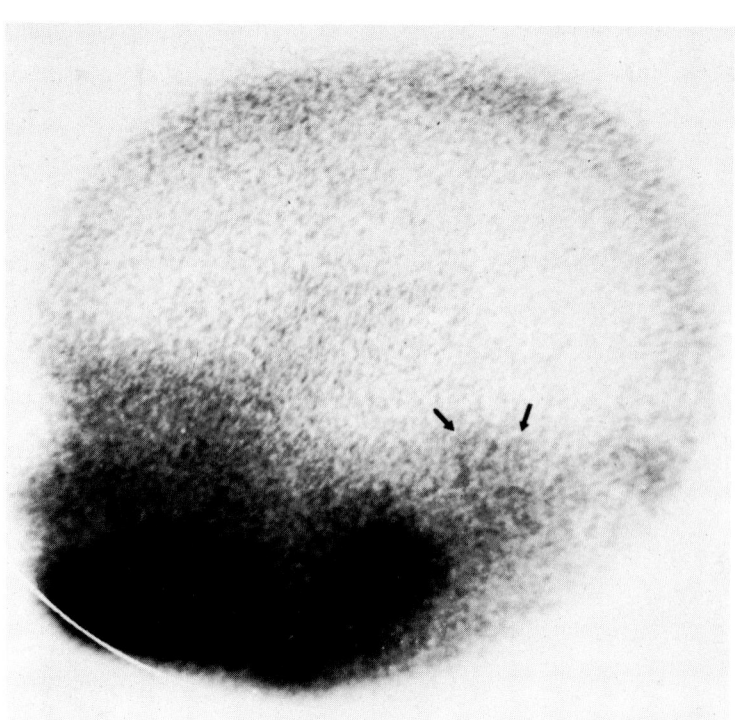

Figure 14-5. Radioactive brain scan, technetium-99m pertechnetate. Uptake of radioactive material within a cerebellar astrocytoma in a five-year-old boy.

pneumoencephalography (lumbar air encephalography) was contraindicated in persons with papilledema or other evidence of increased intracranial pressure. Ventriculography was commonly performed on such patients despite the less informative qualities of this procedure and the greater degree of technical problems. More recent advances in methodology including the use of the fractional, positive pressure technique for pneumography, have reduced the relative hazards of this procedure. If properly performed, lumbar encephalography appears to be as safe as ventriculography in patients with papilledema due to intracranial tumors (Norlén and Wickbom, Prince and Weiner).

More information is generally obtained from pneumography than ventriculography because posterior fossa structures are more reliably demonstrated by this procedure. Also, diagnostic evidence from air located in the extra-ventricular cisterns may result from the lumbar method. While each case must be individualized, most feel there is a place for either procedure, and in certain instances both studies may be needed to accurately localize a tumor. Ventriculography remains a reasonable choice in a child suspected of having a posterior fossa tumor with markedly elevated pressure manifested by lethargy, bradycardia, or high-grade papilledema. Burr holes required for this procedure in children beyond infancy provide a mechanism for rapid decompression if deterioration occurs during the examination.

Pneumoencephalography is the study of choice for tumors suspected within the brain stem and in or above the sella turcica. The procedure is also now widely used in patients with evidence of posterior fossa localization in which papilledema is mild or absent. Air is injected slowly via the lumbar route under pressure without removal of fluid. Serial x-rays are obtained as the air enters and passes through the fourth ventricle and aqueduct.

Neoplasms of the cerebellum or in the fourth ventricle may result in complete obstruction, preventing transmission of air into the ventricular system above. In this case, only the inferior portion of the tumor is outlined by air, and ventriculography may be required to demonstrate the degree of lateral ventricular dilatation and more precisely localize the site of the lesion.

With complete obstruction in the fourth ventricle, the pneumogram may show other abnormalities of importance. The location of the cerebellar tonsils may be demonstrated, either in the normal position or herniated below the foramen magnum. Air may not enter the lateral ventricles but may pass via the basilar cisterns to the pericallosal sulci. Stretching and dilatation of the callosal sulcus indicates ventricular enlargement, thus being consistent with obstructive hydrocephalus when air fails to pass through the fourth ventricle (Pribram, Jacobsen et al.).

With only partial obstruction due to a fourth ventricular or cerebellar tumor, lateral displacement of the fourth ventricle may be apparent on the anteroposterior view. Kinking of the aqueduct above the lesion at the level of the collicular plate on the lateral view is a common finding with cerebellar tumors (Fig. 14-6). Cerebral hemisphere neoplasms may be accurately localized by pneumoencephalography but generally also warrant carotid angiography before a surgical procedure is undertaken.

Pneumoencephalography must be considered a formidable procedure in children. With appropriate precautions, however, the hazards can be reduced considerably. When the procedure is done without general anesthesia, one person performs the test while another closely observes the patient's airway, blood pressure, cardiac rate and rhythm, and pupillary size. It is generally advisable for fluids to be administered intravenously dur-

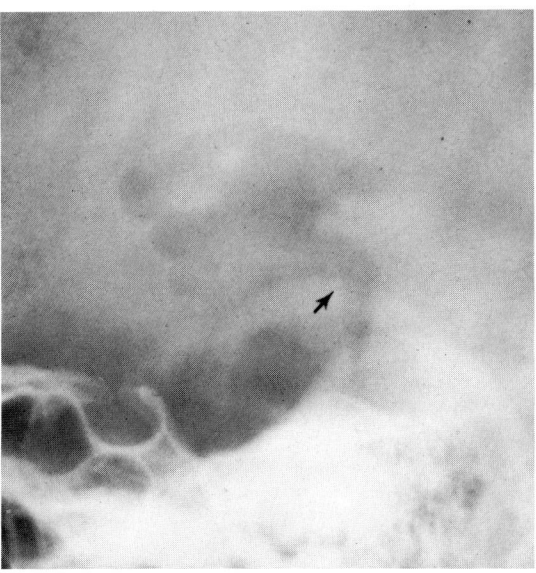

Figure 14-6. Pneumoencephalogram in a 14-year-old boy with a cerebellar astrocytoma. Kinking of the aqueduct (arrow) is indicative of a mass within the posterior fossa.

ing the procedure to provide an available route for other agents if necessary.

Equipment for endotrachial intubation should be available, in addition to a suction machine and face mask and bag attached to an oxygen outlet. This equipment should be examined and proved functional before the air study is started. Drugs available should include diazapam and sodium amytal for control of seizures, and sodium bicarbonate in case of cardiac arrest and subsequent metabolic acidosis. Epinephrine and isoproterenol may also be required if unexpected events occur.

Several potential hazards are present to the child during the performance of a pneumoencephalogram. The infant or young child may become hypothermic if completely unclothed in an air conditioned room, predisposing him to cardiac arrhythmia or acidosis. The sedated child in the sitting position with the neck partially flexed may hypoventilate, culminating in carbon dioxide retention and eventual respiratory or cardiac arrest. This is especially dangerous in younger children with preexistent air-way compromise as occurs with high-arched palate, unilateral choanal atresia, or markedly enlarged adenoids or tonsils.

Other complications of air encephalography include the possibility of air embolism or the accidental introduction of infection. Transient abducens palsies have occurred following pneumoencephalography. Transtentorial or cerebellar tonsillar herniation may occur, but the possibility is reduced by slowly injecting air and by using the positive pressure technique and removing only enough fluid to perform the necessary studies.

Ventriculography is the procedure of choice in the infant with abnormal head enlargement in which intraventricular or posterior fossa tumor is a consideration. Pneumoencephalography may be technically difficult in this age group because the shallowness of the lumbar subarachnoid space allows easy displacement of the needle tip, thereby interfering with further introduction of air. Ventriculography in older children with obstructive lesions in the posterior fossa has the disadvantage that markedly dilated temporal horns filled with air overlay and partially obscure the aqueduct and upper part of the fourth ventricle on the lateral projection (Fig. 14-7).

When this precludes roentgen diagnosis, or other mechanical factors prevent adequate visualization of the site of obstruction below the posterior third ventricle, Pantopaque ventriculography may be helpful. One to 2 ml. of Pantopaque is injected directly into the lateral ventricle and with the patient's face down, the material is collected in the anterior horn. The head is then slowly extended, allowing the material to pass through the

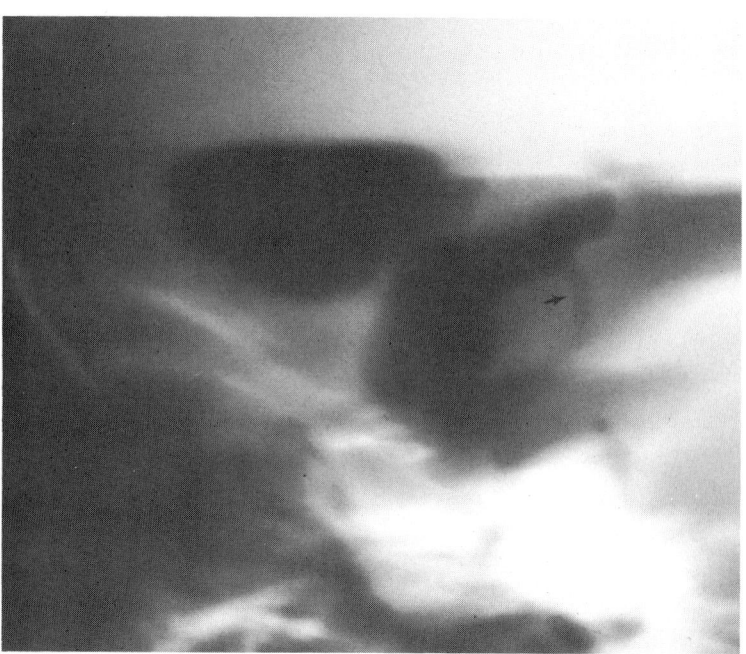

Figure 14-7. Ventriculogram in an eight-month-old child with a medulloblastoma. The aqueduct and fourth ventricle are displaced anteriorly (arrow) but identification is partially obscured by the overlying, distended temporal horn. Confusion of air shadows when the ventricles are markedly enlarged is one of the major disadvantages to ventriculography in patients with posterior fossa tumors.

foramen of Monro and to collect in the third ventricle. The head is then further extended, directing the material into the posterior third ventricle to enter the aqueduct. Serial films demonstrate the site of obstruction and position of the posterior fossa ventricular structures.

Although most patients with midline cerebellar or fourth ventricular tumors have dilated lateral and third ventricles, exceptions exist in which no dilatation is evident on ventriculography (Yashon et al.). This possibility must be kept in mind and is especially subject to erroneous interpretation if the aqueduct and fourth ventricle are inadequately filled with air.

Patients with midline neoplasms above the sella turcica are often subjected to carotid angiography in addition to air encephalography. The relation of the carotid vessels to the neoplasm may be useful information for the surgeon at the time of craniotomy. Angiography may help differentiate gliomas within the anterior hypothalamus from neoplasms that originate above the sella but extrinsic to the hypothalamus. Large aneurysms can occur in the suprasellar region and present as a mass lesion but are distinctly rare in the childhood age group.

Carotid angiography is perhaps the most reliable diagnostic contrast tool for cerebral hemisphere tumors in childhood. Most hemisphere tumors are well localized by this method, which also has the advantage of identification of vascular anomalies masquerading as a mass lesion. Angiography in children is usually done with general anesthesia. Anterior neck swelling following the procedure may produce stridor or other airway problems usually managed by humidification in a croup tent.

Vertebral angiography is a less valuable technique for posterior fossa lesions because localization is more precise with air contrast studies. In certain institutions, however, vertebral angiography is done as a preliminary investigation when a posterior fossa mass is suspected (Wolpert). Inferior cerebellar tumors produce abnormalities mainly in the position of the posterior inferior cerebellar artery, whereas superior cerebellar tumors usually elevate and stretch the superior cerebellar artery.

DIFFERENTIAL DIAGNOSIS

Differential diagnostic considerations include many disorders involving the brain in childhood, although there are a few special problems that closely resemble an intracranial tumor. Pseudopapilledema is an obvious example and must be distinguished from papilledema resulting from increased intracranial pressure. The problem is compounded if the child with pseudochoke is seen because of a headache disorder or because of seizures.

Pseudotumor cerebri manifested by headache, vomiting, and papilledema resembles a midline posterior fossa mass or intraventricular tumor so precisely that only air contrast studies can reliably exclude the latter. Clinical hints suggesting the possibility of pseudotumor cerebri include the appearance of a relative state of well-being despite the presence of papilledema. Also, recent withdrawal of cortiocosteroid therapy, intake of large doses of vitamin A, or obesity in an adolescent girl may be suggestive of this disorder.

Virtually identical symptoms and signs occur in children with obstructive hydrocephalus due to adhesive arachnoiditis obliterating the outlet foramina in the posterior fossa. Mild ataxic signs are often found, further simulating a cerebellar tumor. Ventriculography confirms the existence of obstruction in the posterior fossa, but diagnosis of arachnoiditis is established by craniectomy and visualization of the adhesive process. Dissection and removal of the abnormal meningeal tissue may be sufficient, although some subsequently require a shunt procedure.

Intracranial arachnoid cysts are mass lesions that occur in a variety of locations and produce findings that are indistinguishable from those of neoplastic lesions. They may become symptomatic at any age but most do so in infancy. The pathogenesis of these nonneoplastic, intra-arachnoidal cystic lesions is obscure, although some may be acquired subsequent to inflammatory disorders or head trauma. Starkman et al. postulated that some congenital arachnoid cysts were due to developmental errors during the stage of development of the arachnoid and subarachnoid spaces.

Symptoms and signs depend on the age of the patient and the location of the cyst. They may occur over the convexity of the cerebrum, in the parasagittal region, in or above the sella turcica, in the cisterna ambiens, dorsal to the quadrigeminal plate, or elsewhere in the posterior fossa (Fig. 14-8). Those located in the paracollicular region resemble collicular plate tumor with abnormal ocular signs, obstructive hydrocephalus and a poste-

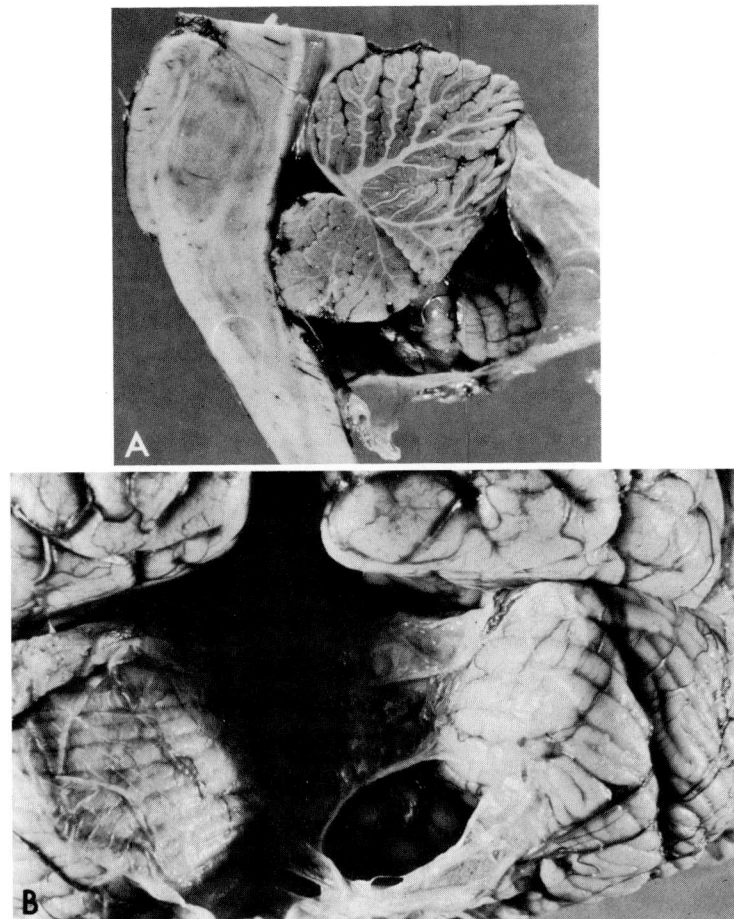

Figure 14–8. Retrocerebellar arachnoid cyst. A, Lesion posterior and inferior to the cerebellum collapsed during removal with escape of clear fluid. During the patient's life, the fluid-filled, benign cyst produced signs of cerebellar dysfunction and increased intracranial pressure due to compression of the fourth ventricle. B, View from posterior surface of the cerebellum reveals the delicate membranes of the collapsed cyst wall and separation of the cerebellar hemispheres by the mass.

rior third ventricle filling defect on air encephalography. This roentgen finding in the infant age group is strong suggestive evidence of an arachnoid cyst (Kruyff) because collicular and pineal neoplasms are unusual at this age.

Optic atrophy, visual field defects, and hypopituitarism secondary to a suprasellar arachnoid cyst are common features shared with the craniopharyngioma as well as other parasellar neoplasms and can be differentiated only by surgical exposure. Arachnoid cysts do not usually communicate with the ventricle or the subarachnoid space and therefore rarely accumulate air on encephalography (Berkman et al.). Although they are unusual, they are important intracranial lesions because of benign qualities, ability to cause pressure on vital structures, and potential curability with surgical treatment.

An occasional child with papilledema and symptoms of increased pressure with mild truncal ataxia is found to have intrinsic obstruction within the aqueduct without its lateral or anteroposterior displacement. This syndrome is usually thought to represent a midline cerebellar tumor until air studies are performed. Aqueductal stenosis or gliosis may remain asymptomatic until adolescence but is not usually considered when symptoms are recently acquired (Schechter and Zingesser). Either complete aqueductal occlusion or marked attentuation of the caliber of the aqueduct may be found on encephalography.

Both ventriculography and lumbar encephalography are usually required to be certain of the level and type of obstruction. The reduced caliber of the aqueduct in these cases may result from congenital stenosis, subependymal gliosis, or ependymitis. A low-grade periaqueductal glioma may also produce aqueductal occlusion without shift. The possibility of tumor in such cases requires periodic observation of the patient after symptoms of pressure have been relieved by a shunt procedure. Patients with a tumor would be expected to develop signs because of local neural dysfunction, whereas those with stenosis should remain well if the shunt functions properly.

Abscess within the cerebrum can be deceptive if the source of infection is not apparent or if fever and leukocytosis are absent. Signs can progress in a fashion suggestive of a neoplastic lesion with the true nature of the process becoming apparent only after surgical exposure. An avascular mass demonstrated by angiography is suggestive evidence of an abscess. Also, a brain scan revealing a circular lesion with a central area devoid of uptake of radioactive material justifies consideration of a brain abscess. Other inflammatory or granulomatous lesions that resemble intracranial neoplasm include tuberculoma, cysticercosis, and sarcoidosis (Goodman and Marqulies, Thompson).

The pronounced increase in intracranial pressure with a gradual, progressive history due to lead poisoning is a possible source of diagnostic errors unless the total picture is cautiously reviewed. Trephenation is potentially hazardous with lead encephalopathy because edematous brain tissue is prone to herniate through the burr holes. The history of pica or exposure to lead, the occurrence of convulsions, and the presence of anemia and proteinuria should indicate the more generalized nature of the illness.

REFERENCES

Berger, H.: Uber das Elektrenkephalogramm des Menschen III. *Arch. Psychiat Nervenkr.*, **94**:16, 1931.

Berkmen, Y. M., Brucher, J., and Salmon, J. H.: Congenital arachnoid cysts. *Amer. J. Roentgen.*, **105**:298–304, 1969.

Gates, G. F., Dore, E. K., and Taplin, G. V.: Interval brain scanning with sodium pertechnetate Tc 99m for tumor detectability. *J.A.M.A.*, **215**:85–88, 1971.

Goodman, S. S., and Marqulies, M. E.: Boeck's sarcoid simulating a brain tumor. *Arch. Neurol. Psychiat.*, **81**:419–423, 1959.

Harrington, D. O.: *The Visual Fields.* St. Louis, C. V. Mosby Co., 1956.

Jacobson, H. G., Zimmer, A. E., Schechter, M. M., and Shapiro, J. H.: The dilated callosal sulcus sign. *Amer. J. Roentgen.*, **94**:547–565, 1965.

Kruyff, E.: Paracollicular plate cysts. *Amer. J. Roentgen.*, **95**:899–916, 1965.

Madsen, J. A., and Bray, P. F.: The coincidence of diffuse electroencephalographic spike-wave paroxysms and brain tumors. *Neurology*, **16**:546–555, 1966.

Martinius, J., Matthes, A., and Lombroso, C. T.: Electroencephalographic features in posterior fossa tumors in children. *Electroenceph. Clin. Neurophysiol.*, **25**:128–139, 1968.

Maynard, C. D., and Kelsey, W. M.: Brain scanning in the pediatric age group. *Develop. Med. Child. Neurol.*, **11**:69–76, 1969.

Mealey, J., Jr.: Brain scanning in childhood. *J. Pediat.*, **69**:399–405, 1966.

Norlen, G., and Wickbom, I.: The relative merits of encephalography and ventriculography for the investigation of intracranial tumors. *J. Neurol. Neurosurg. Psychiat.*, **21**:1–11, 1958.

Overton, M. C., III, Haynie, T. P., and Snodgrass, S. R.: Brain scans in nonneoplastic intracranial lesions. *J.A.M.A.*, **191**:87–92, 1965.

Pribram, H. F. W.: Encephalography in diagnosis of posterior-fossa tumors. *J. Neurosurg.*, **19**:269–276, 1962.

Prince, D., and Wiener, L. M.: Pneumoencephalography in patients with brain tumor. *Neurology*, **14**:677–683, 1964.

Schechter, M. M., and Zingesser, L. H.: The radiology of aqueductal stenosis. *Radiology*, **88**:905–916, 1967.

Starkman, S. P., Brown, T. C., and Linell, E. A.: Cerebral arachnoid cysts. *J. Neuropath. Exper. Neurol.*, **17**:484–500, 1958.

Tefft, M., Jerva, M., and Matson, D. D.: Hg^{197} chlormerodrin for brain scans in children. *Amer. J Roentgen.*, **95**:921–934, 1965.

Thompson, J. R.: Sarcoidosis of the nervous system. Report of a case simulating intracranial tumor. *Amer. J. Med.*, **31**:977–980, 1961.

Wagener, H. P., and Love, J. G.: Fields of vision in cases of tumor of Rathkes pouch. *Arch. Ophth.*, **29**:873–877, 1943.

Wolpert, S. M.: Angiography in posterior fossa tumors of infancy and childhood. *Amer. J. Roentgen.*, **112**:296–305, 1971.

Yashon, D., White, R., Croft, T. J., Becker, D. P., and Jane, J. A.: Midline posterior fossa neoplasms without lateral ventricular enlargement. *J.A.M.A.*, **215**:89–93, 1971.

Chapter Fifteen

POSTERIOR FOSSA TUMORS

Approximately 60 to 70 per cent of intracranial tumors in children occur below the tentorium and the majority of these involve the cerebellum. Thus, evidence of acquired cerebellar dysfunction accompanied or preceded by signs of increased intracranial pressure represent the most common presenting complaints of children with brain tumor.

The neoplasms most often found in the posterior fossa include the medulloblastoma, cerebellar astrocytoma, ependymoma, and brain stem glioma. Hemangioblastoma is an unusual tumor in the pediatric age group, but it is of special interest because of its hematopoietic abilities. With the exception of an intrinsic brain stem tumor, which can usually be recognized by distinctive signs and lack of symptoms of pressure early in the course, most posterior fossa tumors are separable only by histologic examination. Although the clinical manifestations of the "average" case of tumor in this region can be viewed as stereotyped, the exceptions are frequent with a broad range of variations in the mode of presentation and the subsequent clinical course.

Headache is the cardinal symptom of a posterior fossa tumor. The complaint of headache typically is intermittent initially but becomes more frequent and more persistent with the passage of time. The location of headache in such cases is not specific and may be bifrontal or diffuse. In some children, headache may be almost explosive in onset, being precipitated by postural change, coughing, or physical exercise. Paroxysmal headache with systemic hypertension, palpitation, flushing, and tinnitus resembling the manifestations of a pheochromocytoma have also been described with posterior fossa tumors (Cameron and Doig). In cases of this sort, the abruptness of onset and transient quality of symptoms are often explained on the basis of intermittent obstructive hydrocephalus.

MEDULLOBLASTOMA

The medulloblastoma is a malignant, invasive tumor of the cerebellum, which occurs most often between four and ten years of age but also may be found in infancy and early adulthood. It accounts for approximately 20 per cent of childhood brain tumors and most commonly originates in the vicinity of the roof of the fourth ventricle invading the vermis.

Medulloblastoma was the term proposed by Bailey and Cushing in 1925 and has subsequently been shown to originate exclusively in the cerebellum. The cell type from which this neoplasm develops has been a subject of continuing debate; most authorities favor its derivation from undifferentiated cells with bipotential capacity for both neurogenesis and gliogenesis and referred to as the "indifferent cell" of Schaper.

Embryologic studies by Kershman have confirmed the existence of neuroepithelial cells originating in the roof of the fourth ventricle, which migrate to the external granular layer of the fetal cerebellum. Origin from such primitive cells with bipotential capabili-

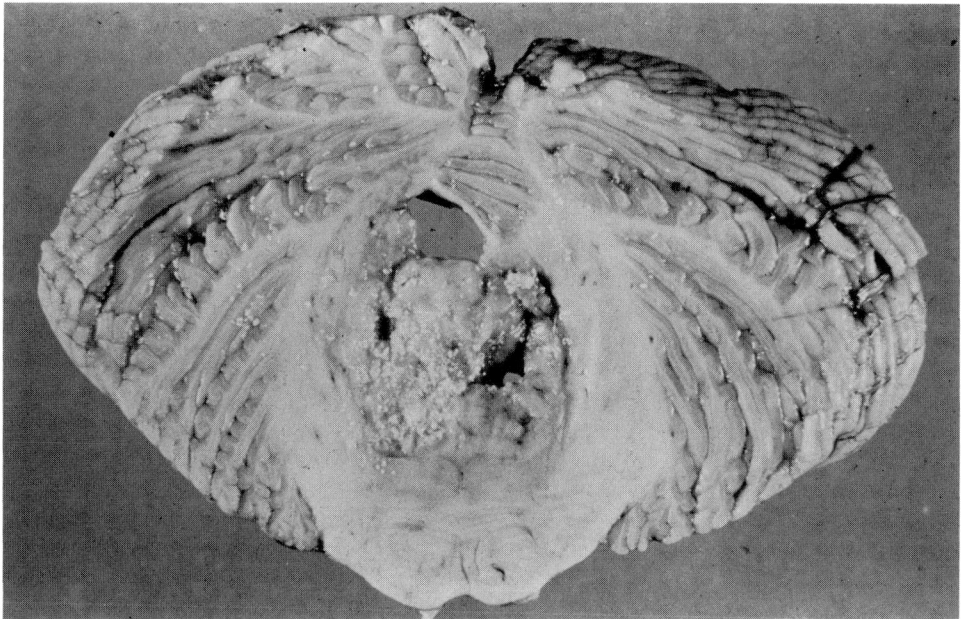

Figure 15–1. Medulloblastoma. Invasive tumor involving mainly the vermis of the cerebellum and almost completely occluding the fourth ventricle.

ties would seem consistent with the finding of maturation within a medulloblastoma to ganglion cell and glial cell forms (Kane and Aronson).

Gross observation of this neoplasm reveals its invasive qualities with growth into the fourth ventricle often with complete obliteration of its lumen (Fig. 15-1). The tumor is relatively noncystic; it may contain areas of necrosis and present a grayish or pink appearance as it projects into the fourth ventricle. It is extremely cellular on microscopic examination and contains sheets of small cells with densely stained nuclei surrounded by scanty, almost imperceptible cytoplasm (Fig. 15-2). Abundant mitoses and rosette or pseudorosette formation are seen in variable degree. As mentioned earlier, in rare instances, neuroblastic differentiation or spongioblastic maturation with the formation of neuroglial fibers may be observed.

The relationship between the medulloblastoma and the "circumscribed arachnoidal cerebellar sarcoma" has been a matter of interest and a point of dispute for many years. Numerous authors developed support for

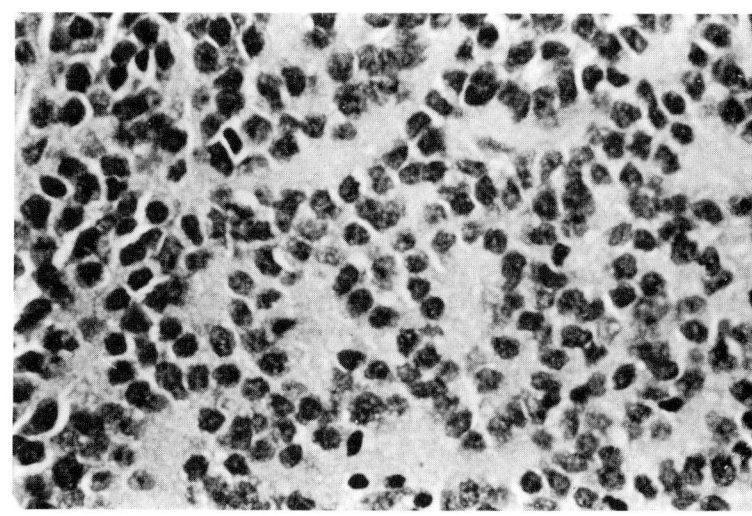

Figure 15–2. Medulloblastoma. Cellular neoplasm composed of small cells with densely stained nuclei surrounded by scanty cytoplasm. Note the circular arrangement of certain cell clusters around homogeneous material.

the existence of a sarcomatous tumor occurring mainly in adolescence and young adults and more often located in the lateral lobes of the cerebellum than in the midline. This tumor was said to be better circumscribed, carried a more favorable prognosis, and contained more reticulin fibers than the classic medulloblastoma. Rubinstein and Northfield attempted to resolve this nosologic conflict by describing transitional forms between these tumors. They preferred to consider the arachnoidal cerebellar sarcoma as a variant of the medulloblastoma and referred to it as a desmoplastic medulloblastoma because of the abundance of connective tissue, a concept we also hold.

Symptoms and Signs

Symptoms and signs of a medulloblastoma are those of obstructive hydrocephalus with increased intracranial pressure, and ataxia, largely truncal. Boys are afflicted with this tumor two to three times as frequently as girls. Headache and recurrent vomiting are the leading initial symptoms and have often been troublesome for one to four months before medical consultation is sought. As a general rule, the duration of symptoms before medical evaluation is shorter in children with medulloblastoma than with other cerebellar tumors, although considerable variation exists.

Recurrent episodes of precipitous vomiting sometimes precede other manifestations by several weeks. The mechanism evoking vomiting prior to other symptoms of pressure remains speculative although some have suggested a brain stem irritative effect. Vomiting is frequently without nausea and usually occurs early in the morning soon after rising. After vomiting, the child may feel well, have breakfast, and attend school without complaints until the episode recurs the following morning. During this phase, gastrointestinal disease may be suspected, accounting for the frequency with which upper gastrointestinal series are performed on such children.

Headaches soon develop and school performance, desire to participate in after-school play, and span of interest, decrease progressively. Ease of fatigue, listlessness, and personality change superimposed upon vomiting and headache may provide the stimulus for parents to seek medical attention for the child. Ataxia, especially involving the gait, may have been noticed by the child's parents but often is not recognized until neurologic examination is performed. Certain children exhibit only minimal or no truncal ataxia despite the presence of the tumor within the cerebellum. Diplopia may occur either early or late during the illness and is secondary to abducens paresis, which represents a false localizing sign due to increased pressure.

Medulloblastoma, like other posterior fossa tumors, is more diagnostically elusive when it develops in infancy. Irritability as a sign of intracranial hypertension is less specific than are complaints of headache in older children and thus is less easily analyzed. Also, ataxia is less readily recognized in the infant or toddler in whom tremulousness of the trunk or outstretched arms may be the best evidence of cerebellar dysfunction. Head enlargement, tense fontanel, and suture spread suggest hydrocephalus, with the true nature of the problem becoming apparent only with ventriculography.

Medulloblastoma usually afflicts previously healthy children; however, there are conditions in which a predisposition for this tumor exists. Medulloblastoma is one of several neurologic complications associated with the basal cell nevus syndrome (Berlin, Gorlin et al.). Ataxia-telangiectasia, better known for its relationship with lymphoreticular malignancy, has been described in association with medulloblastoma (Shuster et al.).

Evidence of recent weight loss and signs of increased pressure, including papilledema and often lateral rectus paresis, are noted on examination. Ataxia is apt to involve mainly the truncal structures, thus primarily disturbing the child's gait because the medulloblastoma tends to be located in or near midline structures. If gait incoordination is mild, it may be best demonstrated by observing the child while turning to walk in the opposite direction or while attempting to walk a line with the heel of one foot placed in front of the toes of the other foot.

Frequent yawning suggests high-grade increased pressure and, as with several types of posterior fossa tumors, may be accompanied by resistance to forward flexion of the neck. One frequently notices either head turning or a head tilt, with one ear directed toward the shoulder on the same side. In some patients, head turning or tilting is compensatory for double vision; in other children with posterior fossa tumors, the reason remains unclear.

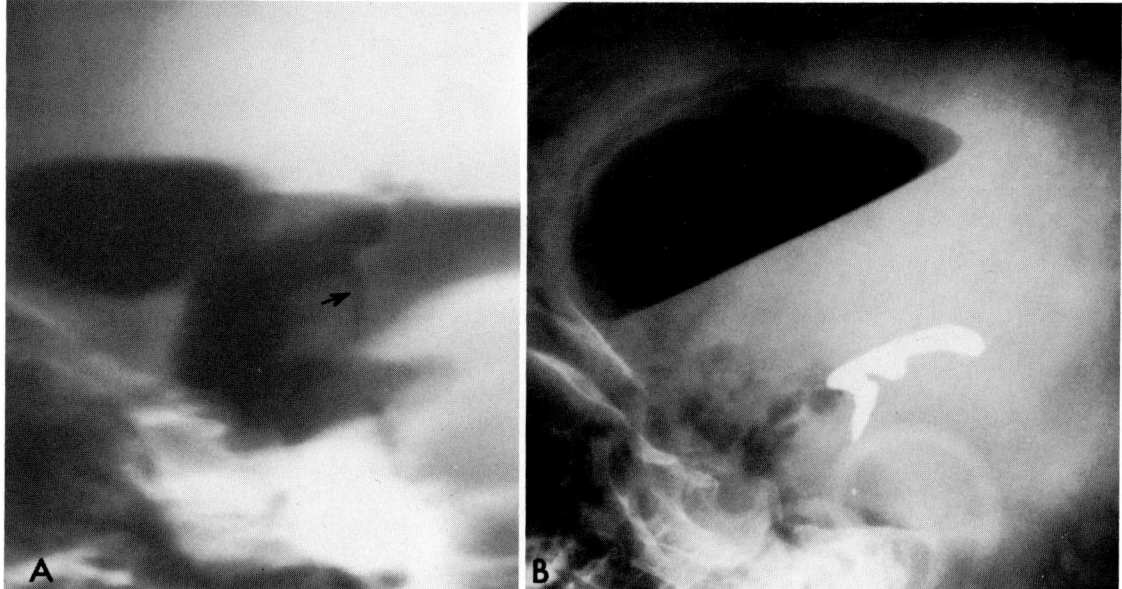

Figure 15–3. Medulloblastoma. Eight-month-old boy with three-week history of irritability, vomiting, and lethargy. Physical signs included head circumference of 50 cm., papilledema, and bilateral sixth nerve palsies. *A,* Air ventriculography revealed intraventricular obstructive hydrocephalus with forward displacement of the aqueduct (arrow) but without precise localization of the site of obstruction. *B,* Positive contrast ventriculography demonstrates radiopaque material in the posterior third ventricle and aqueduct with complete obstruction to its flow at the level of the superior aspect of the fourth ventricle.

Muscle tone and stretch reflexes in the limbs are either normal or diminished. Horizontal nystagmus is much more prominent with laterally placed cerebellar tumors and may be absent in patients with vermis lesions. Certain children with vermis tumors have limited upward ocular gaze, apparently a false localizing sign due to increased pressure. Rarely, massive bleeding into a medulloblastoma may antedate other obvious clinical manifestations producing sudden coma, decerebration, and usually a rapidly fatal outcome (McCormick and Ugajin).

Laboratory studies are generally not helpful but ancillary examinations, including skull x-rays, electroencephalogram, and brain scan, are consistent with a posterior fossa mass. Despite the histologic similarity to the neuroblastoma of sympathetic origin, urinary catecholamine excretion in children with medulloblastoma is usually normal (Drachman et al.). Air contrast studies confirm the diagnosis of a posterior fossa tumor, leading to decisions regarding the best mode of therapy (Fig. 15-3).

Treatment

Opinions differ in regard to the sequence and type of therapeutic approach. In patients with high-grade papilledema, some surgeons elect to place decompressing subgaleal shunts at the time of the ventriculogram and to proceed with craniectomy two or three days later. Others recognize hazard in delay following air study and perform surgery immediately thereafter. Surgical exposure and biopsy is necessary, however, because one cannot otherwise differentiate the partially resectable medulloblastoma from the removable cystic astrocytoma. When a medulloblastoma is identified, enough tumor is resected to establish patency of the fourth ventricle if possible. The need for a more permanent shunt is decided at the time of operation.

Postoperative irradiation therapy is indicated for medulloblastoma and is usually initiated 8 to 12 days following operation. Treatment is directed to the tumor site as well as the entire neural axis because of the tendency for seeding to occur throughout the subarachnoid space. Subarachnoid dissemination of tumor is believed by some to be enhanced by the operative procedure and may result in cranial nerve deficits, seizures due to cortical irritation, or spinal cord or cauda equina syndromes (Fig. 15-4).

In addition to its ability to spread throughout the subarachnoid pathways, extracranial metastases of medulloblastoma are well known (Drachman et al., Lassman et al.,

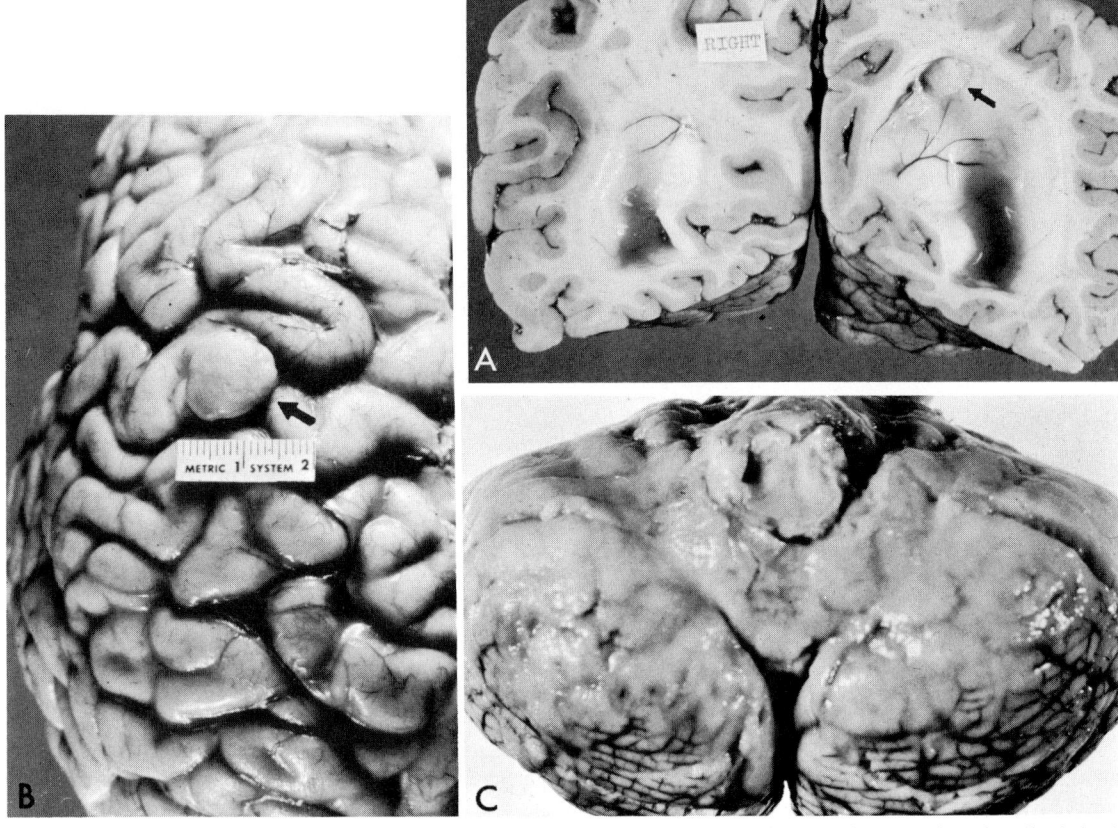

Figure 15–4. Medulloblastoma with subarachnoid dissemination. *A*, Seeding to the ependymal wall of the left lateral ventricle from a cerebellar medulloblastoma. Note the marked hydrocephalus secondary to ventricular obstruction in the posterior fossa. *B*, Metastatic nodule on the surface of the cerebral hemisphere. *C*, Glistening, white opacification of the basilar leptomeninges due to diffuse subarachnoid seeding from a vermis medulloblastoma.

Gyepes and D'Angio). Anemia secondary to bone marrow invasion, and bone pain due to periosteal involvement are potential complications. Makeever and King referred to a child with spread to the lungs via a ventriculovenous shunt.

Seeding to the spinal subarachnoid space may be treated by additional local irradiation to the suspected site or by daily intrathecal injection of methotrexate in a dosage of 0.25 mg. per kilogram of body weight for five days. Extracranial metastases to bone, lymph nodes, or other structures, as well as local recurrence within the cerebellum, have been treated with systemic vincristine sulfate (Lampkin et al., Lassman et al.) or a combination of vincristine and cyclophosphamide (Hagler et al.).

Prognosis

The prognosis for children with medulloblastoma remains guarded, but an attitude of total pessimism is no longer warranted. Bailey and Cushing recognized the limitations of radical surgery when dealing with this tumor, not to mention the relatively high operative mortality rate. Among patients who survived surgery and received no other form of treatment, the average duration of life postoperatively was 5.6 months (Faust et al.).

Awareness of the remarkable radiosensitivity of this anaplastic tumor promoted more aggressive treatment methods by radiation therapists, with gradual improvement in longevity resulting. In 1953, Paterson and Farr reported 7 of 13 and Richmond 7 of 14 patients living three years following radiation treatment. Subsequent advances have further improved the outlook, with the possibility of cure now within grasp. In 1969, Bloom et al. described a 39 per cent five-year survival rate among 82 children with medulloblastoma treated surgically and with postoperative irradiation. Additional improvement in treatment methods may come from further understanding of the most profitable uses of chemotherapy combined with surgery and irradiation.

The medulloblastoma is perhaps the most susceptible of all the common primary intracranial tumors in childhood to the effects of chemotherapeutic agents. The recognized proclivity of this tumor to be disseminated during operative manipulation might be inhibited by intraventricular methotrexate instilled immediately prior to the procedure. Other uses of these agents need further consideration and can possibly further improve longevity and reduce the mortality rate from this disease.

CEREBELLAR ASTROCYTOMA

This tumor presents a more optimistic outlook than does the medulloblastoma because many are completely removable, resulting in cure. This is especially true of those located within one cerebellar hemisphere with a large cyst containing a smaller mural nodule. Cerebellar astrocytomas represent approximately 20 per cent of childhood intracranial tumors (Matson) and thus occur at about the same frequency as the medulloblastoma. Certain authors have found it to be slightly more common than the medulloblastoma (Bailey et al., 1939; Cushing, 1931).

There may be little to differentiate these two tumors from the clinical standpoint because there is considerable overlap of symptoms and signs. The probability of a cerebellar astrocytoma, however, is greater when symptoms extend several months to a year, when it occurs in an older group in childhood, and when the signs point to involvement of one cerebellar hemisphere.

Cerebellar astrocytomas vary from those in the cerebrum by tendency to be better circumscribed and to be more often grossly cystic. Cystic changes may be in the form of microcystic degeneration within an apparently solid lesion. More often, there is a single large cyst containing xanthochromic fluid of high protein content with the solid tumor in the form of a smaller mural nodule along one portion of the circumference of the cyst. In one series of 75 cerebellar astrocytomas, 82 per cent were cystic and 18 per cent were solid (Gol).

Microscopic features of this tumor are variable with pilocytic, fibrillary and protoplasmic astrocytic changes, often associated with secondary and degenerative alterations. Transitional forms within a single tumor are not uncommon and foci of oligodendroglial cells may be inter-mixed. Rosenthal fibers are often seen but are not specific for this tumor or even for neoplastic disease. These fibers are densely stained, eosinophilic masses within the cytoplasm of tumor cells and may be found in glial tumors in varous locations. Leptomeningeal invasion by tumor cells adjacent to the lesion may occur.

Symptoms and Signs

Cerebellar astrocytomas may be located predominantly in the vermis, may occupy the vermis with extension into one hemisphere, or may be located entirely within the cerebellar hemisphere. Although these tumors are often thought of as laterally placed, in Matson's series, only 12 of 34 were limited entirely to one cerebellar hemisphere. The symptoms, and especially the neurologic signs, depend on the site of the tumor within the cerebellum. Those in the vermis differ little symptomatically from medulloblastoma, with headache, vomiting, papilledema, and truncal ataxia being common to both.

The cystic astrocytoma of the cerebellar hemisphere is usually also associated with manifestations of pressure but is more distinctive because of homolateral signs of cerebellar dysfunction. Horizontal nystagmus is most pronounced on gaze toward the same side as the lesion. Dysmetria, dyssynergia, and adiadokinesis are present in the arm and leg on the same side as the tumor. Hypotonia, hyporeflexia, and past pointing are also noted on the same side. A positive Romberg test and ataxia of gait may be evident but are overshadowed by the unilaterality of the coordination disturbances. Morning vomiting may occur weeks or months before other symptoms.

Some children with posterior fossa mass lesions describe a feeling of light-headedness, but true vertigo is unusual and usually suggests end-organ or nerve disease. In a minority of cases, cerebellar abnormalities and signs of obstructive hydrocephalus are accompanied by cranial nerve signs secondary to extension of tumor into or along the brain stem. In other cases, a cerebellar hemisphere astrocytoma may extend into the cerebellopontine angle simulating an angle tumor.

Roentgenographic Findings

Skull x-rays may be normal or show evidence of increased intracranial pressure. In children under 10 years of age, suture spread may be noted. In rare cases, mineralization within the tumor may be evident on x-ray. With long-standing increased pressure, erosion or thinning of the posterior clinoid process and erosion with concavity of the clivus may be evident. Asymmetry of the occipital bone is occasionally observed with thinning and outward bulging of the occipital squama on the same side as the tumor.

When high-grade pressure is obvious, air ventriculography is the diagnostic procedure of choice (Fig. 15-5). Fractional, positive pressure pneumoencephalography may be used when pressure signs are minimal or absent. When ventriculography does not satisfactorily demonstrate the posterior fossa structures, an attempt should be made to document the location of the tumor by fractional pneumography or Pantopaque ventriculography prior to the performance of a craniectomy.

The existence of a burr hole for decompression and injection of only a small volume of air via the lumbar route decreases the relative danger of the procedure. Some believe that if clinical findings are consistent with a cerebellar tumor, a positive brain scan and a retro-grade brachial angiogram are sufficient to warrant posterior fossa exploration without confirmation by ventriculography (Geissinger and Bucy).

Treatment

The cerebellar astrocytoma has been described as the most favorable of all intracranial tumors in childhood for surgical removal. Matson judged that complete removal was accomplished in 27 of 34 patients subjected to operation. Total excision is facilitated by the presence of a large cyst with a mural tumor nodule; however, even some solid tumors may be entirely removable. In those with extensive cerebellar infiltration or with extension via the cerebellar peduncles into the brain stem, only partial resection is possible. Postoperative irradiation treatment is indicated in these cases and long-term survival may follow. Adhesive arachnoiditis has been described as an infrequent postoperative complication with posterior fossa tumors and may require a shunt procedure (Matson).

EPENDYMOMA OF THE FOURTH VENTRICLE

Ependymomas may develop at any site within the nervous system where ependymal tissue is present but the region of the fourth

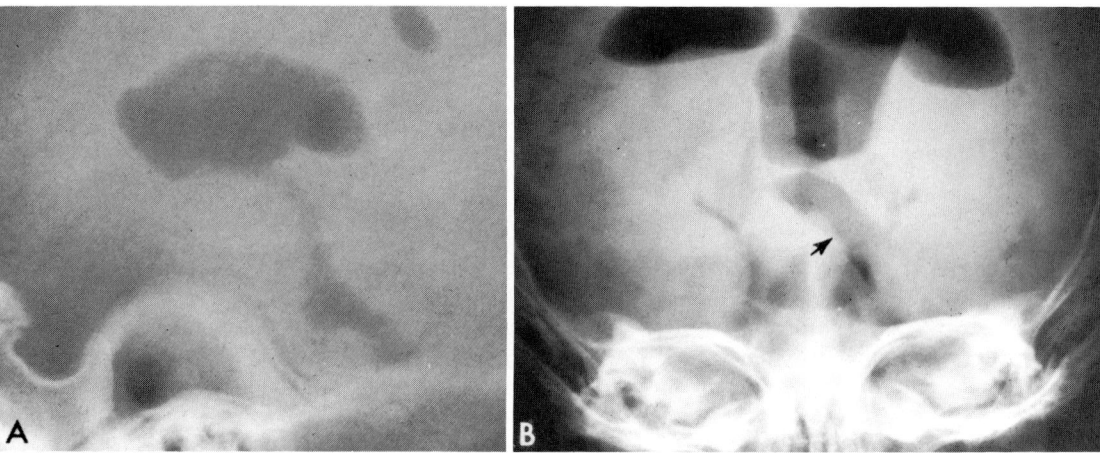

Figure 15-5. Cerebellar hemisphere astrocytoma. One-year-old boy with history of vomiting and irritability for six weeks. Physical signs included paralysis of the abducens and facial nerves on the right in addition to hearing loss on the same side. Cerebellopontine angle syndrome in children is often the result of a glioma within the lateral hemisphere of the cerebellum. *A,* Ventriculogram, lateral view. The third ventricle is distended and there is complete obstruction in the midportion of the fourth ventricle. *B,* Posteroanterior view shows enlarged lateral and third ventricles. The fourth ventricle (arrow) is displaced from its normal midline location to the site opposite of the tumor.

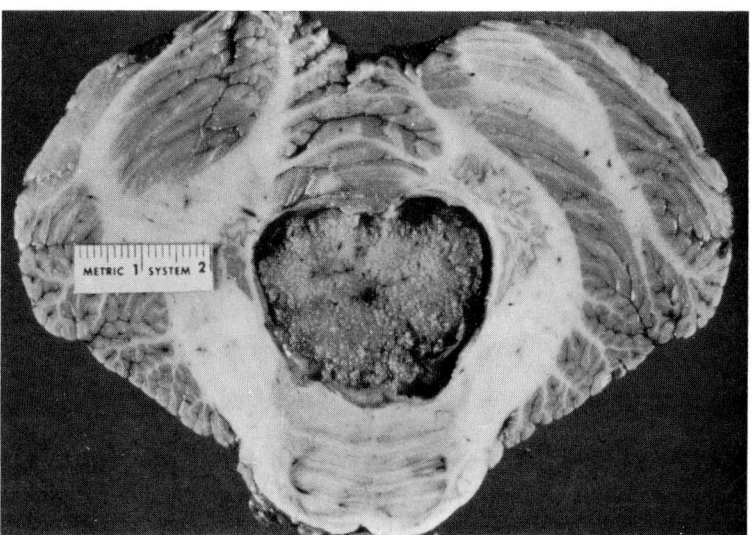

Figure 15–6. Ependymoma of the fourth ventricle at the level of the pons. The neoplasm has caused distention of the fourth ventricle and virtually fills its lumen, producing intraventricular obstructive hydrocephalus.

ventricle is the most common location. Its origin is more often from the floor of the fourth ventricle than elsewhere, and thus its attachment to the dorsal surface of the brain stem precludes its total removal. Less commonly, the ependymoma originates from the lateral medullary velum, a thin band of glial-containing tissue of the lateral recess of the fourth ventricle. Originating from this site, the tumor occupies the cerebellopontine angle, causing compression of the cranial nerves within this region in addition to ipsilateral ataxia and signs of increased pressure (Chusid et al., Kernohan et al.).

The ependymoma of the fourth ventricle is usually solid rather than cystic, is reddish gray, soft, and highly vascular (Fig. 15-6). Children with this tumor present no clinical features distinguishing it from other more common midline posterior fossa neoplasms. Identification therefore is usually based on histologic examination following craniectomy in a child recognized to have a fourth ventricular tumor. Age distribution is of little help because this tumor may occur at any age from infancy to adulthood.

Because of the location within the lumen of the fourth ventricle, signs of obstructive hydrocephalus represent the primary complaints in most cases. In certain patients, headaches, vomiting, and papilledema are the only abnormalities present, a situation that provides little localizing information and which may be misinterpreted as pseudotumor cerebri. Headache may be sudden in onset lasting only minutes and followed by a symptom-free interval until the next paroxysm. Some describe episodes of dizziness or light-headedness, perhaps precipitated by changes in posture. True vertigo, however, is uncommon.

Neck stiffness is sometimes found in children with fourth ventricular tumors and may be due to cerebellar tonsillar herniation or to extension of the mass into the region of the foramen magnum. It is imperative not to attempt forceful flexion of the neck in children with posterior fossa tumors because medullary compression and respiratory failure may result. Truncal ataxia reflects extension into the vermis and certain cranial nerve palsies may develop, either secondary to increased pressure or by direct brain stem infiltration.

The ependymoma developing in the posterior fossa may spread by subarachnoid pathways to remote sites. Cerebral, cranial nerve, spinal cord, or cauda equina syndromes may result from the diffuse spread of tumor cells.

Lumbar puncture is not indicated in a child suspected of harboring a fourth ventricle tumor, but when it is performed, one may be misled by the presence of lymphocytes within the fluid. The lymphocytic response may be erroneously interpreted as evidence of an inflammatory process, especially when neck stiffness is present.

Calcification within the tumor is rarely observed on skull x-ray. Ventriculography, demonstrating a fourth ventricular tumor, is followed by posterior fossa craniectomy with biopsy and resection to a degree permitted on the basis of the operative findings. If possible, the fourth ventricle is decompressed but many require a shunt procedure for relief of pressure symptoms and to prevent visual loss secondary to chronic papilledema. Complete removal can be accomplished only rarely. Irradiation therapy is indicated in instances of subtotal or partial removal.

HEMANGIOBLASTOMA

This tumor occurs rarely in childhood; most are found in the adult population. It is of particular interest, however, because of its potential hematopoietic properties and because of its occasional relationship with the genetic condition referred to as the von Hippel–Lindau syndrome. The hemangioblastoma may occur in a variety of visceral structures of the body and within the spinal cord. Intracranially, it is largely confined to the posterior fossa. Some have occurred in the pons or medulla but most are situated within the cerebellum. Here it may be in the vermis or one hemisphere, may be single or multiple, may be cystic or solid, or may be cystic with a small mural nodule.

Most hemangioblastomas are solitary lesions without associated erythrocytosis and without other stigmas of the von Hippel-Lindau syndrome. Microscopically, the tumor is composed of multiple blood channels lined by endothelial cells and separated by sheets of large cells with vacuolated cytoplasm and with oval nuclei. Large cysts are often located adjacent to the solid portion of the mass and contain deeply xanthochromic fluid, in part probably from bleeding from the highly vascular solid lesion (Fig. 15–7). The source of the fluid within a neoplastic cyst has been a matter of speculation, but studies suggest it is a plasma filtrate resulting from diffusion from capillaries of the tumor (Cumings, Gardner et al.).

The cerebellar hemangioblastoma has been described in association with pheochromocytoma (Chapman and Diaz-Perez, Nibbelink et al.), but its position within the von Hippel–Lindau syndrome is better known. This condition, inherited as an autosomal dominant trait, consists of retinal angiomatosis, cystic lesions of the pancreas, liver, or kidney, and hemiangioblastoma of the cerebellum or spinal cord. Although only the minority of patients with hemangioblastoma appear to be in this category, identification of this tumor warrants search for the other features of the syndrome. The solitary hemangioblastoma without other organ system involvement also may occur in several members of a family (Bonebrake and Siqueira).

Erythrocytosis is found in patients with cerebellar hemangioblastoma on rare occasion (Ward et al., Blumberg and Myerson). Only the red cell count and hemoglobin level are elevated while the white cell count and platelet levels remain normal. Solid tumors are more likely to be associated with this finding than are cystic ones within the cerebellum. Several theories have been presented to account for erythrocytosis in these patients, but the cause remains speculative. Some have suggested a pressure effect on the diencephalon; others have postulated respiratory depression with bone marrow stimulation from hypoxia. The most attractive postulate is that the tumor produces erythropoietin or

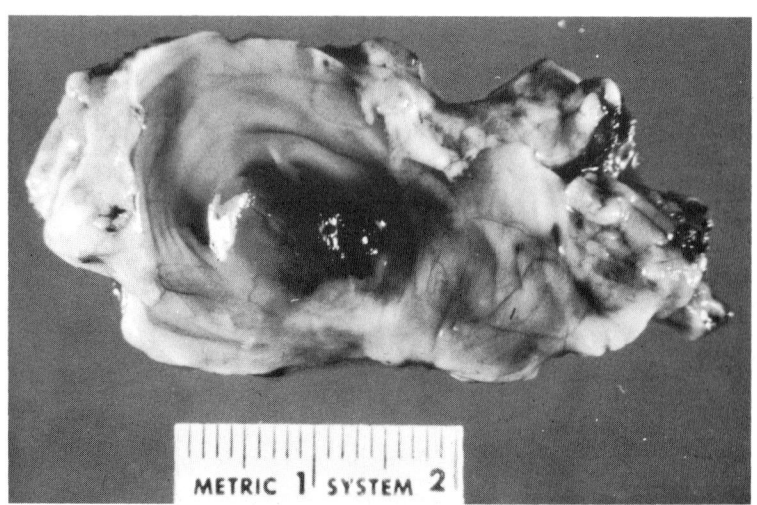

Figure 15–7. Hemangioblastoma of the cerebellum. Neoplasm consists of a hemorrhagic mural nodule surrounded by a large, solitary cyst.

similar substance that simulates the bone marrow to produce and release red cells (Brody and Rodriguez). After surgical removal of the tumor, the red cell count and the hemoglobin level return to normal in these cases.

Symptomatically, the cerebellar hemangioblastoma resembles other benign tumors in the same location. The suspicion of this particular tumor is raised preoperatively only by an associated erythrocytosis, retinal angiomatosis, or the presence of previously identified cerebellar tumors in other family members. Ventriculography or fractional pneumography is the diagnostic procedure of choice, although vertebral angiography is of value if hemangioblastoma is suspected.

Angiography demonstrates the vascularized portion of the tumor while a cystic component is evident by vessel displacement (Wolpert). Total surgical removal is often possible, especially in laterally placed cystic tumors with a small mural nodule.

BRAIN STEM GLIOMA

Tumors of the brain stem occur more often in childhood than in adults but any age may be affected. Most are found between three and eight years, with the peak being at six years of age (Bray et al.). It is unusual for symptoms of this neoplasm to develop in infancy. Luse and Teitelbaum described a new-

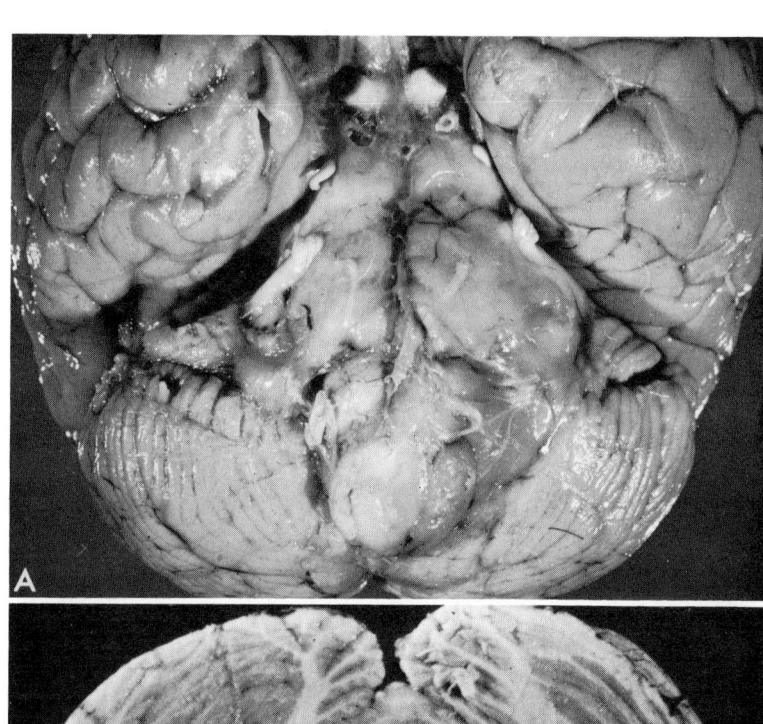
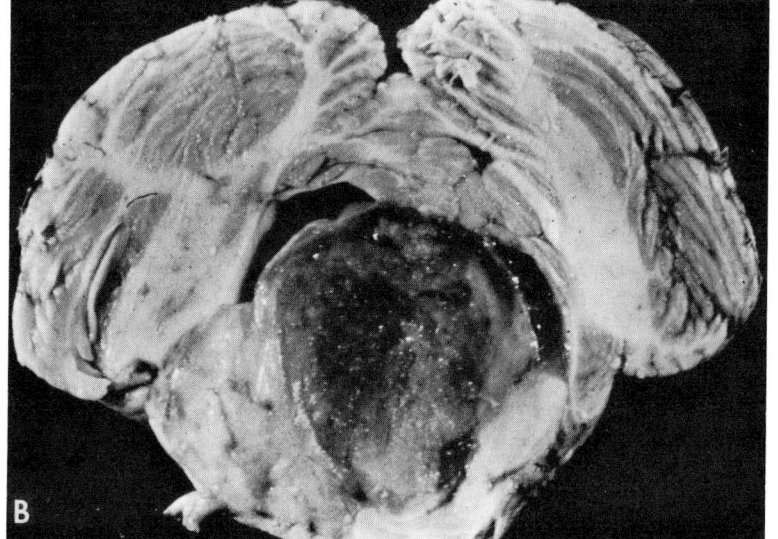

Figure 15–8. Pontine glioma. *A*, Neoplasm has resulted in asymmetrical enlargement of the pons with a nodular appearance in the region of the left cerebellopontine angle. The tumor also extends along, and involves, the left side of the medulla. *B*, Section at the level of the pons shows extensive neoplastic transformation with virtually no normal pontine tissue being present. Note the posterior displacement of the fourth ventricle, which represents the characteristic pneumoencephalographic finding in patients with this tumor.

born with respiratory distress and vocal cord paralysis resulting from a mixed glioma of the medulla. It is estimated that gliomas of the brain stem represent 10 to 15 per cent of intracranial tumors in childhood. The clinical triad of a progressive illness with multiple cranial nerve palsies, long tract signs, and ataxia is well known as one signaling the presence of a brain stem tumor. However, the exceptions to the rule plus more prompt request for medical evaluation for less advanced symptoms have enhanced the diagnostic complexities relative to this lesion.

Brain stem gliomas are predominately pontine in location but eventually may extend to the mesencephalon or downward into the medulla. Primary origin within the medulla or midbrain is less common and results in different presenting symptoms. Cells of this tumor characteristically infiltrate between existing neural structures separating them without causing destruction. Consequently, the tumor can attain remarkable size and produce surprisingly few symptoms or signs. Function eventually is compromised, however, and worsening of signs may occur in rapid fashion.

Viewing the brain from the basal surface, one observes marked enlargement of the pons in these cases (Fig. 15-8). Considerable asymmetry of the two sides of the pons may be evident with irregularity or even nodularity of the surface and with the basilar artery grooving the midline. In years past, this bulbous distention of the pontine region was descriptively referred to as hypertrophy of the pons.

The majority of brain stem gliomas are astrocytic in origin with different grades of malignancy sometimes being present within a single tumor. Most are fibrillary astrocytomas. Some contain histologic features consistent with the more malignant glioblastoma multiforme. The term spongioblastoma polare has been applied to tumors with elongated bipolar cells of astrocytic derivation.

Symptoms and Signs

The initial symptoms in children with pontine gliomas are variable. Although abnormalities of neurologic function probably most often develop slowly, it is not uncommon that they are abruptly recognized by parents or other observers and described as being of sudden onset. In some, a cranial nerve palsy is observed as the first abnormality; in others, staggering gait or clumsiness is the initial complaint. Seventh nerve involvement producing peripheral facial paresis is the most common cranial nerve deficit and is followed by a myriad of other disturbances of cranial nerve function.

Diplopia due to abducens nerve involvement, facial numbness or loss of the corneal reflex secondary to fifth nerve dysfunction, and dysarthria or dysphagia may subsequently become apparent. Horizontal and vertical nystagmus are frequently found. Other ocular signs that may occur include paralysis of conjugate gaze, or internuclear ophthalmoplegia due to invasion of the medial longitudinal fasciculus.

With the exception of trigeminal pathways, sensory fibers within the lemniscal system in the brain stem seem peculiarly resistant to the pressure effects of this tumor. Sensory deficits of the trunk or limbs are seldom identified until late in the course of the illness.

In addition to cranial nerve signs, most children with this neoplasm are ataxic with a combination of gait incoordination and limb dyssynergia. Bilateral long tract signs are usually elicited, although occasionally a hemiparetic syndrome is seen. The combination of ipsilateral facial and lateral rectus paralysis with contralateral hemiparesis is referred to as the Millard-Gubler syndrome, a pontine syndrome of highly localizing significance. Deep tendon reflexes are almost always exaggerated, especially in the lower extremities, and extensor plantar responses are usual.

Manifestations of increased intracranial pressure are not common in children with pontine gliomas but may develop with continued growth of the tumor. Lassman and Arjona found evidence of increased pressure in 6 of 27 children with pontine tumors; Bray et al. identified papilledema in 17 of 48 cases. Headaches may be present without increased pressure. Personality changes have been notable in some series and need not be the result of increased pressure (Panitch and Berg).

Gliomas of the medulla are less common than those in the pons and provoke lower cranial nerve deficits combined with long tract signs. Recurrent vomiting, sometimes precipitated by postural changes, vertigo, dysarthria, dysphagia, nystagmus, and atrophy or fasciculations of the tongue are findings common to this tumor.

Midbrain gliomas provoke variable symptoms depending on the mesencephalic structures involved. Those in the tectum of the midbrain resemble pineal tumors symptomatically, with ocular signs being outstanding. Upward gaze may be deficient because of superior colliculus dysfunction along with dilated pupils that respond poorly to light. Convergence paresis may also be present. Ophthalmoparesis, including ptosis, unilateral or bilateral, may be associated with these signs and result from oculomotor and trochlear involvement. Obstructive hydrocephalus due to aqueductal occlusion is more common with tumors here than within the pons.

Neoplastic involvement of certain combinations of midbrain structures may produce syndromes with eponymic designations. A unilateral third nerve paralysis with contralateral hemiplegia indicates involvement of the oculomotor nerve traversing the cerebral peduncle and is referred to as Weber's syndrome. Benedikt's syndrome is characterized by ipsilateral oculomotor paralysis with contralateral limb ataxia and tremor resulting from third nerve involvement as it passes through the red nucleus.

The foregoing descriptions of symptoms and signs represent the usual examples generally seen in children with brain stem gliomas. Some cases are far less clearcut, however, and one may not consider neoplastic disease until progression of signs has become evident. For example, abnormalities may be first noticed during or immediately after a systemic febrile illness leading one to suspect postinfectious encephalomyelitis. In others, multiple abnormalities of function may have been suddenly recognized and thus described as being of sudden onset, leading one to consider a demyelinating disorder. Rarely, the combination of signs of increased pressure and hemiparesis points to a cerebral hemisphere lesion until bilateral signs become evident or until air studies localize the tumor within the pons.

Another diagnostic pitfall occurs when portions of the tumor extend into the cerebellopontine angle, implicating the fifth through eighth cranial nerves on one side plus ipsilateral ataxia. The primary site of origin within the brain stem may not become evident in this case until craniectomy is performed.

Diagnostic Studies

Skull x-rays, electroencephalogram, and brain scan are generally of little diagnostic assistance in the child with a brain stem glioma because they are usually normal. Spinal fluid examination likewise is not revealing unless the pressure is elevated, in which case it may be misleading. The protein content may be modestly increased but usually is normal, and infrequently a few lymphocytes may be visualized in the fluid.

Pneumoencephalography is the most definitive diagnostic procedure for brain stem gliomas (Fig. 15-9). Lateral tomograms during the initial part of the procedure are of special value, facilitating the outline of the aqueduct and fourth ventricle. Diagnostic features of the air study include posterior displacement and bowing of the fourth ventricle, posterior and superior displacement of the aqueduct, and narrowing of the cisterna pontis with the anterior surface of the enlarged pons encroaching on the clivus. Occasionally, upward displacement of the posterior third ventricle is also noted. Despite its displacement posteriorly, the fourth ventricle is usually patent, allowing entry of air into the lateral ventricles, which are normal in size and shape. In rare cases, adequate air filling of the fourth ventricle cannot be accomplished. Visualization may be successful in such instances by Pantopaque ventriculography with injection of the opaque material into the lateral ventricle through a frontal burr hole.

Vertebral angiography may reveal a variety of distinctive changes in both arterial and venous phases in cases of pontine tumor (Huang and Wolf). Angiography, however, is technically more difficult and less reliable as a diagnostic tool for posterior fossa neoplasms.

Treatment

Except in unusual cases, neurologic signs localizing disease to the brain stem and the characteristic deformity on pneumoencephalography can be accepted as diagnostic evidence of a brain stem tumor. Surgery is ordinarily not indicated either for biopsy or therapy. Lassiter et al., however, have recommended surgical exploration in the hope of identifying a cystic lesion within the tumor. These authors operated upon 34 patients with gliomas of the brain stem and found neoplastic cysts of significant size in five which could be evacuated. Long-term survival occurred in four of these patients and was in part attributed to the operative procedure.

A ventriculoatrial shunt is warranted to al-

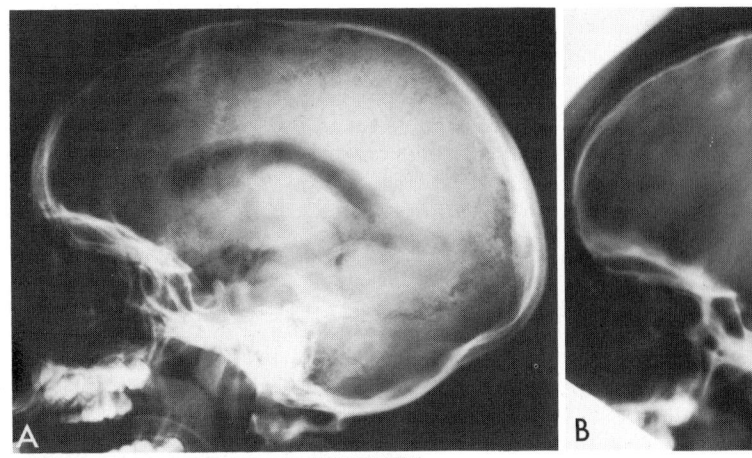
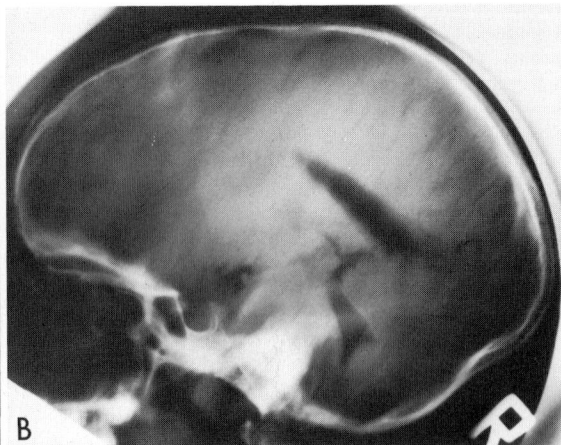
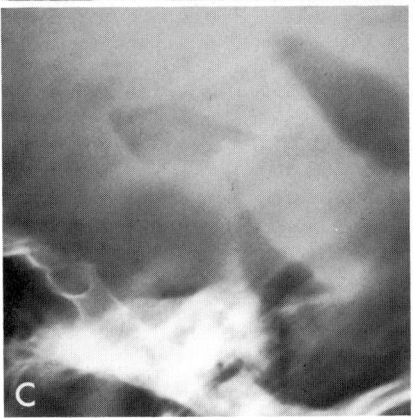

Figure 15–9. Brain stem glioma. Seven-year-old girl with multiple and bilateral cranial nerve signs, ataxia, and diffuse hyperreflexia. Symptoms and signs of increased intracranial pressure were not present. *A*, Pneumoencephalogram, lateral view. The lateral ventricular system is normal. Diagnosis cannot be made from this view in the absence of air within the fourth ventricle. *B*, Filling film showing the characteristic posterior displacement of the fourth ventricle and concavity of its anterior surface. *C*, Normal fourth ventricle for comparison.

leviate headache and vomiting in patients with obstructive hydrocephalus. Irradiation therapy is currently the most widely used treatment for the brain stem glioma. The tumor is invariably fatal, although symptomatic improvement may be expected with x-ray treatment. Improvement may be apparent within two or three weeks after initiation of treatment, but often it does not become evident for several weeks after completion. Lassman and Arjona found that survival time after diagnosis without therapy averaged four months, whereas in those receiving radiation it was 15 months. Survival in the series studied by Panitch and Berg averaged 15 months in the untreated group and 47 months in those given irradiation. An occasional child may survive for as long as five years after irradiation therapy (Redmond).

In the late stages of the illness, the child with a brain stem tumor becomes lethargic, intensely spastic with neurogenic bladder and bowel dysfunction, and with bulbar signs that prevent fluid or food intake. The child may linger in this stage for a surprisingly long period of time, requiring attention for the prevention of bed sores and nasogastric feeding for nutrition and hydration. Life-supporting measures beyond this are usually not indicated. Death comes from respiratory failure, from aspiration pneumonia, or from hemorrhage into the tumor with cardiorespiratory failure.

REFERENCES

Bailey, P., Buchanan, D. N., and Bucy, P.: *Intracranial Tumors of Infancy and Childhood.* Chicago, University of Chicago Press, 1939.

Bailey, P., and Cushing, H.: Medulloblastoma cerebelli: a common type of midcerebellar glioma of childhood. *Arch. Neurol. Psychiat.,* **14**:192–223, 1925.

Berlin, N. I.: Basal cell nevus syndrome. *Ann. Intern. Med.,* **64**:403–421, 1966.

Bloom, H. J. G., Wallace, E. N. K., and Henk, J. M.: The treatment and prognosis of medulloblastoma in children. *Amer. J. Roentgen.,* **105**:43–62, 1969.

Blumberg, B., and Myerson, R. M.: Erythrocytosis associated with cerebellar hemangioblastoma. *Neurology,* **7**:367–369, 1957.

Bonebrake, R. A., and Siqueira, E. B.: The familial occurrence of solitary hemangioblastoma of the cerebellum. *Neurology*, **14**:733–743, 1964.

Bray, P. F., Carter, S., and Taveras, J. M.: Brainstem tumors in children. *Neurology*, **8**:1–7, 1958.

Brody, J. I., and Rodriguez, F.: Cerebellar hemangioblastoma and polycythemia (erythrocythemia). *Amer. J. Med. Sci.*, **242**:579–584, 1961.

Cameron, S. J., and Doig, A.: Cerebellar tumors presenting with clinical features of pheochromocytoma. *Lancet*, **1**:492–494, 1970.

Chapman, R. C., and Diaz-Perez, R.: Pheochromocytoma associated with cerebellar hemangioblastoma. *J.A.M.A.*, **182**:1014–1017, 1962.

Chusid, J. G., de Gutierrez-Mahoney, C. G., and Garvey, T. O., Jr.: Ependymoma of the cerebellopontine angle in an infant. *Neurology*, **6**:152–156, 1956.

Cumings, J. N.: Chemistry of cerebral cysts. *Brain*, **73**:244–250, 1950.

Cushing, H.: Experiences with cerebellar astrocytomas. *Surg. Gynec. and Obst.*, **52**:129–204, 1931.

Drachman, D. A., Winter, T. S., and Karon, M.: Medulloblastoma with extracranial metastases. *Arch. Neurol.*, **9**:518–530, 1963.

Faust, D. S., Tatem, H. R., Brady, L. W., Olsen, A. K., Osterholm, J. L., Kazem, I., and Mancall, E. L.: Radiation therapy in the management of medulloblastoma. *Neurology*, **20**:519–522, 1970.

Gardner, W. J., Collis, J. S., Jr., and Lewis, L. A.: Cystic brain tumors and the blood-brain barrier. *Arch. Neurol.*, **8**:291–298, 1963.

Geissinger, J. D., and Bucy, P. C.: Astrocytomas of the cerebellum in children. *Arch. Neurol.*, **24**:125–135, 1971.

Gol, A.: Cerebellar astrocytomas in children. *Amer. J. Dis. Child.*, **106**:21–24, 1963.

Gorlin, R. J., Vickers, R. A., Kellen, E., and Williamson, J. J.: Multiple basal-cell nevi syndrome. *Cancer*, **18**:89–104, 1965.

Gyepes, M. T., and D'Angio, G. J.: Extracranial metastases from central nervous system tumors in children and adolescents. *Radiology*, **87**:55–63, 1966.

Hagler, S., Currimbhoy, Z. E., and Tinsley, M.: Cerebellar medulloblastoma. Chemotherapeutic remission with vincristine, cyclophosphamide and methotrexate. *Cancer*, **21**:912–919, 1968.

Huang, Y. P., and Wolf, B. S.: Angiographic features of brain stem tumors and differential diagnosis from fourth ventricle tumors. *Amer. J. Roentgen.*, **110**:1–30, 1970.

Kane, W., and Aronson, S. M.: Gangliogliomatous maturation in cerebellar medulloblastoma. *Acta Neuropath.*, **9**:273–279, 1967.

Kernohan, J. W., Woltman, H. W., and Adson, A. A.: Gliomas of the cerebellopontine angle. *J. Neuropath. Exper. Neurol.*, **7**:349–367, 1948.

Kershman, J.: The medulloblast and the medulloblastoma. *Arch. Neurol. Psychiat.*, **40**:937–967, 1938.

Lampkin, B. C., Mauer, A. M., and McBride, B. H.: Response of medulloblastoma to vincristine sulfate: A case report. *Pediatrics*, **39**:761–763, 1969.

Lassiter, K. R. L., Alexander, E., Jr., Davis, C. H., Jr., and Kelly, D. L., Jr.: Surgical treatment of brain stem gliomas. *J. Neurosurg.*, **34**:719–725, 1971.

Lassman, L. P., and Arjona, V. E.: Pontine gliomas of childhood. *Lancet*, **1**:913–915, 1967.

Lassman, L. P., Pearce, G. W., Banna, M., and Jones, R. D.: Vincristine sulfate in the treatment of skeletal metastases from cerebellar medulloblastoma. *J. Neurosurg.*, **30**:42–29, 1969.

Luse, S. A., and Teitelbaum, S.: Congenital glioma of the brain stem. *Arch. Neurol.*, **18**:196–201, 1968.

Makeever, L. C., and King, J. D.: Medulloblastoma with extracranial metastasis through a ventriculovenous shunt. *J. Clin. Path.*, **46**:245–249, 1966.

Matson, D. D.: Cerebellar astrocytoma in childhood. *Pediatrics*, **18**:150–158, 1956.

Matson, D. D.: Intracranial tumors. *In* Farmer: *Pediatric Neurology*, New York, Hoeber, 1964.

McCormick, W. F., and Ugajin, K.: Fatal hemorrhage into a medulloblastoma. *J. Neurosurg.*, **26**:78–81, 1967.

Nibbelink, D. W., Peters, B. H., and McCormick, W. F.: On the association of pheochromocytoma and cerebellar hemangioblastoma. *Neurology*, **19**:455–460, 1969.

Panitch, H. S., and Berg, B. O.: Brain stem tumors of childhood and adolescence. *Amer. J. Dis. Child.*, **119**:465–472, 1970.

Paterson, E., and Farr, R. F.: Cerebellar medulloblastoma: treatment or irradiation of whole central nervous system. *Acta Radiol.*, **39**:323–336, 1953.

Redmond, J. S., Jr.: The roentgen therapy of pontine gliomas. *Amer. J. Roengten.*, **86**:644–648, 1961.

Richmond, J. J.: Radiotherapy of intracranial tumors in children. *J. Fac. Radiologists*, **3**:189–199, 1953.

Rubenstein, L. J., and Northfield, D. W. C.: The medulloblastoma and the so-called "arachnoidal cerebellar sarcoma." *Brain*, **87**:379–412, 1964.

Shuster, J., Hart, Z., Stimson, C. W., Brough, A. J., and Poulik, M. D.: Ataxia telangiectasia with cerebellar tumor. *Pediatrics*, **37**:776–786, 1966.

Ward, A. A., Jr., Foltz, E. L., and Knopp, L. M.: "Polycythemia" associated with cerebellar hemangioblastoma. *J. Neurosurg.*, **13**:248–258, 1956.

Wolpert, S. M.: The neuroradiology of hemangioblastomas of the cerebellum. *Amer. J. Roentgen*, **110**:56–66, 1970.

Chapter Sixteen

TUMORS IN THE REGION OF THE PINEAL GLAND

Nowhere in the nervous system is localizing diagnosis of a neoplasm more dependent on correlation with functional anatomy than with tumors in the region of the pineal gland. The strategic position of these tumors in relation to the surrounding structures results in a multiplicity of symptoms and signs as well as distinctive roentgenographic abnormalities.

The term pinealoma has been applied to tumors originating from structures adjacent to the posterior third ventricle since its introduction by Krabbe in 1923. The term has often been erroneously used, however, to include all neoplasms in the region of the pineal gland rather than restricted to those of pineal origin. In addition to the pinealoma, or tumor of the pineal parenchymal cells, neoplasms in this locale include teratomas and a variety of gliomas. The classification of these tumors proposed by Russell in 1944 as follows has found broad acceptance:

1. Teratomas
   A. Typical and teratoid
   B. Atypical
2. Pinealomas
   A. Pineoblastoma
   B. Pineocytoma
3. Glial tumors and other forms
4. Cysts

Although the natural history and prognosis may vary with different histologic types, the signs of local neural dysfunction are similar with all varieties of tumor present in this region. In addition, because most tumors located in the pineal region are not approached surgically, histologic diagnosis is rarely obtained in life. The designation of "posterior third ventricular tumor," therefore, is perhaps the most accurate and noncommittal term for these lesions.

Teratomas developing in this region may replace the pineal gland, compress it, or leave it essentially intact. Some contain tissues derived from all three germinal layers, including cartilage, bone, cuboidal epithelium, and muscle. The so-called "atypical" teratoma has caused the greatest controversy regarding its position within the group and is perhaps the commonest tumor in the pineal region (Russell and Rubinstein).

The two-celled population characteristic of this tumor has been held by some as evidence of its pineal origin. However, the presence of other tissue components places it in the teratoma category. The two cell types include spheroidal cells with vacuolated cytoplasm inter-mixed with clumps of small cells resembling lymphocytes. The pinealoma originates from pineal parenchymal cells, which may appear poorly differentiated or may be mature. The poorly differentiated lesions resemble the medulloblastoma because of the extreme cellularity. The more highly differentiated tumors are less cellular and resemble more closely the normal pineal morphology.

Separation of tumors that contain proliferating pineal tissue from those that compress or destroy it is important in regard to postulated normal function of the pineal gland.

Although the precise regulatory influence of the pineal gland remains unclear, certain aspects of its function have been gradually unraveled. Descartes, in 1662, regarded the pineal gland as the seat of the soul; this was a generous proposal but one unsupported by subsequent knowledge of neural and psychic function.

In 1898, Heubner described a child with a pineal tumor who exhibited precocious puberty. This observation led to a correlation between pineal function and gonadal development. Several additional reports appeared of young males with premature sexual development with "pineal" tumors. The literature, therefore, came to include precocious puberty as one manifestation of the pinealoma. Some investigators believed that precocious sex development in these patients resulted from a substance liberated from the pineal tumor; others attributed it to compression of the hypothalamus, resulting in excessive release of gonadotropins from the anterior pituitary.

In 1954, Kitay reviewed the relationship between precocious puberty and pineal tumors. He made the interesting observation that pineal parenchymal tumors were only rarely associated with early sex development, but tumors in this region that destroyed the pineal gland more often produced precocious puberty. This led to the concept that the pineal gland perhaps could secrete a hormone that inhibited the development of puberty up to a certain time and that removal of this inhibiting substance allowed pubertal changes to occur prematurely.

The nature of the postulated substance remained unknown, but in 1958, Lerner and colleagues succeeded in isolating an indole from the pineal gland, which they called melatonin. Giarman and Day subsequently demonstrated that the pineal gland contained large amounts of serotonin, a precursor of melatonin. Synthesis of melatonin within the pineal gland has been shown to be related to light stimulation, which eventually influences the pineal gland by its innervation via the sympathetic nerves originating from the superior cervical ganglia (Cohen et al.). The demonstration that melatonin produced in the pineal gland can inhibit gonadal function (Wurtman et al.) seemed consistent with the observations by Kitay regarding type of tumor and effect on sex maturation.

In view of our present information, one may postulate that a pinealoma, or tumor of pineal parenchymal cells, may be associated with delayed sexual maturation because of hyperactivity of cell function with elaboration of greater than normal levels of gonadal-inhibiting melatonin. Conversely, a tumor in the region of the pineal gland that destroys pineal function might be expected to be associated with precocious sexual development in childhood.

Much of the basis for these physiologic concepts rests on experimental studies in animals and remains to be documented in humans. The concepts appear sound, however, and are reasonably consistent with past clinical experiences. It should be added that most often tumors in the pineal region in childhood are not associated with any abnormality of sexual maturation that is apparent.

PINEALOMA

The pinealoma is a rare intracranial tumor that develops inferior to the splenium of the corpus callosum, dorsal to the quadrigeminal plate, and posterior to the hypothalamus and third ventricle. Tumors with morphology resembling pineal tissue may develop elsewhere, especially in the chiasmatic region, and are designated ectopic pinealomas. Seeding to the suprasellar area from the primary site of origin may occur in rare cases, resulting in diabetes insipidus, visual field defects, or hypopituitarism.

Symptoms and Signs

The symptoms and signs of the pinealoma are evident from knowledge of the anatomy adjacent to its site of origin. Obstructive hydrocephalus due to aqueductal compression occurs early in most cases, leading to headache, vomiting episodes, and papilledema. Blurred vision is described by some patients with high-grade papilledema. Diplopia may occur because of lateral rectus paresis secondary to increased pressure. Ataxia of gait is a common early sign and is caused by compression of the superior cerebellar peduncle within the brain stem.

A rare neurologic finding in children with a pinealoma is mild chorea, the cause of which is unknown. Most children afflicted by this tumor have no abnormalities of sex development but theoretically, delayed pubertal change might be expected in some patients as discussed previously.

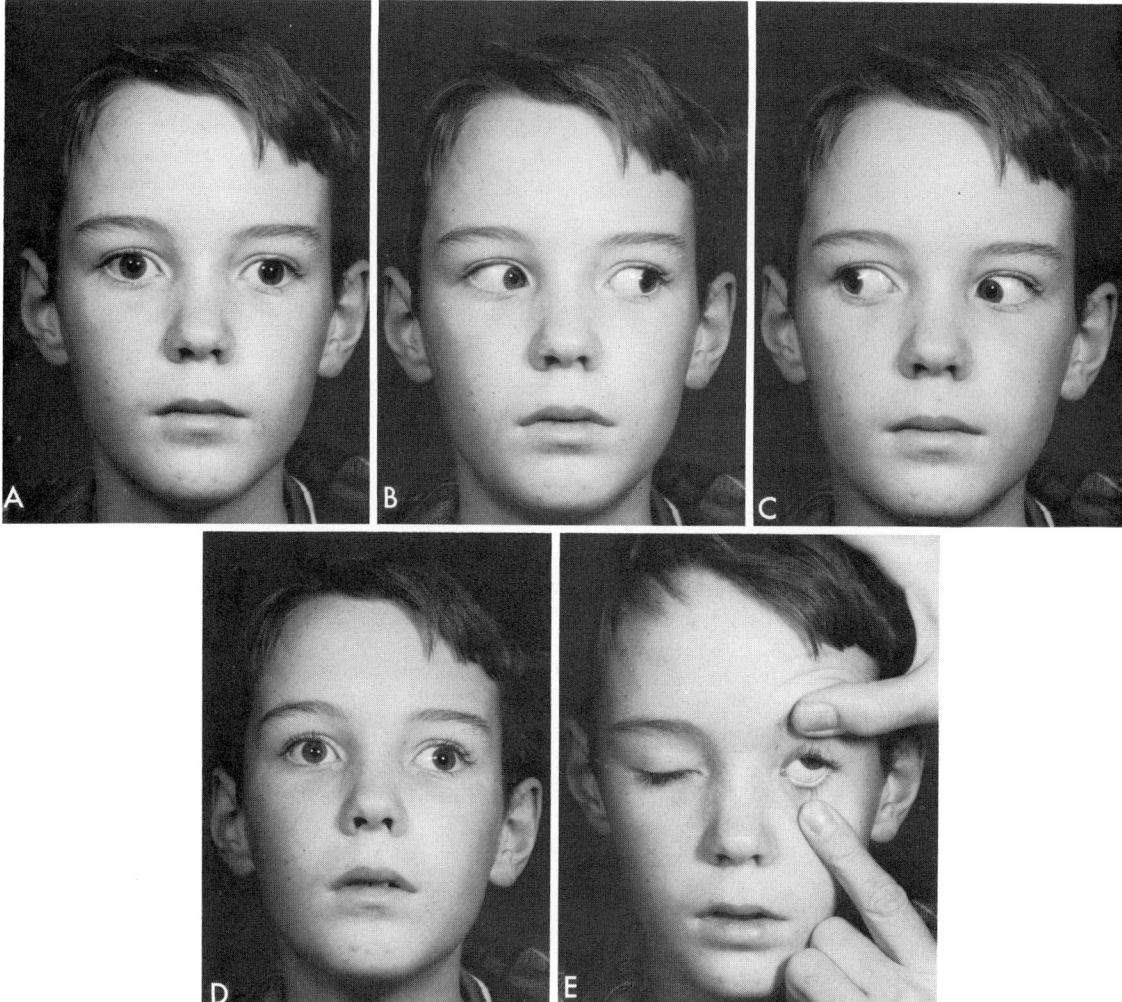

Figure 16–1. Pinealoma. Fourteen-year-old boy with ocular signs indicative of a tumor in the region of the posterior portion of the third ventricle. *A*, Gaze directly forward. Mild pupillary dilatation is present despite bright illumination for photography. *B*, Normal horizontal gaze to the left. *C*, Essentially normal horizontal gaze to the right except for slight deviation downward of the left eye. *D*, Attempted gaze upward demonstrates nearly complete paralysis of upward movement (Parinaud's syndrome). *E*, With forced eyelid closure, the left eye is noted to rotate upward (Bell's phenomenon), indicating the central origin of the upward gaze paralysis demonstrated in *D*.

The most definitive localizing signs in a child with a pineal tumor are those pertaining to ocular function and pupillary disturbance (Fig. 16-1). Paralysis of vertical conjugate gaze upward occurs in most such patients. Its supranuclear origin is apparent when following upward gaze is absent but when upward deviation of the eyes is demonstrated during forced eyelid closure, or the so-called Bell's phenomenon.

The mechanism of this defect of vertical conjugate gaze has been eloquently described by Crosby. Fibers form occipital areas eighteen and nineteen from internal corticotectal fibers, which project to the rostromedial portions of the paired superior colliculi of the dorsal midbrain. Tecto-oculomotor fibers therefrom pass to portions of the oculomotor nuclei innervating muscles that result in elevation of the eyes. Thus, compression of the dorsal and medial surfaces of the superior colliculi disrupts this fiber system, causing bilateral upward gaze paralysis and mild ptosis. This complex of findings is the Parinaud syndrome and is suggestive but not diagnostic of neoplastic disease involving the dorsal midbrain.

Following movements in the horizontal

plane are not disturbed because occipital fibers related to horizontal ocular movement are collected in the corticotegmental pathways passing ventrally to bypass the collicular plate. It has been said that extension of the tumor to involve the caudolateral portion of the superior colliculi will cause paralysis of conjugate gaze downward (Crosby), but this must be infrequent.

The pupils are usually symmetrically dilated in these patients and react poorly to light, if at all. This pupillary disturbance is attributed to compression of the pretectal nuclei and the interconnection through the posterior commissure. Fibers in the optic tract concerned with light reflexes synapse in the ipsilateral pretectal nucleus in the dorsal mesencephalon. From the pretectal nucleus, connections are made with Edinger-Westphal nuclei of the oculomotor complex. Fibers then pass to the ciliary ganglion where postganglionic fibers are relayed to the sphincter of the iris, resulting in pupillary constriction from light stimulation. Interruption of this pathway at the pretectal level causes dilated pupils that are unresponsive to light but may constrict on accommodation. Analysis of ocular gaze abnormalities may become

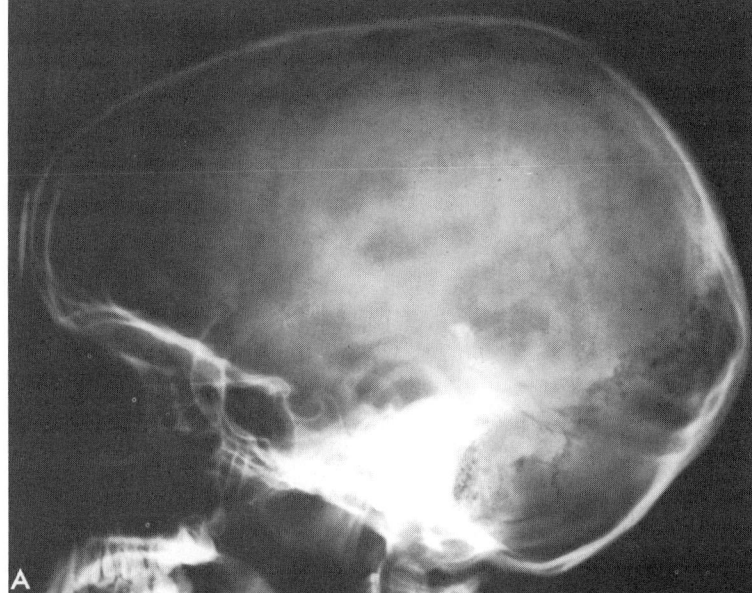

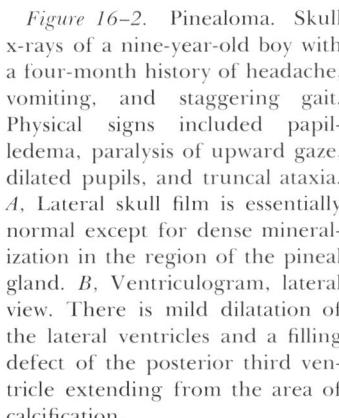

Figure 16–2. Pinealoma. Skull x-rays of a nine-year-old boy with a four-month history of headache, vomiting, and staggering gait. Physical signs included papilledema, paralysis of upward gaze, dilated pupils, and truncal ataxia. *A*, Lateral skull film is essentially normal except for dense mineralization in the region of the pineal gland. *B*, Ventriculogram, lateral view. There is mild dilatation of the lateral ventricles and a filling defect of the posterior third ventricle extending from the area of calcification.

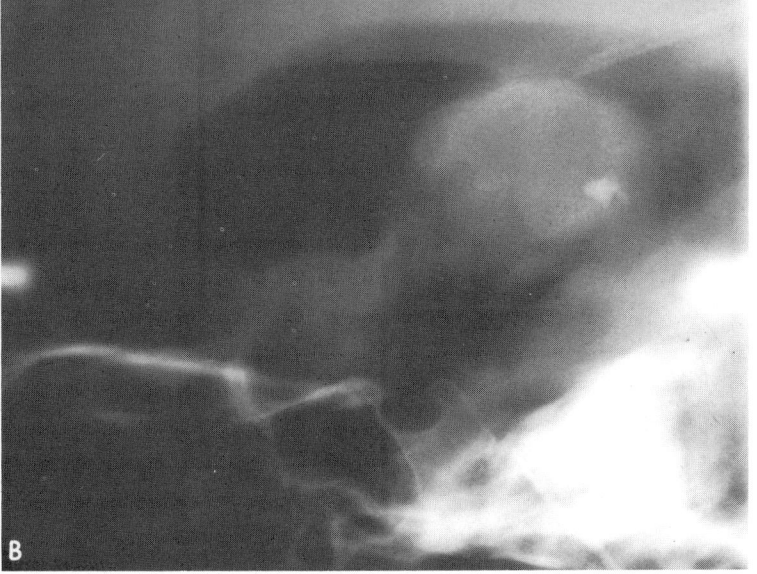

complicated if an abducens palsy results from pressure or if oculomotor paralysis occurs from neoplastic infiltration of the oculomotor nuclear complex.

Additional unusual signs that have been noted in children with pineal tumors include convergence spasm, nystagmus retractorium, and hearing loss. The hearing loss is attributed to spread of the tumor inferiorly to the inferior colliculi, an important way station for auditory impulses passing to the cerebral cortex. Long tract signs manifested by hyperreflexia and pathologic toe signs may occur but are not common.

Roentgenographic Findings

Skull x-rays may be normal but usually show evidence of increased intracranial pressure. Mineralization of the pineal gland in children less than 10 years of age is sufficiently unusual that it is regarded as presumptive evidence of a neoplastic process (Fig. 16-2). Pineal teratomas are more apt than parenchymal pinealomas to show calcification on x-ray.

Clinical evidence of a pineal tumor should be confirmed by ventriculography. The brow-down lateral and tomogram lateral views reveal a posterior third ventricular filling defect, usually with obstruction of the aqueduct and ventricular distention. The suprapineal recess is almost always obliterated. Carotid angiography is generally not necessary or indicated, but if it is performed, the bowed sweep of the anterior cerebral vessels reflects the underlying lateral ventricular dilatation. On the venous phase, the vein of Galen is displaced superiorly with distortion of its normal curvature.

Treatment

Treatment of a pineal tumor includes a procedure to circumvent increased pressure and application of irradiation therapy to the tumor site. In past years, surgeons attempted to remove tumors of the posterior third ventricle through the splenium of the corpus callosum but with a high mortality rate. Horrax emphasized the hazards of surgery in this region either for biopsy or removal of the tumor and advocated irradiation therapy accompanied by subtemporal decompression. Others recommended third ventriculostomy for decompression. More recently, most authorities prefer either a ventriculoatrial shunt or ventriculocisternostomy to relieve manifestations of pressure. Ventriculoatrial shunt is technically less difficult, but ventriculocisternostomy has fewer late complications to beset its function.

Pineal tumors are now usually treated with irradiation therapy without biopsy confirmation and with fair to good results regarding long-term survival (Cummins et al., Poppen and Marino). The response to irradiation is variable, but some patients improve greatly and remain well for many years.

REFERENCES

Cohen, R. A., Wurtman, R. J., Axelrod, J., and Snyder, S. H.: Some clinical, biochemical, and physiological actions of the pineal gland. *Ann. Intern. Med.*, **61**:1144–1161, 1964.

Crosby, E. C.: *In* Kahn, E. A., Bassett, R. C., Schneider, R. C., and Crosby, E. C.: *Correlative Neurosurgery*, Springfield, Ill., Charles C Thomas, 1955, pp. 197–204.

Cummins, F. M., Taveras, J. M., and Schlesinger, E. B.: Treatment of gliomas of the third ventricle and pinealomas. *Neurology*, **10**:1031–1036, 1960.

Descartes, R.: De Homine, 1662. Cited by Rolleston, H. D.: *The Endocrine Organs in Health and Disease*. New York, Oxford University Press, 1936.

Giarman, N. J., and Day, M.: Presence of biogenic amines in the bovine pineal body. *Biochem. Pharmacology*, **1**:235, 1959.

Heubner, O.: Tumor der glandula pinealis. *Deutsch. Med. Wschr.*, **24**:214, 1898.

Horrax, G.: Treatment of tumors of the pineal body. *Arch. Neurol. Psychiat.*, **64**:227–242, 1950.

Kitay, J. I.: Pineal lesions and precocious puberty. A review. *J. Clin. Endocr.*, **14**:622–625, 1954.

Krabbe, K. H.: The pineal gland, especially in relation to problem of its supposed significance in sexual development. *Endocrinology*, **7**:379–414, 1923.

Lerner, A. B., Case, J. D., Takahashi, Y., Lee, T. H., and Mori, W.: Isolation of melatonin, pineal gland factor that lightens melanocytes. *J. Amer. Chem. Soc.*, **80**:2587, 1958.

Poppen, J. L., and Marino, R., Jr.: Pinealomas and tumors of the posterior portion of the third ventricle. *J. Neurosurg.*, **28**:357–364, 1968.

Russell, D. S.: Pinealoma: its relationship to teratoma. *J. Path. Bact.*, **56**:145–150, 1944.

Russell, D. S., and Rubinstein, L. J.: *Pathology of Tumors of the Nervous System*. London, Edward Arnold, 1971.

Wurtman, R. J., Axelrod, J., and Chu, E. W.: Melatonin, a pineal substance: effect on the rat ovary. *Science*, **141**:277, 1963.

Chapter Seventeen

PARAPITUITARY, PITUITARY AND HYPOTHALAMIC TUMORS

Neoplasms above the sella turcica and those within the hypothalamus collectively represent 10 to 15 percent of childhood intracranial tumors. Combinations of fundus and visual field disturbances, neuroendocrine dysfunction, and distinctive roentgen abnormalities permit accurate topical diagnosis in most instances. The tumors that occur in this region in children include the craniopharyngioma, the optic nerve glioma, gliomas of the hypothalamus, and the ectopic, or teratomatous, pinealoma.

Age factors are important regarding tumors in this area because certain types are rare in children. Meningioma, aneurysm, pituitary adenoma, and cholesteatoma are notable lesions in or above the sella in the adult population but are infrequent in childhood. Tumors developing primarily within the third ventricle also are rare in childhood. A curious syndrome has been described with third ventricular cysts in childhood with a bobbing movement of the head and trunk reminiscent of that in dolls with weighted heads resting on a coiled spring (Benton et al.). This has been referred to as "the bobblehead doll syndrome" but is not specific for mass lesions because it has also been observed in a child with hydrocephalus secondary to aqueductal stenosis (Nellhaus).

Endocrinologic Evaluation

An important aspect of neoplasms located in or above the sella is the effect on endocrine function, either by pressure directly on the pituitary or secondarily by disturbing function of the hypothalamus. Adequate evaluation of the endocrine status is essential, not only because of the diagnostic implications but also because replacement therapy may be necessary before surgery is performed.

Diabetes insipidus is evident from polyuria, polydipsia, and inability to concentrate urine during water deprivation. A useful screening test is the determination of the urine specific gravity of the first morning urine specimen after a night's sleep. If the specific gravity is greater than 1.020, diabetes insipidus is probably not present and further tests are not necessary.

When random urine specimens consistently show low specific gravities, a controlled eight-hour water deprivation test should be performed. The test should be begun at approximately 8 A.M. so that its course can be closely observed. Specimens should be obtained at the beginning of the test for urine osmolarity and specific gravity, and serum osmolarity. Body weight and temperature should also be recorded.

During the eight-hour test, the body weight and temperature should be periodically measured and urine output carefully determined. Loss of 3 per cent or more of body weight and significant temperature elevation indicate dehydration and warrant termination of the test. Specimens are again obtained for determinations of osmolarities and urine specific gravity at the conclusion of the test.

An elevation of serum osmolarity and persistent output of urine of low specific gravity is indicative of antidiuretic hormone insufficiency, or diabetes insipidus. If urine specific gravity is less than 1.008 at the end of the examination, pitressin should be administered in safe dosage. Urine output and specific gravity are measured thereafter at intervals for the next 48 hours. Inability to concentrate urine during water deprivation but response to pitressin confirms the diagnosis.

Anterior pituitary function is evaluated by observation of the patient's physical stature, by measurement of the effects of its trophic hormones, and by estimation of growth hormone release with provocative stimulation. Growth failure is the hallmark of long-standing panhypopituitarism in children but may be absent in those with acquired pituitary failure due to neoplastic disease (Fig. 17–1). In patients with growth failure, the proportions of the body are usually near normal for chronological age. Height age is often more abnormal than is weight age. The excessive subcutaneous fat characteristic of these children results in an immature or a doll-like facial appearance. Skeletal maturation also is usually retarded but tends to be less so than height age.

Thyroid-stimulating hormone (TSH) function is assessed by determination of serum levels of TSH (normal = less than 10 micrograms per milliliter), T_4 (normal = 4 to 11 nanograms per milliliter), and measurement of the radioactive iodine uptake. In certain children with panhypopituitarism, the T_4 may be low normal while the iodine uptake is profoundly reduced. Thus, both studies should be done.

Adrenocorticotropic hormone (ACTH) secretion is evaluated by estimation of 17-hydroxycorticosteroids in a 24-hour urine specimen. The procedure has limited value in younger children because of the wide range of normal values. The estimation of pituitary reserve by the metyrapone test provides a more reliable indication of ACTH activity. A 24-hour urine collection is made for 17-

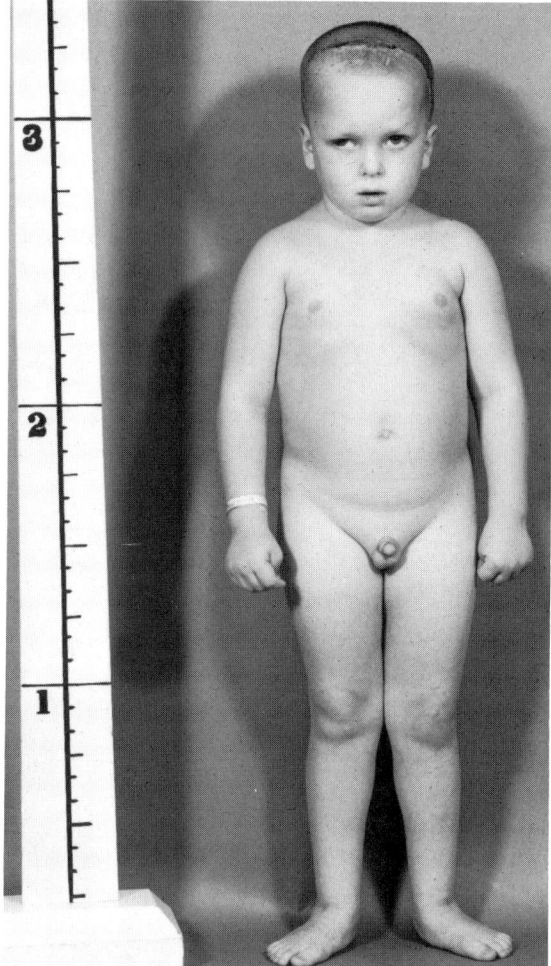

Figure 17–1. Panhypopituitarism. Eight-year-old boy with craniopharyngeal duct cyst. Diabetes insipidus was noted at six months of age and visual loss secondary to optic atrophy was found soon thereafter. Somatic growth was slow from the first few months of life. Pneumoencephalography at eight years of age revealed an anterior third ventricle filling defect. At surgery, a cystic lesion within and above the sella turcica was removed.

Note the small stature for age but with normal upper-to-lower segment ratios. The face is immature or "doll-like" and subcutaneous fatty tissue is generous, characteristic of the appearance with anterior pituitary deficiency. At a chronological age of eight years, his weight age and bone age were five years, and height age was four years.

hydroxycorticosteroids, and metyrapone is then given orally in total dosage of 2500 mg. per square meter of body surface area in 6 divided doses. Another 24-hour urine collection is made the following day. An increase in excretion of 17-hydroxycorticosteroids of 200 per cent or greater over the baseline level indicates adequate pituitary reserve. In children less than 12 years of age, tests for gonadotropin deficiency are of little value because of the extremely low levels present in normal children before puberty.

Radioimmunoassay of growth hormone has recently been developed, providing another valuable estimate of pituitary function in children with suprasellar tumors. Since growth hormone concentration varies from 1 to 10 micrograms per milliliter in normal children, random blood specimens are of little use for this determination. Growth hormone is liberated with provocative agents and advantage of this response is taken for its determination.

Hypoglycemia induced by insulin administration is one stimulus to the secretion of growth hormone. A single dose of regular insulin, 0.1 unit per kilogram of body weight, is given and followed by serial determinations of blood glucose and growth hormone over the subsequent 90 minutes. Patients with pituitary insufficiency are markedly sensitive to insulin and therefore must be carefully observed during this test.

Because of the danger of insulin-induced hypoglycemia, most prefer arginine as a provocative agent for growth hormone analysis. Arginine is infused intravenously in a dose of 0.5 gram per kilogram of body weight (up to 30 grams) over a period of 30 minutes. Preinfusion specimens are obtained for glucose and growth hormone and are again obtained at 30, 45, 60, and 90 minutes. A normal response consists of an increase of growth hormone greater than 5 micrograms per milliliter above the fasting level. Pubertal girls normally show a greater rise than boys of equal age, presumably because of estrogens enhancing growth hormone responsiveness to arginine stimulation (Sperling et al.).

CRANIOPHARYNGIOMA

The craniopharyngioma has been given a variety of designations, including Rathke-pouch tumor, hypophyseal duct tumor, and suprasellar epidermoid cyst. It has long been stated that this tumor develops from remnants of the embryonic Rathke's pouch; however, the evidence supporting this concept might justifiably be questioned. Even if the concept is correct, the term craniopharyngioma proposed by Cushing is less than accurate because Rathke's pouch evaginates from the primitive stomatodeum rather than from the pharynx. Clusters of squamous cells in the region of the infundibular stalk as described by Erdheim may well be the site of origin of these neoplasms; however, the derivation of these cells clumps remains questionable.

Most craniopharygiomas are located above the sella (Fig. 17-2) along the pituitary stalk, although some may be chiefly intrasellar (Fig. 17-3). Intrasellar craniopharyngiomas must be differentiated from the non-neoplastic, intrasellar Rathke-cleft cyst, which seems more clearly to be derived from remnants of Rathke's cleft. These cystic structures are usually incidental findings at autospy, but in rare instances, distention of the cleft occurs with cyst-formation causing pituitary compression and visual field deficits (Berry and Schlezinger). Thus, clinically, they bear close similarity to the pituitary adenoma and most are identified in adults. These benign cystic lesions differ from the craniopharyngioma in that the epithelial lining is cuboidal or colum-

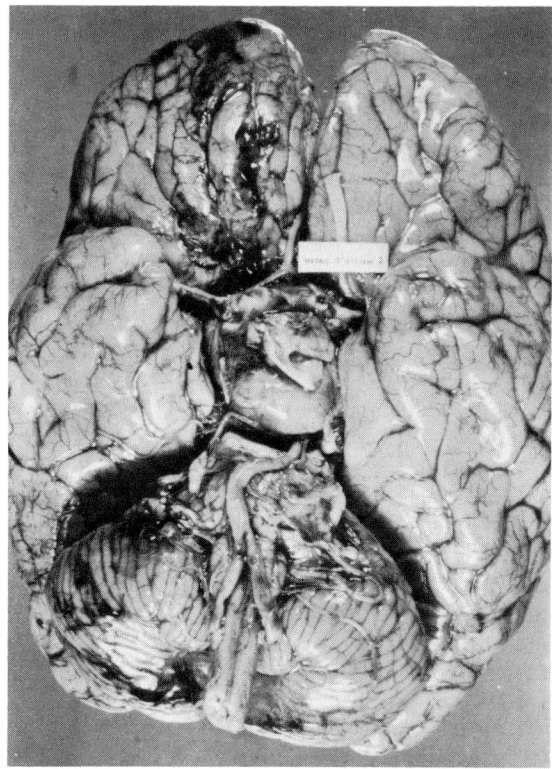

Figure 17-2. Craniopharyngioma. Large, oval mass is evident in the midline extending laterally on both sides almost to the medial temporal lobe structures. Anatomic relationship of the tumor to the optic nerves and chiasm accounts for the visual symptoms usually present in children with this tumor.

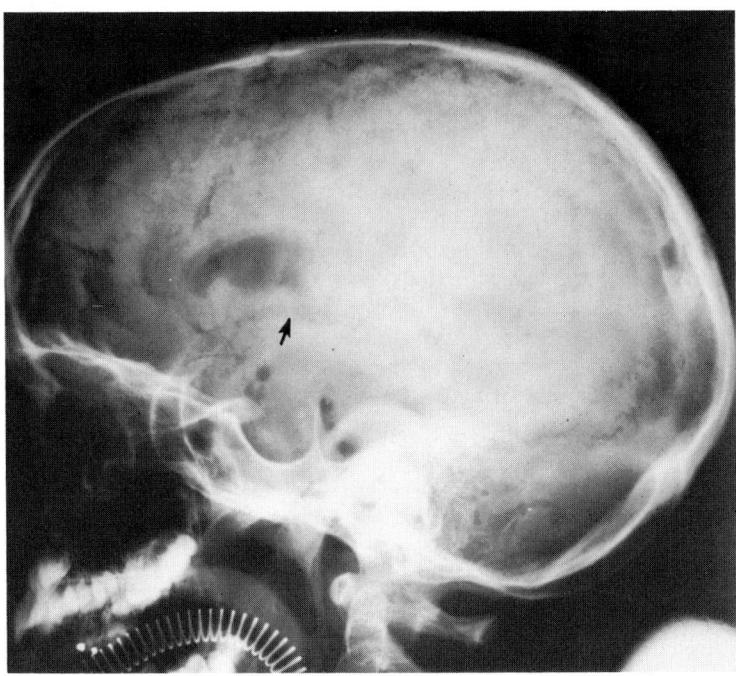

Figure 17–3. Craniopharyngioma. Nine-year-old boy with recurrent headaches, progressive visual loss, and bilateral primary optic atrophy. Somatic growth was normal. The sella turcica is enlarged and intrasellar calcification is present. Suprasellar extension of the cystic tumor is evident by obliteration and elevation of the anterior portion of the third ventricle (arrow). The foramen of Monro is not obstructed and the lateral ventricular size remains normal.

nar while a squamous-cell component is absent.

Craniopharyngioma is usually partially solid, with the cystic component varying from microcystic degeneration to a single large cyst that represents the majority of the tumor (Fig. 17-4). The size of the mass varies greatly from the small lesion that compresses the chiasm to one of enormous size that extends up to the floor of the lateral ventricle and posteriorly to the interpeduncular cistern. Microscopically, nests of squamous cells, cystic spaces lined by squamous or columnar cells, and areas of sparsely cellular connective tissue are intermixed within the tumor. Degenerative changes within the tissue components results in masses of keratin-containing areas of mineral deposition.

The craniopharyngioma is often thought of as a tumor of childhood, although the recorded series illustrate a wide spectrum regarding age of occurrence. Among 49 cases, Northfield found 23 in patients less than 20 years of age and 26 in those between 20 and 56 years of age. The series of 138 cases compiled by Bailey et al. included 66 in patients under 20 years of age and 72 cases in persons over 20 years of age. Several cases have been identified in the elderly (Tiberin et al.).

Certain differences are apparent regarding the clinical manifestations of the craniopharyngioma in children as compared with adults. Papilledema is a more common early finding in the child with this tumor; optic atrophy is more often noted in adults. Calcification within the tumor is usually evident in children but often absent in adults (Kahn). Evidence of gonadotropin failure may be the initial complaint in adults, but it is infrequent in children.

Symptoms and Signs

Craniopharyngiomas in children are associated with a wide range of symptoms and signs. The initial complaints are variable, depending on the intracranial structures implicated and on the astuteness of the parents' observations. Headache, vomiting, and visual impairment lead the list of presenting complaints. Drowsiness, personality change or dementia, and diplopia are other occasional findings resulting from increased pressure. Additional infrequent symptomatic complaints include psychomotor seizures, olfactory hallucinations, and "weak spells" because of orthostatic hypotension.

Compression of the hypothalamus or pituitary gland may result in several endocrine disturbances, the most notable being growth failure. Parents may precisely date the time of onset of the lack of continued normal growth

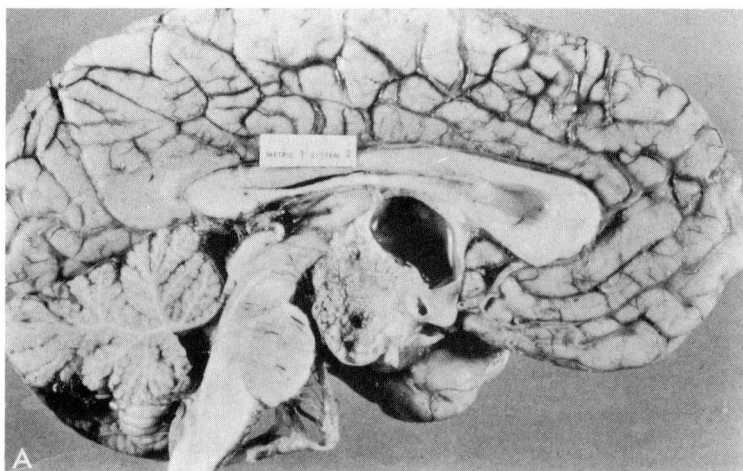

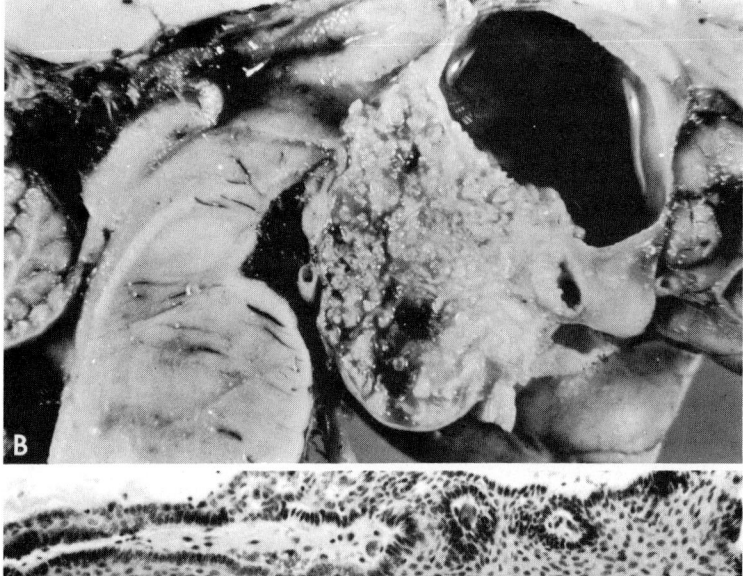

Figure 17–4. Craniopharyngioma. A, Gross appearance of the tumor located in the region of the third ventricle and extending up to the foramen of Monro. There is a single large cyst in addition to a solid component with a granular appearance. The third ventricle is obliterated, although the lateral ventricle does not appear to be distended. B, Close-up of the neoplasm demonstrates the cystic wall and the various components of the solid portion. C, Microscopic view reveals nests of squamous cells and cystic spaces lined by columnar epithelium. A circular mass of material resembling keratin is also present.

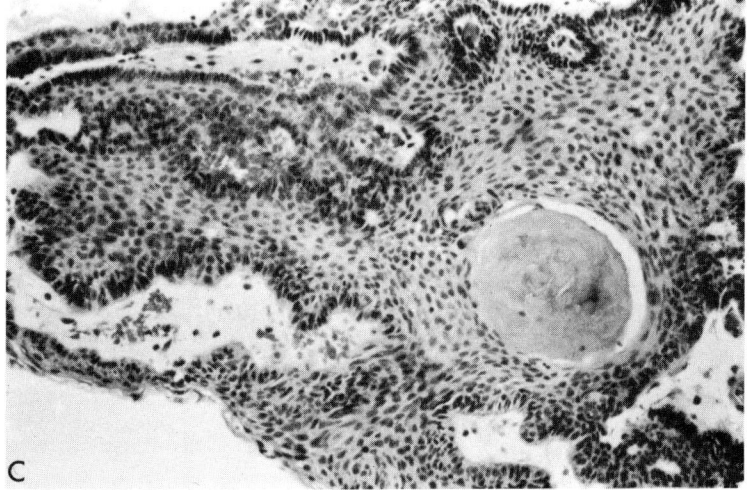

of the child, a statement that indicates its acquired nature, warranting search for an organic cause. Although specific laboratory testing frequently reveals the presence of pituitary insufficiency, the child's physical stature is often normal. Of 57 children with craniopharyngioma, Matson and Crigler found abnormally short stature in only 38 percent. Delay in acquisition of secondary sex characteristics or obesity may also be observed in older children with this neoplasm, but these are rare initial complaints. Diabetes insipidus, likewise, is infrequent before surgery.

Because of the proximity of this tumor to the optic chiasm, ocular symptoms and signs are prominent in a large percentage of patients. Papilledema is frequent; primary optic atrophy is less common. In young children with optic atrophy and visual impairment, searching nystagmus secondary to visual loss may be the first notable abnormality observed by the parents. Regardless of the type of nerve head abnormality present, reduced visual acuity in one or both eyes or visual field defects are frequent. A classic bitemporal hemianopsia is sometimes identified, but a variation thereof with pronounced asymmetry of the temporal field deficits is more characteristic.

Early in the course of chiasmal compression, inferior temporal quadrant defects may occur from pressure by the tumor from above the chiasm. Another pattern that may be observed is unilateral blindness with a temporal field cut in the opposite eye; a finding indicative of pressure atrophy of the optic nerve on the blind side with adjacent compression of the chiasm behind. A more unusual and confusing picture is the presence of bitemporal scotomas due to involvement of the macular fibers near the posterior rim of the optic chiasm. Even incongruous homonymous hemianopsia may occur if the tumor implicates the optic tract on one side posterior to the chiasm.

Combinations of the foregoing neurologic and ocular findings generally permit localization of the lesion to the suprasellar region. The probability that the tumor is a craniopharyngioma is enhanced if suprasellar calcification is present on skull x-ray (Fig. 17-5). This has been found in approximately 85 per cent of childhood cases (McKenzie and Sosman), although one series reported suprasellar calcification in 56 of 57 cases (Matson and Crigler). The sella turcica is often enlarged and the dorsum sellae or clinoid processes are frequently eroded. Large tumors exerting pressure on the sella for a long period of time may result in virtual destruction of the sella.

Reasonable clinical evidence of a suprasellar tumor warrants evaluation of the metabolic and endocrine status of the patient before contrast studies are performed. Serum electrolyte and glucose determinations plus tests for pituitary trophic hormones should be done. Roentgenograms for bone age are indicated if growth retardation is evident, as well as arginine infusion for growth hormone analysis. Daily urine volume and urine specific gravities may either include the possibility of diabetes insipidus or indicate the need for a detailed eight-hour water deprivation test.

Treatment

Confirmation of the location of tumor, the estimation of its size, and the presence of ventricular dilatation is accomplished by either ventriculography or pneumography. In patients with significant increase in pressure, ventriculography is indicated; in patients without marked signs of pressure, pneumography is preferred. Treatment is surgical with the subfrontal approach being the most popular. Some prefer biopsy and partial resection; others favor a more aggressive surgical attack with an attempt to totally excise the tumor whenever possible. Matson stated that of 57 patients operated upon, the lesion was completely excised in 44 of them. This series must be considered exceptional, however, and in certain instances, decompression by removal of cyst fluid and only partial removal of the tumor is advisable.

The cystic contents of this tumor may be very irritative if large amounts are permitted to gain access to the subarachnoid space during the procedure. Aseptic meningitis may result and can be avoided by careful aspiration of the cyst contents under direct vision. Postoperative irradiation therapy is indicated after partial removal of the tumor. Kramer et al. have shown considerable benefit regarding longevity in patients given irradiation treatment.

The most significant factor reducing the surgical mortality rate in children with craniopharyngioma has been the recognition and replacement of endocrine deficits. Those with secondary hypothyroidism should receive

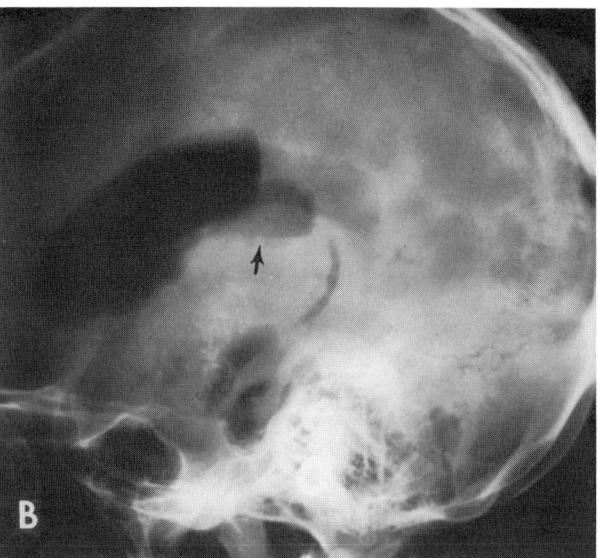
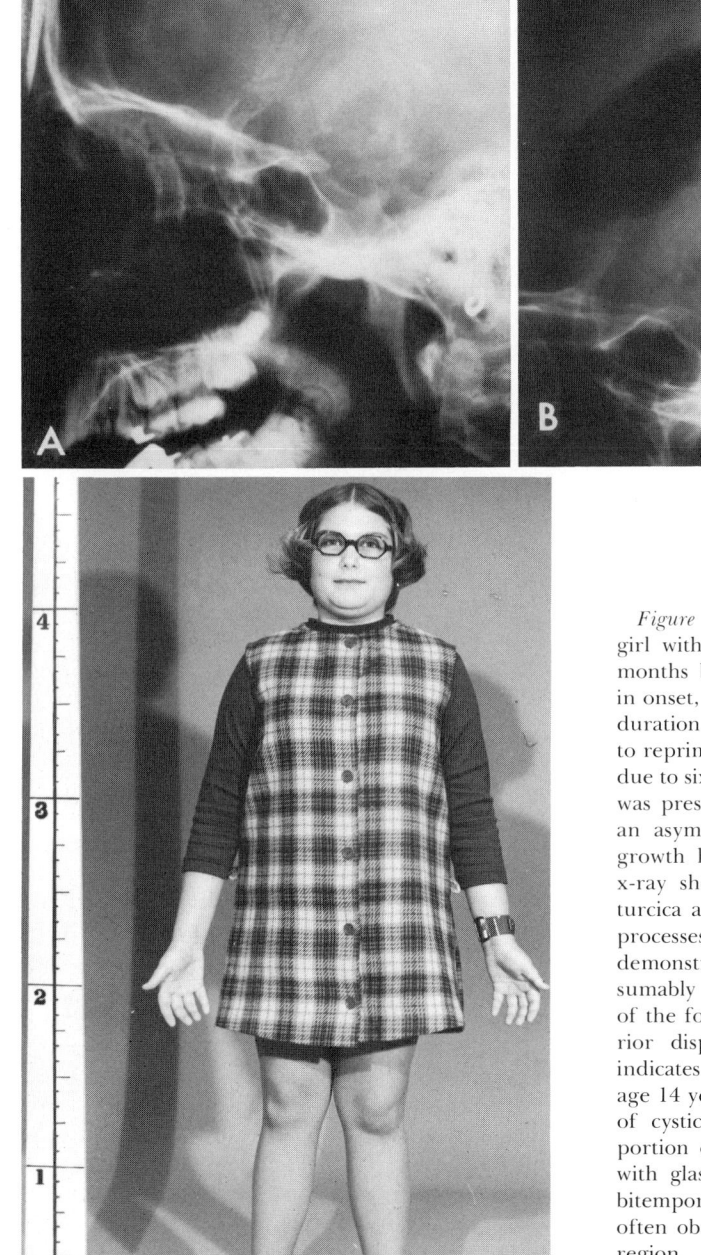

Figure 17–5. Craniopharyngioma. Ten-year-old girl with onset of recurrent, severe headaches six months before admission. Headaches were sudden in onset, associated with vomiting, and often brief in duration. She became more irritable, more sensitive to reprimands, and subsequently developed diplopia due to sixth nerve paralysis. High-grade papilledema was present on admission and visual fields revealed an asymmetrical bitemporal hemianopsia. Somatic growth had remained unaffected. A, Lateral skull x-ray shows extensive calcification above the sella turcica and marked erosion of the posterior clinoid processes and dorsum sellae. B, Ventriculogram demonstrates lateral ventricular dilatation presumably due to partial or intermittent obstruction of the foramen of Monro. The elevation and posterior displacement of the third ventricle (arrow) indicates the size of the cystic tumor. C, Patient at age 14 years, four years after craniotomy, aspiration of cystic fluid, and partial resection of the solid portion of the tumor. Vision is corrected to 20/20 with glasses and the optic discs reveal only slight bitemporal pallor. Note truncal obesity, which is often observed with neoplasms in the hypothalamic region.

thyroid replacement and all should be placed on adrenocorticosteroid therapy. If one calculates the maintenance needs for cortisone acetate at 20 mg. per squre meter of body surface area per day, the child should receive approximately three times this amount during the performance of contrast studies and six times maintenance needs the day of surgery.

Steroid therapy should be continued for several days postoperatively and may be required indefinitely if ACTH insufficiency is documented. Either cortisone acetate or other steroid preparations in equivalent doses may be used. Hydrocortisone, 20 mg. of which is equivalent to 25 mg. of cortisone acetate, is administered intravenously throughout the day of the operative procedure.

During the postoperative period, careful attention to the fluid and electrolyte balance is critical, in addition to the need for continued steroid therapy. Fluid and electrolyte metabolism may be disrupted by several factors, including diabetes insipidus, excessive insensible loss due to fever, an aldosterone effect with salt retention, and disturbance of the thirst mechanism due to lethargy or hypothalamic dysfunction. Diabetes insipidus is a frequent postoperative complication but may be temporary, lasting days to weeks.

Unless the diabetes insipidus is severe, it may be safer to avoid administering pitressin immediately after surgery but to provide adequate fluid intravenously. A reasonable quantity administered is the sum of the daily urine output plus 500 ml. per square meter of body surface area to replace insensible loss. When urine output cannot be accurately measured, fluid requirements may be calculated at approximately 1800 ml. per square meter of body surface area per day. With daily electrolytes and frequent urine specific gravity determinations, one can usually maintain water balance until natural factors, including thrist and ADH function, recover. In children with persistent polyuria and dilute urine, pitressin may be used but should be initiated in low dosage, so that the effect can be monitored, and gradually increased as required. In some, pitressin tannate in oil given every second or third day is necessary indefinitely.

Growth hormone insufficiency also may be apparent following surgical removal of these lesions. In some instances, marked improvement in linear growth has been noted after surgery, even though no increase in the amount of growth hormone could be demonstrated by provocative tests (Kenny et al., Holmes et al.). The explanation for such growth spurts with seemingly inadequate quantities of growth hormone remains unexplained.

OPTIC NERVE AND CHIASM GLIOMAS

Gliomas of the anterior visual pathways are infrequent, accounting for approximately 4 per cent of childhood intracranial tumors. Most occur in the pediatric age group and usually in the early childhood years. These tumors are more often located within the optic chiasm than elsewhere but may be restricted to one optic nerve. Gross observation of these lesions reveals a fusiform expansion of the nerve or chiasm (Fig. 17-6). The tumor may extend from the anterior reaches of the optic nerve into the orbit; others originating from the chiasm can protrude upward into the hypothalamus and anterior third ventricle. Microscopic pathology is variable; some resemble low-grade astrocytomas and others contain mixtures of astrocytes and oligodendroglia. Histologic evidence of malignancy is rare and invasiveness in unusual.

There is a relationship between optic gliomas and von Recklinghausen's disease, although the precise association has been disputed. In the series of 56 patients with optic gliomas reported by Chutorian et al., 22 per cent had multiple cafe-au-lait spots but only two of these showed other stigmas of neurofibromatosis. This association with neurofibromatosis along with certain growth characteristics of these tumors has prompted some to assume that they represent congenital hamartomas (Anderson and Spencer) with limited growth potential.

Table 17-1. Relative Potency of Corticosteroid Preparations*

Preparation	Relative Doses
Cortisone acetate	25 mg.
Hydrocortisone	20 mg.
Prednisone	5 mg.
Triamcinolone	4 mg.
Methylprednisolone	4 mg.
Dexamethasone	0.75 mg.

*Cortisone acetate maintenance dose approximately 20 mg. per square meter per day.

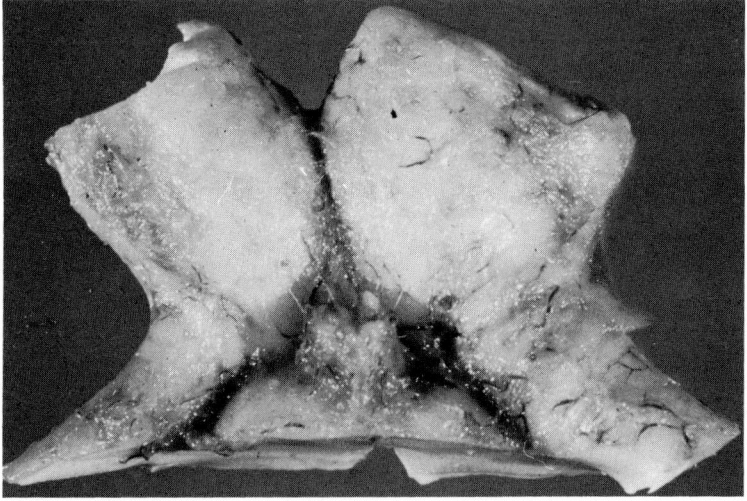

Figure 17-6. Bilateral optic nerve glioma. View from the ventral aspect of the optic pathways demonstrating bulbous enlargement of both optic nerves. The tumor has extended into the left optic tract, resulting in its enlargement also.

The theory that optic gliomas might be congenital is not new because it was postulated by Hudson in his classic monograph in 1912. The hamartomatous concept of this tumor seems out of accord with its recognized ability to enlarge during childhood. Anderson and Spencer demonstrated the accumulation of mucinous material within these tumors and suggested that enlargement of the lesion might be due to this rather than neoplastic proliferation.

Symptoms and Signs

Symptoms and signs of optic gliomas depend on the location and the degree of compression of adjacent structures. Loss of vision is the most common early symptom and is associated with primary optic atrophy (Fig. 17-7). The degree of optic pallor may be less than anticipated when compared with the profound visual loss observed in some cases. Intraorbital gliomas and those developing in

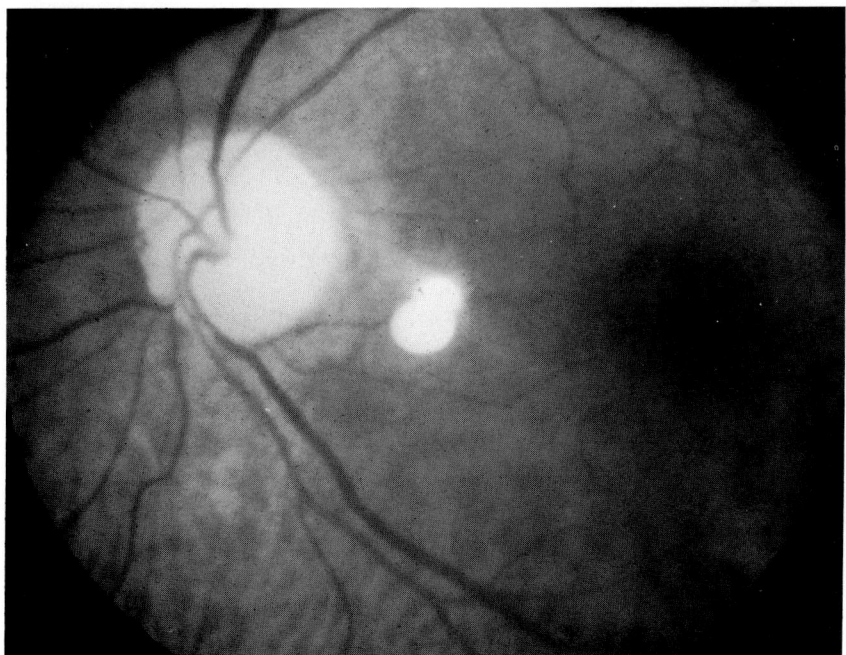

Figure 17-7. Primary optic atrophy in a child with a glioma of the optic chiasm. Nerve head is chalky white, the margins are sharp, and its surface is relatively avascular.

the anterior portion of the optic nerve cause nonpulsatile proptosis with the eye pushed directly forward in most cases. Proptosis is usually mild and with little restriction of the range of motion of the eye.

Searching nystagmus is sometimes the first abnormality observed in young children whose limited vocabulary precludes their description of visual deficits. In others, a routine preschool visual acuity check identifies previously unrecognized loss of vision. Ophthalmologic examination for strabismus, likewise, occasionally leads to the identification of loss of vision and optic atrophy. In patients with tumor confined to one optic nerve, the loss of vision is limited to the involved side.

Gliomas of the chiasm produce bilateral signs, including optic atrophy, and are more often associated with hypothalamic dysfunction. Precocious puberty, obesity, diabetes insipidus, and growth failure are uncommon presenting manifestations but have been reported. In a few patients, headache, vomiting, and papilledema precede other evidence of an optic glioma. Although there are numerous possible presenting symptoms, it is imperative that optic glioma be considered in any child with loss of vision, especially if progressive, combined with primary optic atrophy.

Diagnostic Studies

Visual field abnormalities are variable and not distinctive. Irregular and asymmetrical field defects are expected, but a few patients show bitemporal cuts, scotoma or even homonymous hemianopsia. Roentgenographic studies are of great importance for the identification of this tumor (Holman). Gliomas located within the optic nerve are apt to produce enlargement of the optic foramen without demineralization or erosion of its bony margins (Fig. 17-8). The normal optic foramen measures 6 mm. or less in diameter in children, and the two foramina should not vary more than 1 mm.

Gliomas of the chiasm are less likely to be associated with optic foramen enlargement, but here the lateral skull films usually reveal abnormalities. Elongation of the sella with undercutting of the anterior clinoid processes produces a J-shaped or gourd-shaped sella suggestive of an optic glioma (Fig. 17-9). This altered configuration of the sella results from deepening and enlargement of the chiasmatic sulcus with erosion of the inferior surface of the anterior clinoid process. Suprasellar calcification is not expected, and signs of generalized pressure on x-ray may be present in children with extension of the tumor into the anterior third ventricle.

Pneumoencephalography confirms the localization of the tumor and provides an estimate of its size. The earliest pneumoencephalographic abnormality is a spreading of the chiasmatic and infundibular recesses of the anterior third ventricle along with obliteration of the chiasmatic cistern above the sella. Large tumors extend into the anterior third ventricle, elevating it and displacing it posteriorly. Continued enlargement obstructs the foramen of Monro, with obstructive hydrocephalus and lateral ventricular distention resulting.

Treatment

Treatment of optic gliomas remains a controversial matter, and few absolute guidelines

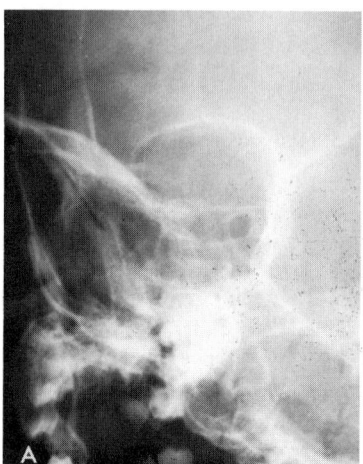
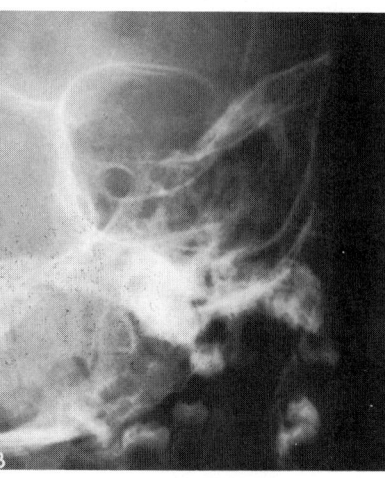

Figure 17–8. Glioma of the right optic nerve. Optic foramina x-rays. A, Normal left optic foramen, which measures 5 mm. B, Enlarged right optic foramen, which measures 7.5 mm. in greatest diameter. Note that despite the enlargement of the bony foramen, the margins retain a normal rim of sclerosis indicative of the chronic nature of this tumor.

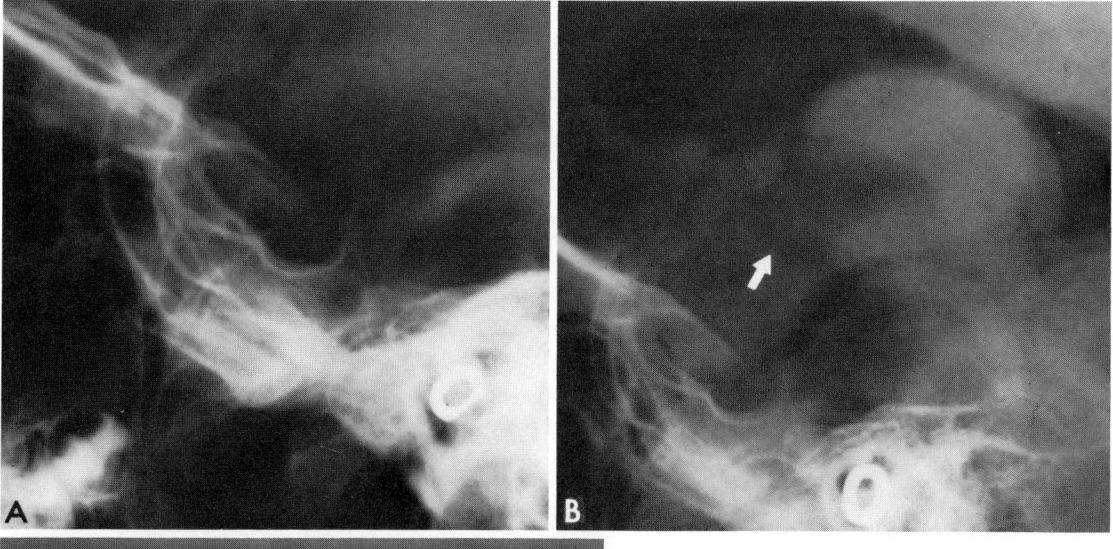

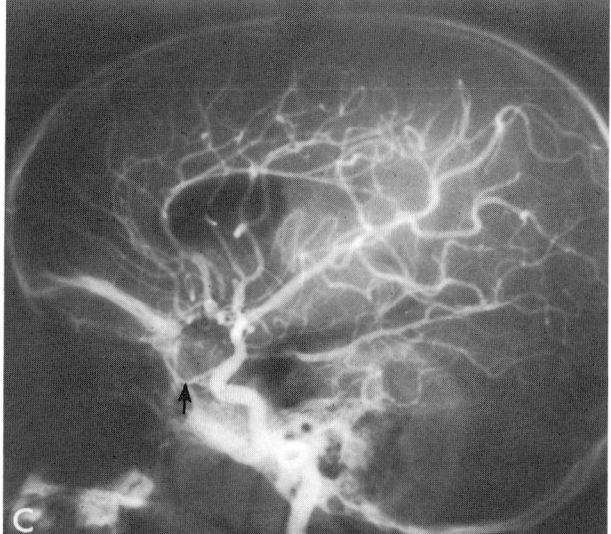

Figure 17–9. Optic chiasm glioma. Six-year-old girl with nystagmus, which was first noticed at age nine months. Optic atrophy in the right eye was observed at age 18 months and in the left eye at age five years. Physical examination was normal except for bilateral optic pallor, poor pupillary response to light, and decreased visual acuity. A, Lateral skull x-ray. The sella turcica is elongated and there is under-cutting of the anterior clinoids. B, Pneumoencephalogram, lateral view. There is obliteration of the chiasmatic and infundibular cisterns of the anterior third ventricle and flattening of its anterior surface (arrow). The lateral ventricles remain normal in size. C, Carotid angiogram reveals displacement inferiorly of the opthalmic artery (arrow).

have been established. Most agree that those of the anterior portion of one optic nerve producing proptosis should be surgically resected. Most also agree that gliomas within the chiasm do not justify radical surgical intervention and some believe that no surgical procedure should be done. In many cases, however, one cannot be certain preoperatively that a suprasellar tumor does develop primarily in the chiasm. Surgery is required in such instances to exclude other lesions that might be safely removed. Hoyt and Baghdassarian have stressed the limited growth tendencies of these tumors and have recommended conservative, nonsurgical management for most.

Numerous patients have been described with a remarkably long and benign course after only partial resection of an optic glioma. Thus, sacrifice of remaining vision by an operative procedure is justifiably questionable when the tumor is extensive. Because of this protracted natural history, surgical procedures for chiasmal gliomas are best limited to either biopsy or to shunt decompressions in children with obstructive hydrocephalus.

The variable but sometimes lengthy natural history of these tumors likewise makes evaluation of irradiation therapy difficult. Taveras and colleagues advocated irradiation treatment and believed it to be of benefit. The advantages of this measure remains unclear but irradiation appears indicated until proved to be of no value.

HYPOTHALAMIC TUMORS

Neoplasms within the hypothalamus are a diverse group both morphologically and clinically. Most are astroglial in origin, the minority are hamartomatous or teratomatous. The clinical manifestations include a complex array of neurologic abnormalities combined with endocrine and metabolic disorders that vary, depending on location within the hypothalamus, age of the child, and adjacent structures implicated. It is unexplained why an astrocytoma of the anterior hypothalamus in the infant produces a syndrome with profound growth failure, while the same lesion in the older child so often results in obesity.

Hypothalamic Tumors In Infancy

In 1951, Russell described five infants with profound emaciation due to anterior hypothalamic neoplasms and coined the term "diencephalic syndrome in infancy." Numerous examples subsequently were reported with strikingly similar clinical manifestations (Dods, Kagan, Braun and Forney, Gareis and Johnson, Torrey and Uyeda, Pitlyk et al., Bain et al., White and Ross). Infants with this disorder are typically described as progressing in normal fashion for the first few months after birth. In a few cases, the onset of symptoms has been delayed until 18 to 24 months of life.

Failure of continued weight gain or even loss of weight is the usual initial symptom. When other signs are not apparent, such babies are often evaluated for "failure to thrive" with leading diagnostic considerations including malabsorption syndrome, cystic fibrosis, renal disease, congenital heart disease, or inadequate caloric intake related to an abnormal maternal-child relationship. Vomiting may be an early symptom, and nystagmus, when present, may be the first definitive finding suggesting neurologic disease.

A remarkable appearance of well-being and alertness despite severe emaciation has often been mentioned in such infants (Russell, Braun and Forney), although some are quite irritable. The facial expression of alertness has been attributed to supranuclear upper eyelid retraction, or Collier's sign, more commonly associated with brain stem lesions (Snyder). Hyperkinesis, tremulousness, facial pallor, hypotension, and hypoglycemia are additional findings present in certain patients. Optic atrophy generally becomes evident during the illness and is associated with loss of vision, apparent in the infant by searching or shimmering nystagmus.

The most striking feature of infants with this tumor is the disturbance in weight gain, which some have claimed to be present despite an adequate caloric intake (Torrey and Uyeda) (Fig. 17-10). This paradox remains unexplained and needs further documentation. In certain cases, caloric loss because of recurrent vomiting may account for lack of growth; in others, hyperactivity may utilize excessive calories. Profound anorexia with an inadequate food intake is obvious in some cases, readily accounting for the state of inanition.

Depletion to virtual absence of subcutaneous fat has been held to be characteristic of this syndrome and may be demonstrated roentgenographically (Poznanski and Manson). Only limited studies on growth hormone secretion in such patients have been performed to date. Pimstone et al. found elevated resting growth hormone levels, which were poorly suppressed by hyperglycemia but which were enhanced by hypoglycemic stress.

Most anterior hypothalamic tumors in infancy with emaciation have been astrocytomas; however, ependymomas and oligodendrogliomas have been identified in some (Torrey and Uyeda). Most have developed primarily within the hypothalamus, but hypothalamic involvement with inanition secondary to tumors of the optic chiasm may also occur (Braun and Forney, Gamstorp et al.).

Laboratory studies are not usually revealing, although the spinal fluid protein content is frequently increased. Suture spread on x-ray may develop later in the illness, but it is apt to be absent early. Radioactive brain scan is a valuable study when anterior hypothalamic glioma is suspected because a positive study strongly supports the diagnosis. The characterisitc anterior third ventricle filling defect on pneumoencephalography is apparent in the majority of cases. As the tumor spreads through the structures of the middle fossa, oculomotor paralysis and other cranial nerve signs develop. Hemiparesis, seizures, and lethargy indicate widespread involvement. Although irradiation therapy following surgical biopsy may impede the rate of growth, the outcome is generally fatal; most children die within three years after the onset of symptoms.

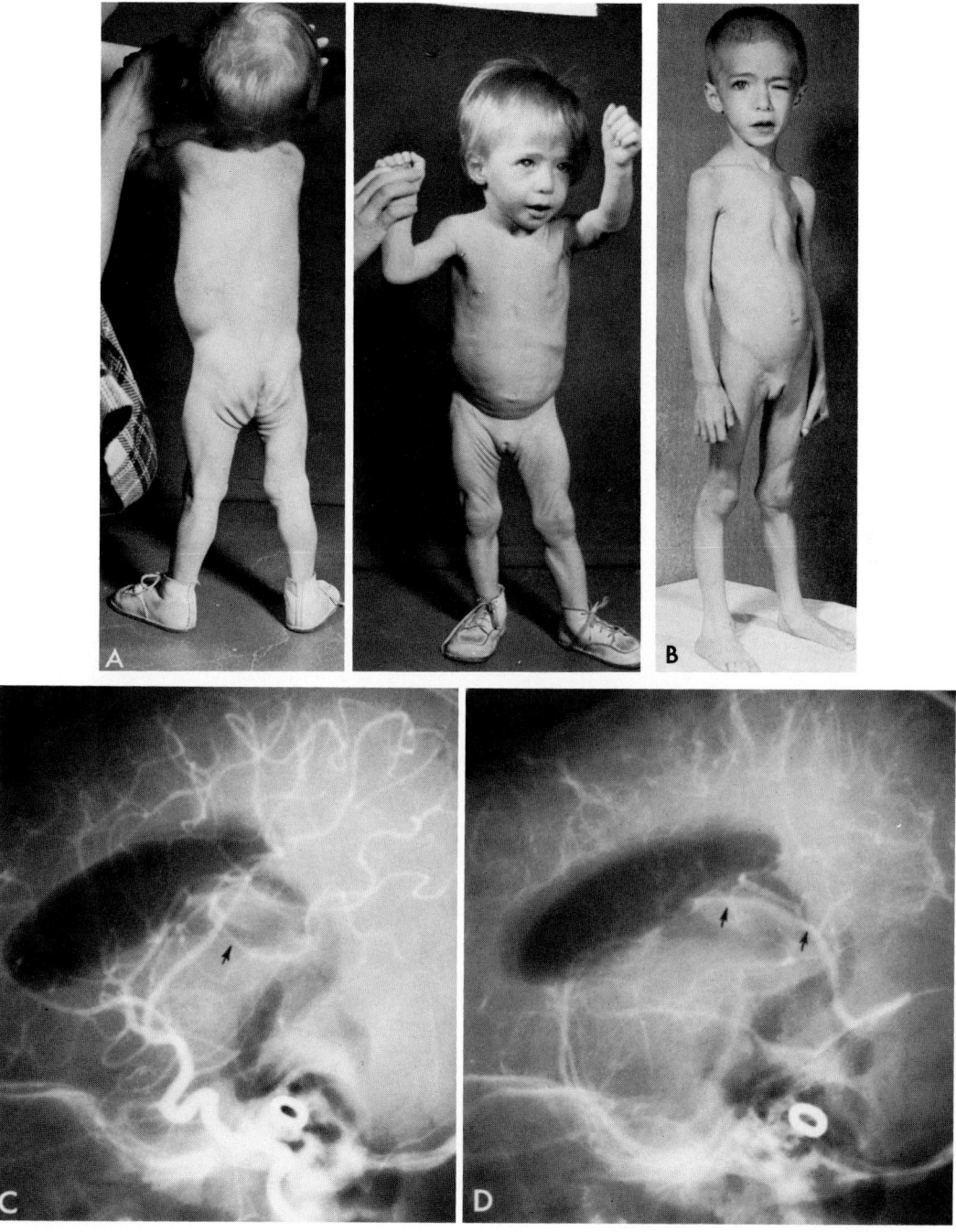

Figure 17-10. Hypothalamic glioma ("diencephalic syndrome"). A, Ten-month-old child with cessation of normal growth at age six months. Weight at age 10 months was 14 lb. Examination revealed horizontal nystagmus, normal fundi, and poor nutritional status. The patient was considered to have malabsorption syndrome although caloric intake was poor. B, At age four years, child's body weight was only 20 lb. Examination disclosed a left third nerve paralysis and right hemiparesis. Papilledema and visual loss were present bilaterally. C, Combined pneumoencephalography and angiography revealed posterior and superior displacement of the third ventricle (arrow). The intracranial portion of the carotid artery is bowed slightly posteriorly and a tumor stain is evident just posterior to the bifurcation of the carotid artery into the anterior and middle cerebral arteries. D, The venous phase demonstrates the superior and posterior displacement of the internal cerebral vein located in the roof of the third ventricle.

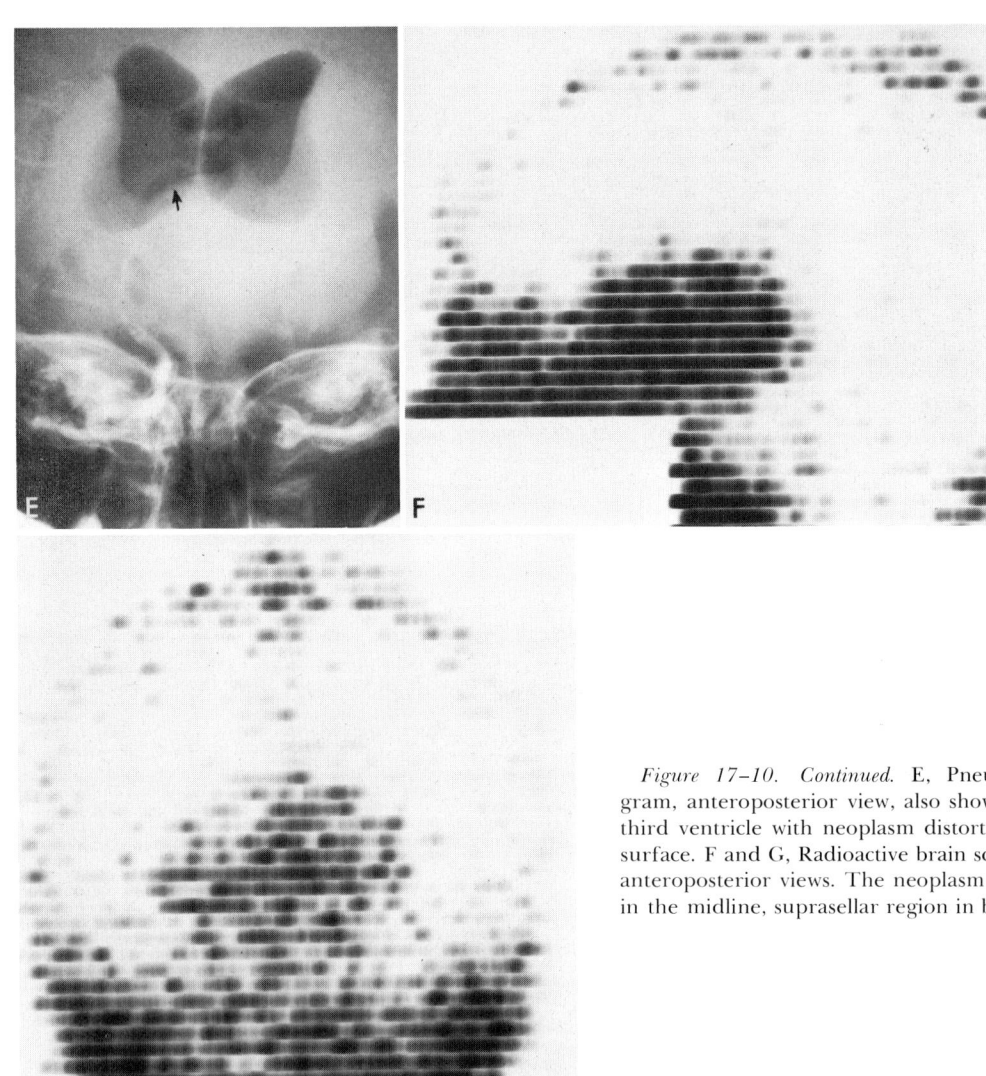

Figure 17–10. Continued. E, Pneumoencephalogram, anteroposterior view, also shows the elevated third ventricle with neoplasm distorting its inferior surface. F and G, Radioactive brain scan, lateral and anteroposterior views. The neoplasm is well defined in the midline, suprasellar region in both views.

Hypothalamic Tumors In Children

In older children, anterior hypothalamic tumors produce symptoms more classically associated with dysfunction of this region. Diabetes insipidus is a common early finding and may be the initial abnormality observed. Obesity is frequently present, in addition to ocular signs, including optic atrophy or papilledema, visual field deficits, or a pressure-induced abducens paralysis (Fig. 17-11). Truncal ataxia may be present and, with signs of increased pressure, can lead one to the erroneous localization to the posterior fossa.

Certain children with gliomas of the anterior hypothalamus have marked serum hyperosmolarity with hypernatremia and hyperchloremia. Several mechanisms may contribute to increased serum osmolarity, and these factors may occur independently or concurrently. The easiest to recognize is diabetes insipidus, in which case hyperosmolarity results from excessive water loss and hypovolemia. The level of blood urea nitrogen is usually elevated, and the electrolyte abnormality is readily corrected by providing adequate amounts of water and pitressin. The thirst mechanism may be disrupted in patients with hypothalamic disease, resulting in insufficient water intake and subsequent dehydration. This metabolic disturbance also is recognized by observation of the patient and provision of sufficient fluid to correct the hyperosmolar state. The most complex condition with hyperelectrolytemia is believed to be due to hypothalamic osmoreceptor dysfunction and has been called neurogenic hyperosmolarity. Serum osmolarity may vary in these cases from 300 to 370 milliosmols per liter and serum sodium from 150 to 180 mEq. per liter.

Hypernatremia is not entirely a result of dehydration in these patients since intravenous fluid administration fails to correct the electrolyte abnormality (Vejjajiva et al.). Excessive fluid administration results in edema and weight gain with only slight decrease in serum sodium and chloride levels. Moreover, children with hypernatremia due totally to dehydration with serum sodium levels in the range of 170 to 180 mEq. per liter are profoundly ill or in shock. Those with similar electrolyte levels resulting from hypothalamic osmoreceptor dysfunction may be ambulatory and conversant but are often confused, disoriented, and ataxic.

Segar described a microcephalic child with chronic hyperosmolarity in which absence of thirst, impaired ability to concentrate urine, and defective hypothalamic osmoregulation all were contributing factors. Whether this disturbance in osmoreceptor function results from the basic pathologic process in the hypothalamus or develops as an alteration of the osmoregulation mechanism to preexistent hypernatremia from dehydration remains unclear.

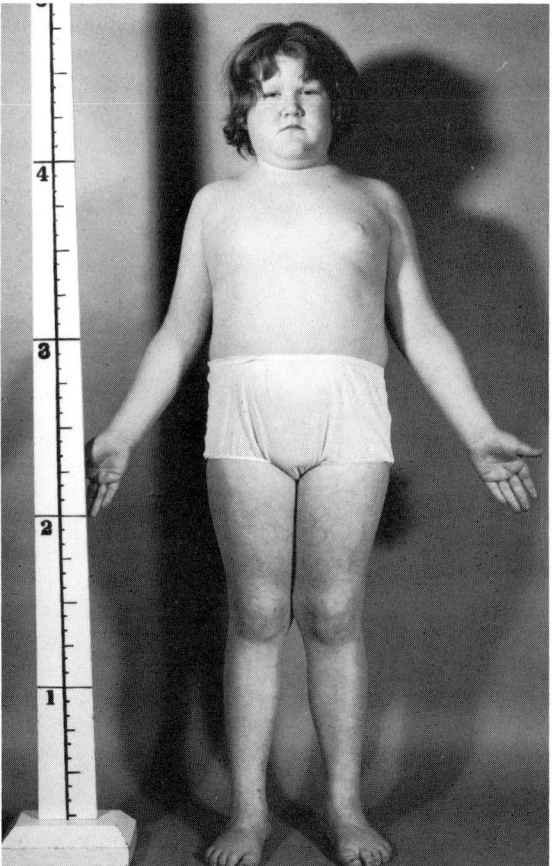

Figure 17–11. Hypothalamic glioma. Ten-year-old girl with history of diabetes insipidus and progressive loss of vision. Findings on hospital admission included bilateral optic atrophy and severe hypernatremia and hyperchloremia. Despite diabetes insipidus, she developed hyperphagia but virtual absence of the thirst mechanism. Note obese features commonly observed in older children with gliomas within the hypothalamus.

Posterior Hypothalamic Tumors

Posterior hypothalamic tumors are far less common than those in the anterior portion

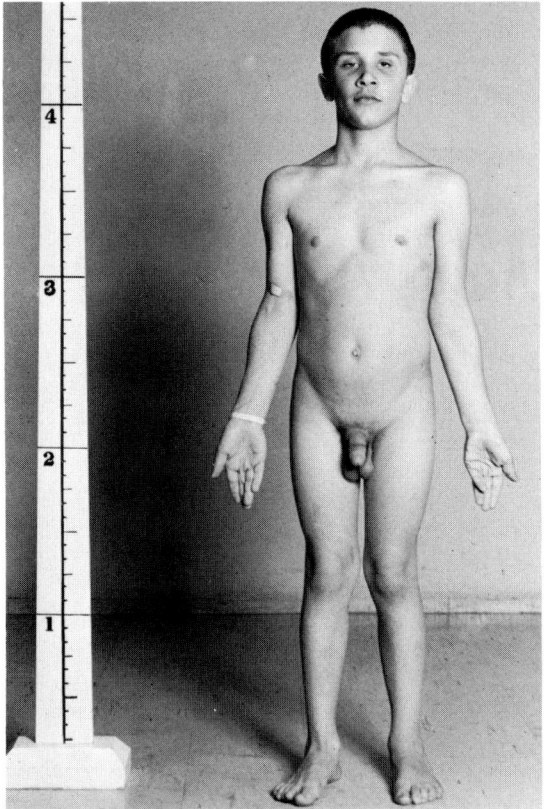

Figure 17–12. Isosexual precocious puberty. Six-year-old boy with testicular and penile enlargement noted at age three years. At chronological age of six years, weight age and bone age were those of a ten-year-old and height age that of a 9-year-old child. Note multiple café-au-lait spots. Bilateral testicular enlargement and increased urinary gonadotropins indicated the neurogenic origin of the premature sex development. These findings in a male child strongly suggest the possibility of a posterior hypothalamic tumor and warrant air studies. Children with neurofibromatosis may exhibit precocious puberty in the absence of an intracranial tumor.

and are notable for their association with isosexual precocious puberty (Papez and Ecker, List et al.) (Fig. 17-12). Most are hamartomas or gangliogliomas, lesions containing neural tissue resembling that normally found in the same region. They are located in the vicinity of the tuber cinereum, which is the portion along the floor of the third ventricle between the infundibular stalk and the mamillary bodies. Some are pedunculated, and if large, may project forward to the chiasm and posteriorly into the interpeduncular cistern.

Precocious sexual development may occur in isolated fashion (Loop) with its neurogenic origin demonstrated by exclusion of adrenal or testicular causes, increased gonadotropins in urine, and a mass evident inferior to the third ventricle on pneumography. Such children usually show abnormally rapid somatic development, advanced bone age, plus premature development of sex characteristics. In addition to penile enlargement and pubic hair, males with neurogenic precocious puberty have symmetrical enlargement of the testes.

It is generally assumed that precocious puberty in children with hypothalamic tumors results from excess releasing factors liberated from the lesion and the adjacent hypothalamic tissue. These substances pass via the portal venous system to the anterior pituitary, producing an excessive liberation of gonadotropins. Other clinical signs may be present, including seizures, behavioral abnormalities and intellectual deterioration.

Seizures in such patients are variable but may include tonic episodes, brief lapse spells resembling petit mal, or more bizarre spells manifested by paroxysmal uncontrolled laughter or cutaneous blushing. Large tumors may compress adjacent cranial nerves or produce obstructive hydrocephalus. Small, pedunculated lesions may be surgically removed, but large masses pose difficult management problems.

ECTOPIC PINEALOMA

Tumors resembling those in the pineal gland may occur in the infundibular region above the sella. In certain instances, this results from seeding or spread from a primary tumor originating within the pineal gland. The ectopic pinealoma, however, has its origin in the suprasellar region without gross or microscopic evidence of disease of the pineal gland. Russell included such ectopic tumors in the category of atypical teratoma and Friedman suggested the term germinoma in view of the similarity to the seminoma of testicular origin.

The germ cell origin of these lesions was based on the concept that primordial germ cells, which are segregated from somatic cells in embryonic life, fail to migrate to the genital ridge. Such cells tend to cluster in midline structures and may develop neoplastic tendencies later in life. The germ cell origin of these suprasellar lesions seems consistent with the seminoma appearance in some and the more malignant, choriocarcinoma features of others. This variation in anaplasia is probably of therapeutic importance because the latter form is more radioresistant than the former.

Ectopic pinealomas have no particular age limitations and are found in both children and young adults. Most, however, have been described in older children between 8 and 16 years of age. Diabetes insipidus is the usual initial symptom and has been present in the majority of patients reported (Kageyama and Belsky). Polyuria and polydipsia may remain the only complaint for months or even years before other signs evolve. Loss of vision is commonly noted and is usually associated with optic atrophy.

Children with large tumors protruding into the anterior third ventricle may have signs of obstructive hydrocephalus. Chiasmal or optic nerve compression results in variable field defects with some patients exhibiting a bitemporal hemianopsia and others with blindness of one eye and field deficits in the other. Pituitary insufficiency is evident by growth failure in children or hypogonadism and other endocrine disturbances in older persons.

In summary, the clinical manifestations of the ectopic pinealoma are usually initiated with diabetes insipidus and followed by the development of visual disturbances and pituitary insufficiency. This constellation of symptoms and signs allows preoperative consideration of this particular histologic diagnosis because it is somewhat different from the pattern of other tumors in this region. This is especially true when skull films are normal because roentgen abnormalities are usually present in children with craniopharyngioma and optic glioma. In addition, preoperative diabetes insipidus is unusual with craniopharyngioma and optic glioma. The only other common tumor in the area in this age group is the hypothalamic glioma, in which pressure signs are more common in the early stages.

Similar to other suprasellar mass lesions, pneumoencephalography is the procedure of choice to demonstrate the site and extent of the tumor. Craniotomy is required to establish the histologic diagnosis. As with any tumor in this location impairing pituitary function, endocrine studies should precede operation and steroid therapy administered before, during, and following the procedure. If frozen section at the time of surgery is consistent with a diagnosis of a suprasellar ectopic pinealoma, only biopsy and an attempt to decompress the chiasm are indicated.

In certain instances, invasion of the optic chiasm produces a bulbous distention of the chiasma resembling an optic glioma. This potential source of diagnostic confusion is avoided by biopsy and frozen section examination.

Rubin and Kramer have emphasized the radiosensitivity of these lesions and suggest that some may be curable by irradiation therapy. The prognosis is variable, however, with some responding well to therapy and others showing a relentlessly progressive course with infiltration into adjacent neural structures and invasion up into the ventricular system.

PITUITARY ADENOMA

The most remarkable aspect of adenomas of the pituitary gland in childhood is the extreme infrequency. Ballooning of the sella in children is much more often the result of chronic increase in intracranial pressure or secondary to an intrasellar craniopharyngioma. The classic subdivision of pituitary adenomas from clinical data into chromophobic, basophilic, and acidophilic types seems undesirable and unjustified to us for several reasons. First, we feel that with proper fixation and staining of pituitary tumor specimens, most can be shown to consist of cells containing granules. Granulation may be sparce but can generally be demonstrated, even in those with clinical evidence of panhypopituitarism (McCormick and Halmi). Formalin fixation is poor for pituitary cytology; fixation in Susa solution provides excellent material for staining. Hematoxylin and eosin stained sections are not ideal, and better stains are now available. Furthermore, pituitary adenomas with mixed-cell populations are not infrequent. Finally, many paradoxical situations have been reported, including acidophilic adenoma without acromegaly or growth excess, and acromegaly (Frasier and Kogut) or Cushing's syndrome (Dingman and Lim) with "chromophobe adenomas." For these reasons, we favor restriction of clinical diagnosis to "pituitary adenoma," with an added description of the type of endocrine disorder produced, if present. Thus, "pituitary adenoma with panhypopituitarism" is more accurate than the time-honored "chromphobe adenoma."

The conventional designation of cell types in the adenohypophysis into agranular chromophobes, basophils, and acidophils has become obsolete with more meticulous study of this gland (Romeis, Ezrin et al., Halmi and

McCormick). Cell types now recognized include alpha cells (acidophils), beta and delta cells (basophils), gamma cells ("amphophils"), and "follicular" cells, seen by electron microscopy. Subdivision of these cell types has been recommended by some, but to date, without general acceptance. The functional significance of the various cells of the adenohypophysis has been only partially delineated. Alpha cells elaborate growth hormone while beta cells are the source of ACTH, MSH (melanocyte-stimulating hormone), and perhaps TSH. Ezrin and colleagues suggested that gamma cells also produce corticotropin and delta cells form and secrete gonadotropins.

The clinical manifestations of pituitary adenomas include a variety of endocrine disorders depending on the functional activity of the tumor and visual disturbances when the optic chiasm is compressed. Headache may be present even with tumors confined to the sella turcica. Visual acuity and visual field abnormalities are of paramount importance in clinical diagnosis. Gradual progressive decline in vision is the usual complaint, but rapid deterioration of vision may also occur.

The characteristic field change induced by a pituitary adenoma is bitemporal hemianopsia. As opposed to the field deficits in patients with the craniopharyngioma, the field cut with pituitary adenoma is usually symmetrical. Since the tumor originates from within the sella, upward extension results in compression of the inferior surface of the chiasm, implicating first the crossing fibers originating from the inferior nasal quadrant of each retina. The earliest field cut, therefore, is in the superior temporal quadrants bilaterally, which is not usually recognized by the patient. With continued enlargement of the tumor, further compression eventually leads to a bitemporal hemianopsia.

Less common forms of field deficits include amaurosis in one eye and a temporal cut in the other. Bitemporal hemianoptic scotomas indicate interference with the posterior rim of the chiasm containing fibers of macular origin. Although it is an uncommon finding in patients with pituitary adenoma, the presence of hemianoptic scotomas is subject to misinterpretation because of its similarity to retrobulbar neuritis.

If a fundus abnormality is present, it is in the form of primary optic atrophy in the majority of patients. It is usually bilateral but not always symmetrical. Optic atrophy may lag behind loss of vision, and visual acuity may decrease considerably before atrophic disc changes are evident on ophthalmoscopy. With advanced optic atrophy, the pupils become dilated and respond poorly to light stimulus. With unilateral optic atrophy, the pupil on the atrophic side is dilated, shows poor or no light response, but reacts consensually.

Parasellar extension of a pituitary tumor into the cavernous sinus is rare but may account for extraocular muscle palsies. Oculomotor paralysis may occur in this fashion or even a "cavernous sinus syndrome" with involvement of the third, fourth, and sixth

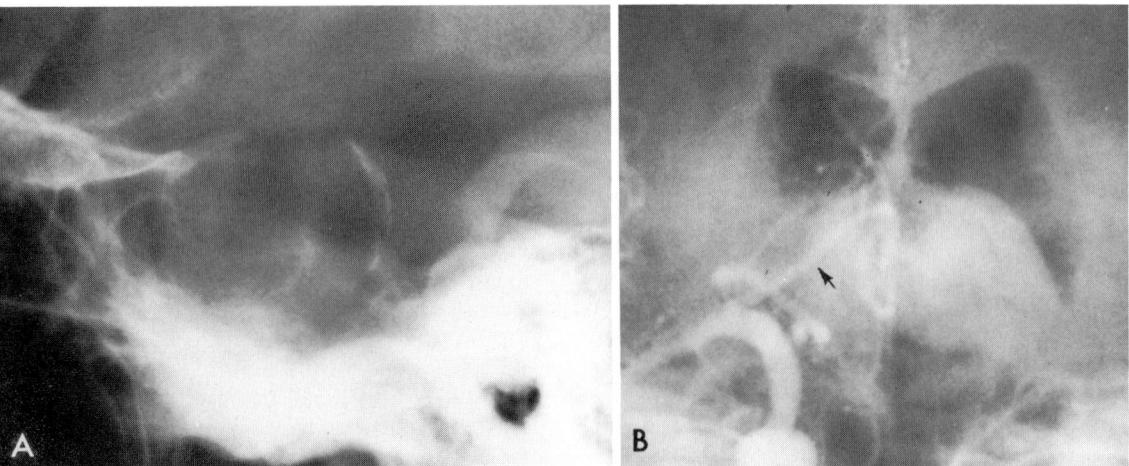

Figure 17–13. Pituitary adenoma, nonfunctional (adult). A, Lateral skull film shows ballooned sella turcica with demineralization of its bony walls and depression of the floor into the sphenoid sinus. B, Carotid angiogram, anteroposterior projection, superimposed on a pneumoencephalogram. Elevation of the first portion of the anterior cerebral artery (arrow) indicates extension of the tumor out of the confines of the sella.

nerves plus facial anesthesia from fifth nerve compression. Such cranial nerve deficits may even be the presenting complaint with a pituitary adenoma (Symonds) but is far less common than symptoms referable to the visual system.

Growth Hormone–Producing Tumors

Growth hormone–secreting pituitary tumors, or acidophilic adenomas, result in gigantism when onset is in childhood before epiphyseal closure, in acromegalic gigantism when onset is in adolescence, and in acromegaly in adulthood. There is a gradual transition of these forms from one to the other depending on age, but even patients with gigantism have certain physical stigmas of acromegaly.

The syndrome of acromegalic gigantism begins with rapid and excessive growth in adolescence. Growth may continue until 25 or 30 years of age and becomes associated with marked enlargement of the hands and feet, coarsening of the external features, prognathism, and kyphoscoliosis. Muscle weakness, ease of fatigue, headache, and pain in the limbs are frequent complaints. Sexual development may proceed in normal fashion, although eventually, panpituitary insufficiency with secondary hypogonadism, hypothyroidism, and hypoadrenalism will occur. A rare complication is sudden, massive hemorrhage within the tumor, which may result in coma, extraocular muscle paralysis, or blindness (Locke and Tyler). This hemorrhagic complication is referred to as pituitary apoplexy. Immediate surgical intervention may be required, and subsequent hormonal inadequacy may follow because of pituitary necrosis (Rigolosi et al.).

The level of serum inorganic phosphorus may be elevated and the glucose tolerance curve is often of the diabetic type in patients with growth hormone–producing tumors. Serum growth hormone levels are markedly elevated and serum insulin content, likewise, may be increased (Elkeles et al.). Most patients show generalized enlargement of the sella turcica on x-ray with demineralization of the anterior and posterior clinoid processes and thinning of the dorsum sellae. The frontal sinuses are enlarged and the supraorbital ridges prominent. Elongation and widening of the vertebral bodies is present as well as many other skeletal abnormalities (Steinbach et al., Lang and Bessler).

Treatment of growth hormone–producing pituitary tumors is controversial but is surgery, irradiation, or a combination of the two. Patients with significant loss of vision or evidence of progressive chiasmal compression are usually managed surgically by a transfrontal approach. Patients without loss of vision have most often been treated with irradiation from an external source, although growth hormone levels remain elevated thereafter (Beck et al.). Roth and colleagues found external irradiation to be comparable to other forms of therapy regarding control of growth hormone secretion.

Visual field and acuity measurements should be recorded every two or three days during irradiation treatment. If deficits appear or markedly progress, therapy should be temporarily delayed and resumed a few days later. Corticosteroid therapy might be of benefit in patients with worsening of vision associated with the initiation of irradiation therapy. Other methods of treatment proposed have included yttrium implantation and cryohypophysectomy (Adams et al.). Substitution therapy with corticosteroids and thyroid preparations is used if target organ failure from pituitary insufficency ensues.

Drug therapy for gigantism and acromegaly shows promise for certain select cases but remains largely investigational. Estrogens antagonize the peripheral effects of growth hormone and may be successful in controlling growth in certain patients (Saxena and Crawford). Progesterone also has been used therapeutically (Lawrence) but appears to have a different mechanism of action. Sherman and Kolodny have demonstrated that, at least in some acromegalic patients, hypersecretion of growth hormone from the pituitary gland is nonautonomous and is influenced by deranged hypothalamic control. Medroxyprogesterone and chlorpromazine may decrease growth hormone release in these patients by suppression of the effects of catecholamines in the hypothalamus thereby inhibiting release of hypothalamic growth hormone releasing factor.

The ACTH-Producing Tumors

The ACTH-producing pituitary tumors resulting in Cushing's disease are rare in childhood. In 1932, Harvey Cushing ascribed to basophilic adenomas the clinical syndrome that included truncal obesity, cutaneous striae, acne, muscle weakness, hirsutism, osteoporosis, hypertension, and disturbances of carbohydrate metabolism. Basophilic tumors have been shown to be the cause of only the minority of cases of Cushing's syndrome. In children, adrenal cortical tumors, especially carcinomas, are the most common cause, except for those iatrogenically produced.

The recognition of adrenal cortical hyperplasia in adults with Cushing's syndrome shifted emphasis on the primary site of the functional disturbance from the pituitary to the adrenal glands. Recent evidence, however, has renewed interest in the role of the hypothalamus with inappropriate control of corticotrophin-releasing factor acting through the anterior pituitary gland leading to cortisol excess from the adrenal glands (Rovit and Duane, Hunder).

An interesting association has been repeatedly reported of Cushing's syndrome in patients with "chromophobe adenomas" of the pituitary gland (Cloutier et al., Myerson and Hingston, Nelson et al., Dingman and Lim, Scholz et al.). In some patients the pituitary tumor did not become apparent until after subtotal adrenalectomy. Although the precise cause-and-effect relationship remains unclear, it may be that the agranular character of these pituitary tumors results from intense stimulation from the hypothalamus, leading to degranulation from continued secretory activity (Rovit and Duane).

Basophilic adenomas of the pituitary gland are usually small lesions and therefore do not often cause enlargement of the sella or visual field defects. These tumors may be found incidentally within the pituitary gland at autopsy.

REFERENCES

Adams, J. E., Seymour, R. J., and Earll, J. M., Tuck, M., Sparks, L. L., and Forsham, P. H.: Transsphenoidal cryohypophysectomy in acromegaly: clinical and endocrinological evaluation. *J. Neurosurg.*, **28**:100–104, 1968.

Anderson, D. R., and Spencer, W. H.: Ultrastructure and histochemical observations of optic nerve gliomas. *Arch. Ophthal.*, **83**:324–335, 1970.

Bailey, P., Buchanan, D. N., and Bucy, P.: *Intracranial Tumors of Infancy and Childhood*. Chicago, University of Chicago Press, 1939.

Bain, H. W., Darte, J. M. M., Keith, W. S., and Kruyff, E.: The diencephalic syndrome of early infancy due to silent brain tumor: With special reference to treatment. *Pediatrics*, **38**:473–482, 1966.

Beck, P., Schalch, D. S., Parker, M. L., Kipnis, D. M., and Daughaday, W. H.: Correlative studies of growth hormone and insulin plasma concentrations with metabolic abnormalities in acromegaly. *J. Lab. Clin. Med.*, **66**:366–379, 1965.

Benton, J. W., Nellhaus, G., Huttenlocher, P. R., Ojemann, R. G., and Dodge, P. R.: The bobble-head doll syndrome. *Neurology*, **16**:725–729, 1966.

Berry, R. G., and Schlezinger, N. S.: Rathke-cleft cysts. *Arch. Neurol.*, **1**:48–58, 1959.

Braun, F. C., Jr., and Forney, W. R.: Diencephalic syndrome of early infancy associated with brain tumor. *Pediatrics*, **24**:609–615, 1959.

Chutorian, A. M., Schwartz, J. F., Evans, R. A., and Carter, S.: Optic gliomas in children. *Neurology*, **14**:83–95, 1964.

Cloutier, M. D., Hayles, A. B., and Sprague, R. G.: Pituitary tumor and Cushing's syndrome. *Amer. J. Dis. Child.*, **112**:596–599, 1966.

Cushing, H.: The basophil adenomas of the pituitary body and their clinical manfestations. *Johns Hopkins Med. J.*, **50**:137–195, 1932.

Dingman, J. F., and Lim, N. Y.: Cushing's syndrome due to an ACTH-secreting chromophobe adenoma. *New Eng. J. Med.*, **267**:696–699, 1962.

Dods, L.: A diencephalic syndrome of early infancy. *Med. J. Aust.*, **2**:689–691, 1957.

Elkeles, R. S., Wright, A. D., Lowy, C., and Fraser, T. R.: Serum-insulin in acromegaly. *Lancet*, **2**:615–618, 1969.

Erdheim, J.: Uber hypophysenganggeschwulste und hirncholesteatome. *Sitzungsb. d. k. Akad. d. Wissenschaft*, **113**:537–582, 1904.

Ezrin, C., Swanson, H. E., Humphrey, J. G., Dawson, J. W., and Hill, F. M.: Beta and delta cells of the human adenohypophysis: Their response to adrenocortical disorders. *J. Clin. Endocr.*, **19**:621–631, 1959.

Frasier, S. D., and Kogut, M. D.: Adolescent acromegaly: Studies of growth hormone and insulin metabolism. *J. Pediat.*, **71**:832–839, 1967.

Friedman, N. B.: Germinoma of the pineal; its identity with germinona ("seminoma") of testis. *Cancer Res.*, **7**:363–368, 1947.

Gamstorp, I., Kjellman, B., and Palmgren, B.: Diencephalic syndromes of infancy. Report of 3 children with emaciation syndrome and disproportionately large hands and feet. *J. Pediat.*, **70**:383–390, 1967.

Gareis, F. J., and Johnson, J. A.: Inanition in infants associated with diencephalic neoplasms. *Amer. J. Dis. Child.*, **109**:349–352, 1965.

Halmi, N. S., and McCormick, W. F.: The delta cell of the human hypophysis in childhood. *J. Clin. Endocr.*, **29**:1036–1041, 1969.

Holman, C. B.: Roentgenologic manifestations of glioma of the optic nerve and chiasm. *Amer. J. Roentgen.*, **82**:462–471, 1959.

Holmes, L. B., Frantz, A. G., Rabkin, M. T., Soeldner, J. S., and Crawford, J. D.: Normal growth with subnormal growth-hormone levels. *New Eng. J. Med.*, **279**:559–566, 1968.

Hoyt, W. F., and Baghdassarian, S. A.: Optic glioma of childhood. *Brit. J. Ophthal.*, **53**:793–798, 1969.

Hudson, A. C.: Primary tumors of the optic nerve. *Roy. London Ophthal. Hosp. Rev.*, **18**:317–439, 1912.

Hunder, G. G.: Pathogenesis of Cushing's disease. *Mayo Clin. Proc.*, **41**:29–39, 1966.

Kagan, H.: Anorexia and severe inanition associated with a tumor involving the hypothalamus. *Arch. Dis. Childh.*, **33**:257–260, 1958.

Kageyama, N., and Belsky, R.: Ectopic pinealoma in the chiasma region. *Neurology*, **11**:318–327, 1961.

Kahn, E. A.: Some physiologic implications of craniopharyngiomas. *Neurology*, **9**:82–90, 1959.

Kenny, F. M., Iturzaeta, N. F., Mintz, D., Drash, A.,

Garces, L. Y., Susen, A., and Askari, H. A.: Iatrogenic hypopituitarism in craniopharyngioma: Unexplained catch-up growth in three children. *J. Pediat.*, **72**:766–775, 1968.

Kramer, S., McKissock, W., and Concannon, J. P.: Craniopharyngiomas. Treatment by combined surgery and radiation therapy. *J. Neurosurg.*, **18**:217–226, 1961.

Kramer, S., Southward, M., and Mansfield, C. M.: Radiotherapy in the management of craniopharyngioma: Further experiences and late results. *Amer. J. Roentgen.*, **103**:44–52, 1968.

Lang, E. K., and Bessler, W. T.: The roentgenologic features of acromegaly. *Amer. J. Roentgen.*, **86**:321–328, 1961.

Lawrence, A. M.: Medical treatment of acromegaly with progestins. *Clin. Res.*, **17**:289, 1969.

List, C. F., Dowman, C. E., Bagchi, B. K., and Bebin, J.: Posterior hypothalamic hamartomas and gangliogliomas causing precocious puberty. *Neurology*, **8**:164–174, 1958.

Locke, S., and Tyler, H. R.: Pituitary apoplexy. *Amer. J. Med.*, **30**:643–648, 1961.

Loop, J. W.: Precocious puberty. Pneumoencephalography demonstrating a hamartoma in the absence of cerebral symptoms. *New Eng. J. Med.*, **271**:409–411, 1964.

Matson, D. D., and Crigler, J. F., Jr.: Management of craniopharyngiomas in childhood. *J. Neurosurg.*, **30**:377–390, 1969.

McCormick, W. F., and Halmi, N. S.: Absence of chromophobe adenomas from a large series of pituitary tumors. *Arch. Path.*, **92**:231–238, 1971.

McKenzie, K. G., and Sosman, M. C.: The roentgenological diagnosis of craniopharyngeal pouch tumors. *Amer. J. Roentgen.*, **11**:171–176, 1924.

Myerson, R. M., and Hingston, W. L.: Cushing's syndrome associated with chromophobe adenoma of pituitary. *Arch. Intern. Med.*, **109**:609–611, 1962.

Nellhaus, G.: The bobble-head doll syndrome: A "tic" with a neuropathologic basis. *Pediatrics*, **40**:250–253, 1967.

Nelson, D. H., Meakin, J. W., and Thorn, G. W.: ACTH-producing pituitary tumors following adrenalectomy for Cushings syndrome. *Ann. Intern. Med.*, **52**:560–569, 1960.

Northfield, D. W. C.: Rathke-pouch tumors. *Brain*, **80**:293–312, 1957.

Papez, J. W., and Ecker, A.: Precocious puberty with hypothalamic tumor (infundibuloma). Case report. *J. Neuropath. Exper. Neurol.*, **6**:15–23, 1947.

Pimstone, B. L., Sobel, J., Meyer, E., and Eale, D.: Secretion of growth hormone in the diencephalic syndrome in childhood. *J. Pediat.*, **76**:886–889, 1970.

Pitlyk, P. J., Miller, R. H., and Johnson, G. M.: Diencephalic syndrome of infancy presenting with anorexia and emaciation. *Mayo Clin. Proc.*, **40**:327–333, 1965.

Poznanski, A. K., and Manson, G.: Radiographic appearance of the soft tissues in the diencephalic syndrome of infancy. *Radiology*, **81**:101–106, 1963.

Rigolosi, R. S., Schwartz, E., and Glick, S. M.: Occurrence of growth-hormone deficiency in acromegaly as a result of pituitary apoplexy. *New Eng. J. Med.*, **279**:362–364, 1968.

Romeis, B.: *In* Mollendorff, W.: *Handbuch der microskopischen Anatomik des Menschen.* Vol. VI, Part 2. Berlin, Springer Verlag, 1940.

Roth, J., Gordon, P., and Brace, K.: Efficacy of conventional pituitary irradiation in acromegaly. *New Eng. J. Med.*, **282**:1385–1391, 1970.

Rovit, R. L., and Duane, T. D.: Cushing's disease and pituitary tumors. *Amer. J. Med.*, **46**:416–427, 1969.

Rubin, P., and Kramer, S.: Ectopic pinealoma: A radiocurable neuroendocrinologic entity. *Radiology*, **85**:512–523, 1965.

Russell, A. A.: A diencephalic syndrome of emaciation in infancy and childhood. *Arch. Dis. Childh.*, **26**:274, 1951.

Russell, D. S.: "Ectopic pinealoma": Its kinship to atypical teratoma of the pineal gland. Report of a case. *J. Path. Bact.*, **68**:125–129, 1954.

Saxena, K. M., and Crawford, J. D.: Acromegalic gigantism in an adolescent girl. *J. Pediat.*, **62**:660–665, 1963.

Scholz, D. A., Gastineau, C. F., and Harrison, E. G., Jr.: Cushing's syndrome with malignant chromophobe tumor of the pituitary and extracranial metastasis. *Mayo Clin. Proc.*, **37**:31–42, 1962.

Segar, W. E.: Chronic hyperosmolarity. *Amer. J. Dis. Child.*, **112**:318–327, 1966.

Sherman, L., and Kolodny, H. D.: The hypothalamus, brain-catecholamines, and drug therapy for gigantism and acromegaly. *Lancet*, **1**:682–685, 1971.

Snyder, R. D.: Diencephalic neoplasms—letter to the editor. *Amer. J. Dis. Child.*, **110**:109, 1965.

Sperling, M. A., Kenny, F. M., and Drash, A. L.: Arginine-induced growth hormone responses in children. Effect of age and puberty. *J. Pediat.*, **77**:462–465, 170.

Steinbach, H. L., Feldman, R., and Goldberg, M. B.: Acromegaly. *Radiology*, **72**:535–549, 1959.

Symonds, C.: Ocular palsy as the presenting symptom of pituitary adenoma. *Johns Hopkins Med. J.*, **3**:72–82, 1962.

Taveras, J. M., Mount, L. A., and Wood, E. H.: The value of radiation therapy in the management of gliomas of the optic nerves and chiasm. *Radiology*, **66**:518–528, 1956.

Tiberin, P., Goldberg, G. M., and Schwartz, A.: Craniopharyngiomas in the aged. *Neurology*, **8**:51–54, 1958.

Torrey, E. F., and Uyeda, C. I.: The diencephalic syndrome of infancy. *Amer. J. Dis. Child.*, **110**:689–696, 1965.

Vejjajiva, A., Sitprija, V., and Shaungshoti, S.: Chronic sustained hypernatremia and hypovolemia in hypothalamic tumor. *Neurology*, **19**:161–166, 1969.

White, P. T., and Ross, A. T.: Inanition syndrome in infants with anterior hypothalamic neoplasms. *Neurology*, **13**:974–981, 1963.

Chapter Eighteen

CEREBRAL HEMISPHERE TUMORS

The incidence of neoplasms involving the cerebral hemispheres in children and in adults differs. Children have a higher percentage of gliomas and a lower percentage of metastatic tumors and glioblastomas. In addition, there is a greater tendency for parenchymal cerebral tumors in childhood to possess bizarre histologic characteristics, at times sufficient to prevent accurate morphologic classification. Cerebral tumors in childhood usually occur in sporadic fashion, unassociated with other diseases. On occasion, however, they develop in patients with recognized familial disorders, including neurofibromatosis, tuberous sclerosis, Wiscott-Aldrich syndrome (Brand and Marinkovich, ten Bensel et al.), and familial polyposis (Baughman et al., Turcot et al.) (Fig. 18-1).

Most cerebral hemisphere tumors in children are gliomas, with astrocytoma being the most common type. Low and colleagues reported 115 histologically proved cerebral hemisphere tumors in patients 16 years of age or younger of which 46 per cent were astrocytomas, 12 per cent glioblastomas, 12 per cent oligodendrogliomas, and 8 per cent ependymomas. In several of these categories, certain components of other glial forms were present. Of the series of 97 cerebral gliomas of Miller et al., 51 per cent were astrocytomas graded 1 through 4, 25 per cent were ependymomas, and 11 per cent were oligodendrogliomas. The parietal lobe was the most common site of tumor in this group, followed by the temporal and frontal lobes.

Although the clinical signs and ancillary studies may suggest localization to one particular lobe, it is not uncommon that adjacent lobes are involved. Total hemisphere replacement by tumor has been described with congenital neoplasms (Oberman) (Fig. 18-2). Cerebral tumors in children are usually solitary and may be either cystic or solid. Multicentric, primary cerebral gliomas are uncommon at any age but most have been described in adults (Courville, Batzdorf and Malamud, Elam and McLaurin, Solomon et al.).

The explanation for the occurrence of two or more primary gliomas unrelated by continuity remains speculative but may be germane to the pathogenesis of neoplastic transformation in general. Some have championed the "field theory" of Willis which, when applied to the brain, presupposes that tumors originate from a field of diffuse gliosis, or gliopathy (van Der Horst). De-differentiation of cell groups within fields results in progressive neoplastic transformation and thus might account for multiplicity of lesions described in rare instances.

Symptoms and signs of cerebral hemisphere tumors are generally related to the location of the lesion. Localization is not always precise, however, because expected signs in reference to the lobe involved may be absent and signs that are present may have misleading implications. For example, grand mal convulsions may occur with a tumor in any lobe of the brain. Page et al. commented on the occurrence of brief lapses or akinetic seizures with bilateral electroencephalographic discharges in children who only after several years developed localizing manifestations indicative of cerebral gliomas.

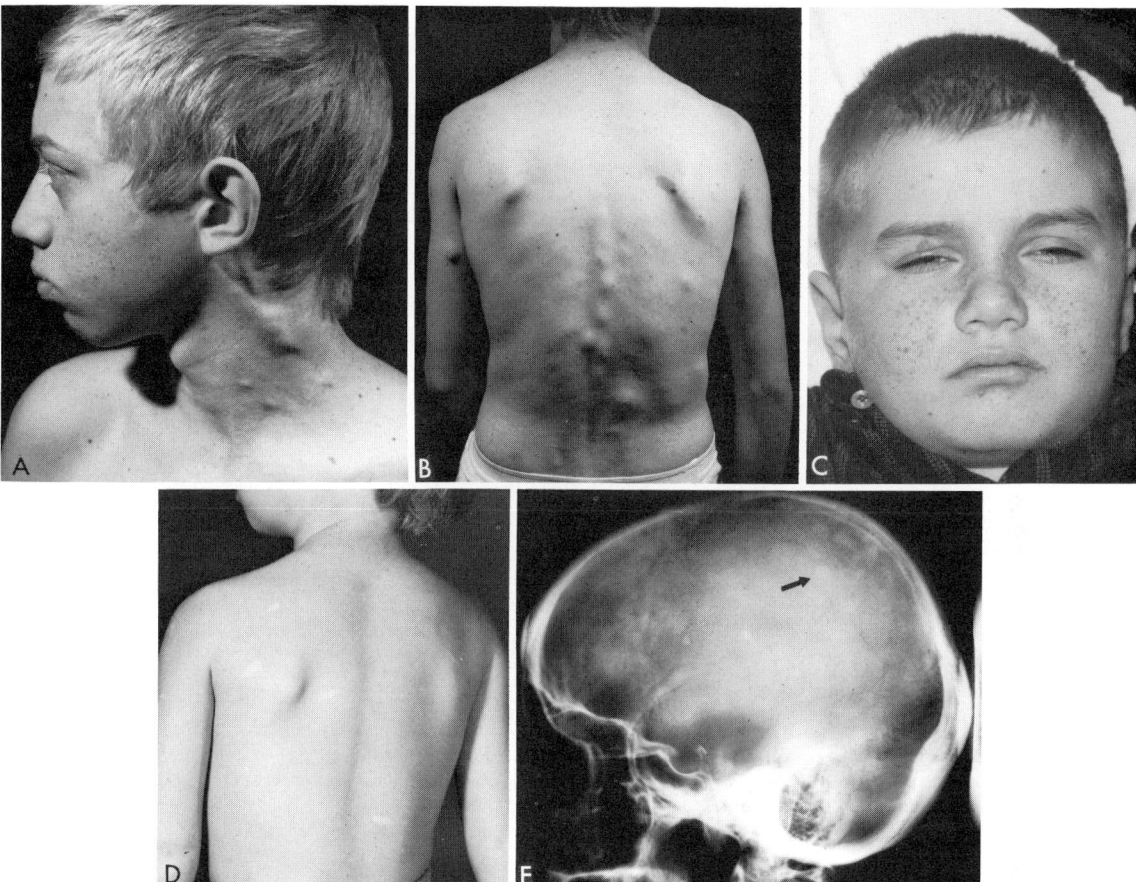

Figure 18–1. Neurocutaneous syndromes. A and B, Neurofibromatosis. Multiple subcutaneous nodules of various sizes and café-au-lait spots. The incidence of intracranial tumors in patients with neurofibromatosis is higher than in general population. Children may develop cystic or solid cerebral hemisphere gliomas, optic chiasm gliomas, or neoplasms within the brain stem. In adults with this disease, gliomas likewise may occur, but meningiomas or acoustic neurinomas are more characteristic. C, Tuberous sclerosis. Eight-year-old boy with a history of seizures in infancy followed by evidence of developmental and mental retardation. Angiofibromas ("adenoma sebaceum") of the face are the most characteristic cutaneous lesions of children with this disease but may not become evident until three to five years of age. D, Four-year-old girl with myoclonic seizures in infancy and developmental retardation. Multiple depigmented nevi, evident here, were present at birth. Angiofibromas of the face and intracranial calcifications were noted at age three years, confirming the diagnosis of tuberous sclerosis. The depigmented lesions, D, are often observed in infancy with this disorder and can serve as a hint to the diagnosis when they are associated with infantile seizures or developmental retardation. E, Skull x-ray of a 14-year-old boy with tuberous sclerosis. There are intracranial calcifications in addition to areas of hyperostosis of the skull (arrow). These patches of increased bone density are frequently observed two or three years before parenchymal calcification is apparent on roentgenographic examination.

The child with tuberous sclerosis also may develop one of a variety of intracranial tumors, in addition to the cerebral "tubers" characteristic of the disease. The predisposition to the formation of brain tumors (other than "tubers"), however, is considerably less in patients with tuberous sclerosis than in those with neurofibromatosis. Gemistocytic astrocytoma, subependymal giant cell astrocytoma, mixed glioma, spongioneuroblastoma, and ganglioglioma are morphologic types that have been described in association with tuberous sclerosis.

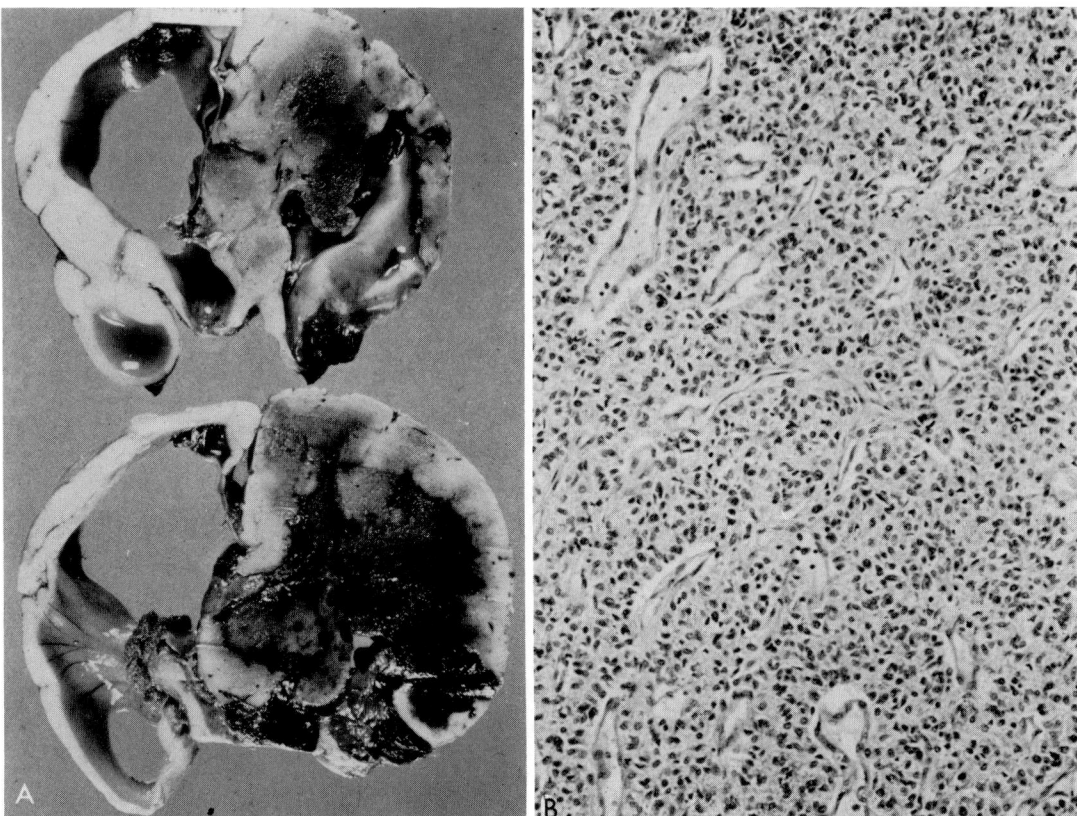

Figure 18–2. Congenital cerebral hemisphere glioma. A, The neoplasm virtually replaces the entire hemisphere and extends into the upper portion of the brain stem. Central hemorrhage into the tumor is extensive and parts have become necrotic. Marked distention of the lateral ventricle on the opposite side is due to obstruction at the level of the foramen of Monro and of the aqueduct. B, Microscopically, the lesion is a moderately vascular, highly cellular glial neoplasm.

Signs of increased pressure and ataxia are clearly suggestive of a posterior fossa lesion but can be observed with frontal lobe tumors. Factors related to the age of the child also enhance the diagnostic complexities of hemisphere tumors. Irritability and a negative attitude toward examination precludes the identification of minor motor or sensory deficits in toddlers. Description of sensory seizures, of visual field defects, or even of headaches is not available in many younger children, permitting the illness to progress until more easily recognized signs become apparent.

FRONTAL LOBE TUMORS

Frontal lobe tumors in children result in variable signs, including those of increased pressure, behavioral or personality changes, and seizures in a significant percentage of patients. Seizures may be akinetic or grand mal, although focal motor or Jacksonian motor seizures are of greater localizing significance. Tumors located in or extending to the posterior frontal region commonly result in a contralateral spastic hemiparesis, which may be associated with a central facial paresis on the paretic side. Papilledema may be found, although in younger children, spread of cranial sutures may delay the appearance of nerve head edema for months or years after the onset of symptoms. Visual field abnormalities are not common with frontal lobe neoplasms except for enlarged blind spots when papilledema is present.

PARIETAL LOBE TUMORS

Parietal lobe tumors may be deceptively silent with symptoms only of headache, vom-

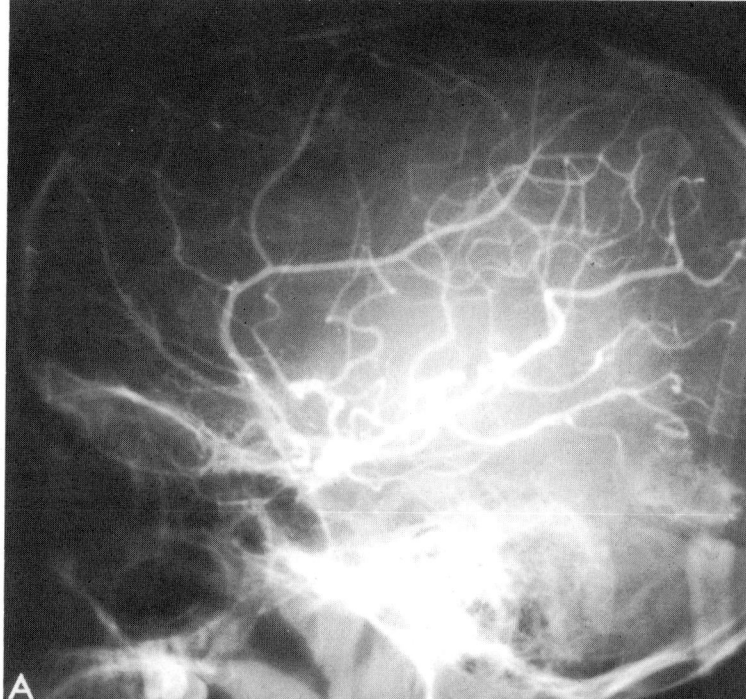

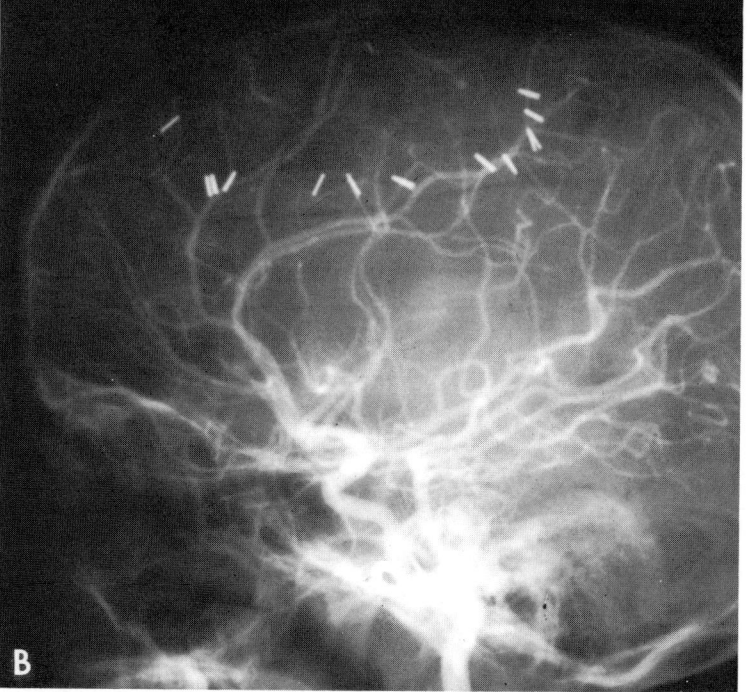

Figure 18–3. Frontal lobe astrocytoma, 12-year-old boy. A, Preoperative carotid angiogram. There is flattening and depression of the pericallosal branch of the anterior cerebral artery in addition to stretching of its distal branches around the tumor. B, Carotid angiogram four months after surgical resection of the neoplasm. The anterior cerebral artery now assumes its more normal distribution. Subsequent x-rays showing separation or displacement of the metallic clips may be used as an indicator of regrowth of the tumor or accumulation of cyst fluid.

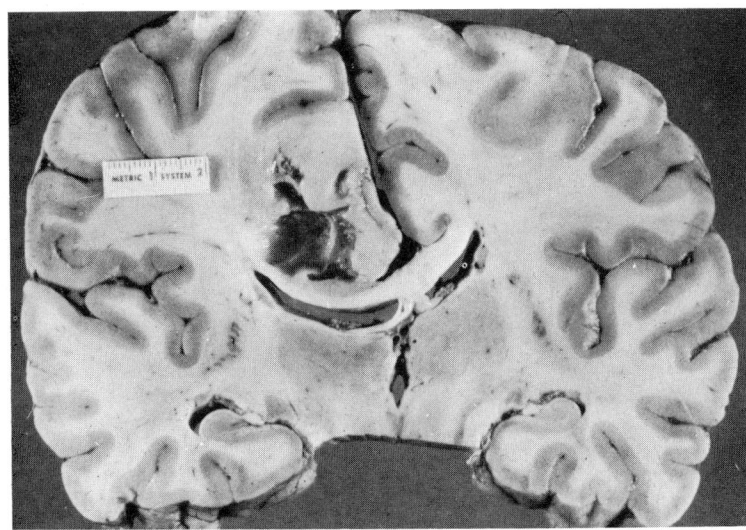

Figure 18–4. Parietal lobe cystic glioma. Demarcation between neoplastic tissue and normal brain tissue is indistinct and cannot be determined by gross examination. There is flattening and depression of the lateral ventricle beneath the tumor and shift of the position of the opposite lateral ventricle.

iting, and increased pressure. Anterior parietal lobe lesions often extend to the motor strip of the frontal lobe, leading to a combination of tingling, mild pin and touch diminution, and limb paresis on the side opposite the tumor. With parietal cortical lesions, the sensory loss to exteroceptive stimuli is only partial. Sensory impulses arriving in the parietal lobe are distributed from the thalamus, which is the seat of conscious awareness of these modalities. Thus, parietal lobe disease may be associated with alterations of sensory stimuli, but complete analgesia or anesthesia does not occur.

Tumors developing in the parasagittal parietal region produce tingling that begins in the foot on the side opposite the tumor; those lower along the postcentral gyrus cause sensory alterations of the face and hand. Focal sensory seizures are described by some patients with tumors in this location and may be associated with a Jacksonian march.

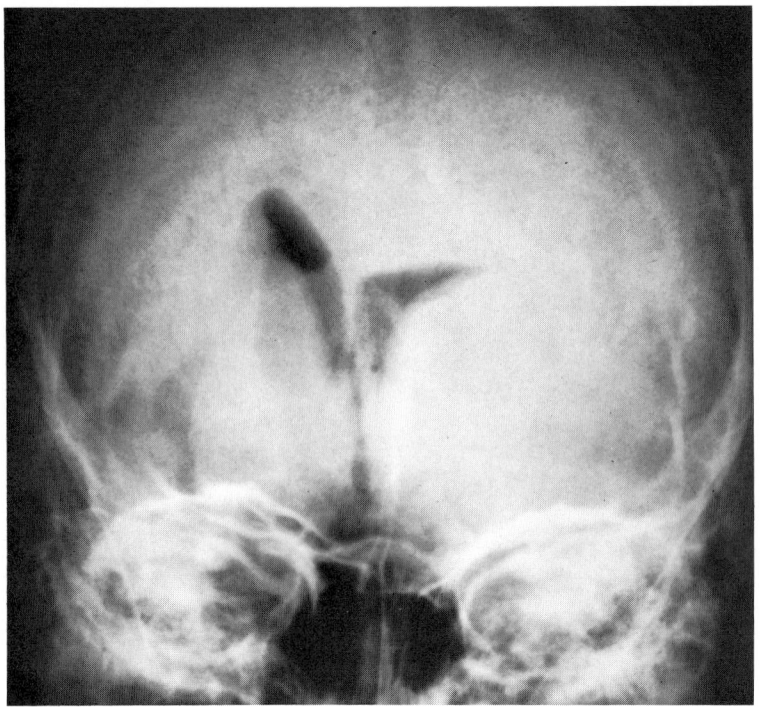

Figure 18–5. Parietal lobe astrocytoma in 12-year-old girl. Pneumoencephalogram, anteroposterior view. There is shift of the lateral ventricles to the opposite side and straight shift of the third ventricle. Flattening of the roof of the lateral ventricle on the side of the tumor is the result of herniation beneath the falx cerebri.

The characteristic sensory deficits of parietal lobe disease are those of higher discriminative functions rather than simple appreciation of tactile stimulation. Astereognosis, or the perception of form and structure of objects by tactile stimulation, can be recognized only if exteroceptive sensation in the hand being tested is intact. Graphesthesia, the ability to recognize numbers or letters written on the skin surface, two-point discrimination, and the recognition of the position of the limbs in space (proprioception) are other perceptual disturbances of parietal lobe disease. Apraxia, anosognosia, and Gerstmann's syndrome are additional parietal lobe manifestations but are rarely seen in children.

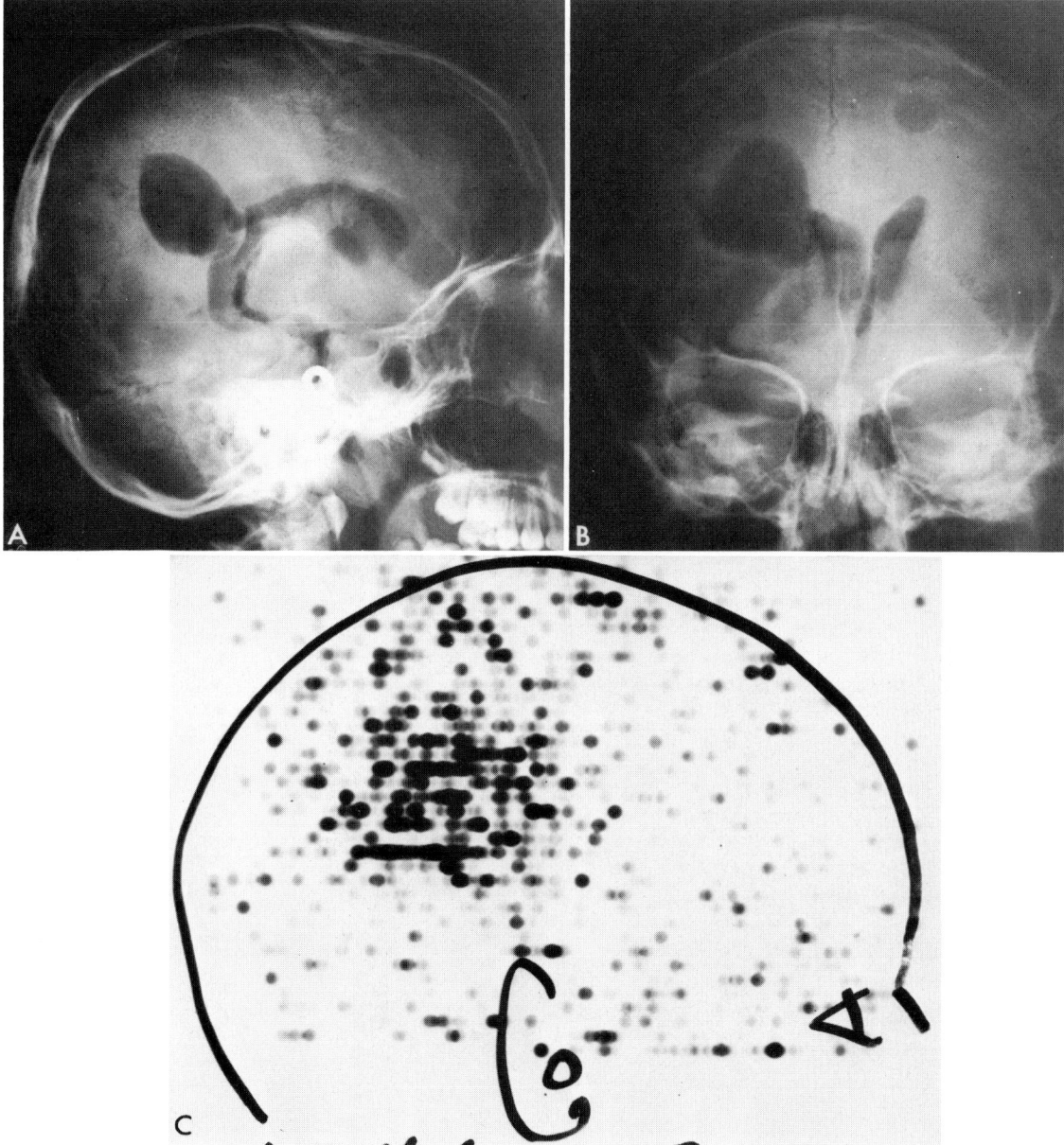

Figure 18-6. Parietal cystic astrocytoma, 12-year-old girl. A, Ventriculogram, lateral view. Cystic cavity was entered first by the penetrating needle and did not communicate with the ventricular system. Advancement of the needle and instillation of air then filled the ventricular system. Note the indentation and depression of the posterior portion of the right lateral ventricle by the neoplastic cyst. B, Ventriculogram, anteroposterior view. The lateral ventricles are shifted to the opposite side and there is a straight shift of the third ventricle, characteristic of parietal lobe tumors. C, Radioactive brain scan demonstrating neoplasm that encircled the cystic mass.

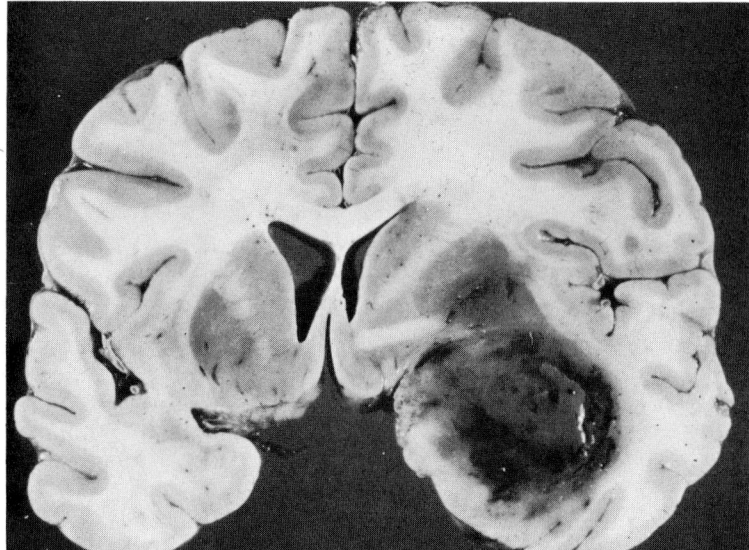

Figure 18–7. Temporal lobe malignant glioma. The entire hemisphere on the same side as the tumor is larger than the opposite hemisphere and there is ventricular shift away from the lesion. The neoplasm is invasive and contains necrosis and hemorrhage.

Tumors in the parietal region that invade white matter to reach the geniculocalcarine fibers cause visual field abnormalities. Inferior homonymous quadrant defects have significant localizing value in this regard but are not often identified in childhood. A complete, or nearly complete, homonymous hemianopsia is more often observed and may be identical to that produced by an occipital lobe tumor. Optikokinetic nystagmus induced by a rotating drum is abnormal in some patients with parietal tumors, especially those of the angular and supramarginal gyri. Decrease or absence of induced nystagmus occurs with rotation of the drum toward the side with the lesion.

TEMPORAL LOBE TUMORS

Temporal lobe neoplasms are characterized by signs of increased pressure if the

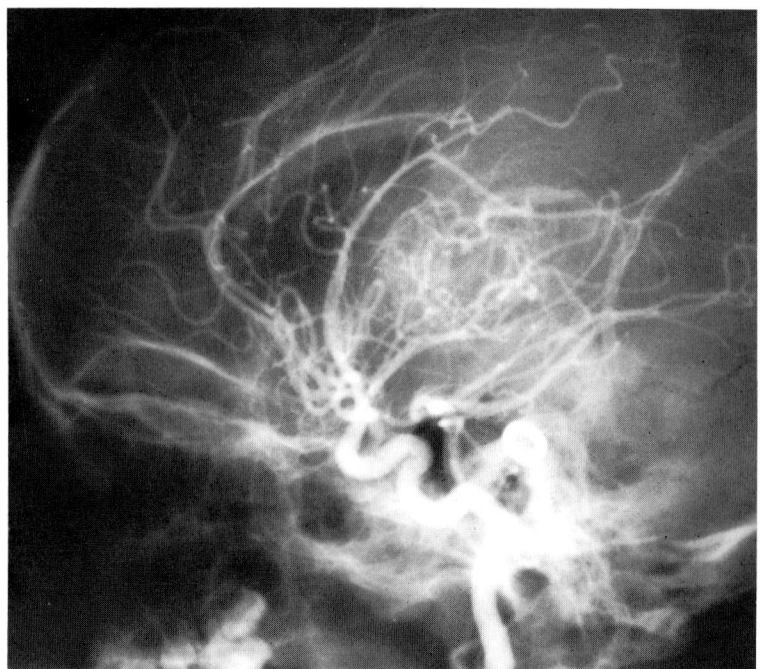

Figure 18–8. Temporal lobe and deep-seated glioblastoma, six-year-old girl. Carotid angiogram demonstrates the abnormal vascularity within the tumor. The middle cerebral artery is elevated so strikingly that it assumes a vertical course. The bowed depression of the posterior cerebral artery indicates transtentorial hippocampal herniation.

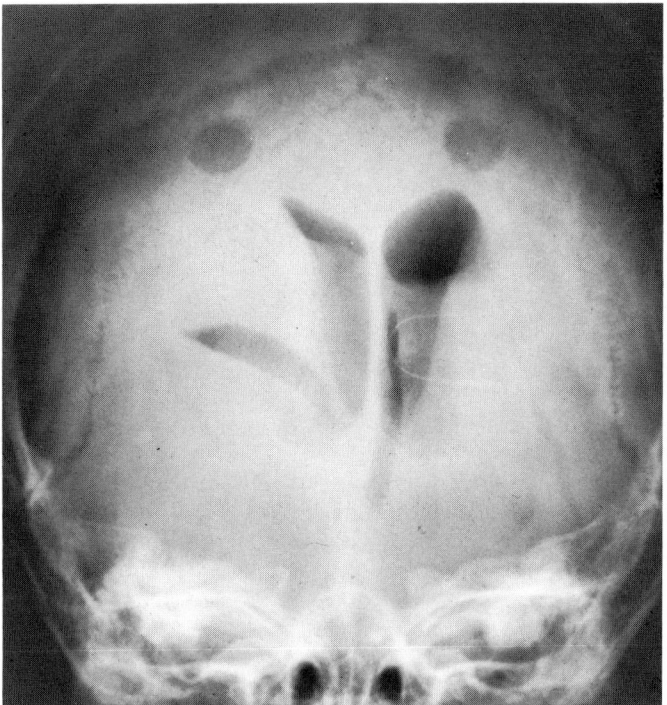

Figure 18-9. Temporal lobe glioma, five-year-old boy. Ventriculogram shows medial and superior displacement of the temporal horn and bowed shift of the third ventricle to the opposite side.

tumor is large. Smaller lesions may be associated with few localizing symptoms except for recurrent psychomotor seizures. Uncinate seizures, or hallucinations of olfaction, sometimes precede a psychomotor episode or may occur in isolated fashion. Organized visual distortions, such as micropsia or macropsia, may also be associated with other epileptic temporal lobe phenomena. Central facial paresis or focal motor seizures on the opposite side of the body indicate extension of the lesion to the posterior inferior frontal region.

Aphasic disorders from tumors of the temporoparietal region of the dominant hemisphere are seen more often in adults than in children. An incongruous homonymous hemianopsia may be present, but of greater localizing value is a superior homonymous quadrantanopsia. This selective type of quadrant defect is indicative of temporal lobe disease and is due to infiltration of the inferior portion of the calcarine fibers passing around the ventricle in the temporal lobe.

OCCIPITAL LOBE TUMORS

Tumors of the occipital lobe are less common than those in any other lobe of the cerebrum. Few specific neurologic signs are evident in children with occipital lobe tumors except for those due to increased intracranial pressure and those pertaining to vision. A symmetrical, or congruous, homonymous hemianopsia is the most characteristic visual disturbance but does not differentiate tumors of the occipital lobe from those of the parietal or temporal regions. Some report recurrent visual hallucinations manifested by unformed patterns, such as moving lines or flickering lights or spots. Younger children may be frightened by episodes of visual disturbances of this type and respond by covering the eyes with the hands or by crying. Although such visual hallucinations occurring in the hemianoptic field are highly localizing to the contralateral occipital lobe, their importance is restricted by their rare occurrence. Grand mal convulsions may occur in patients with occipital tumors and may be preceded by a visual abnormality suggestive of an occipital discharge.

DIAGNOSTIC STUDIES

Recognition of the possibility of a cerebral hemisphere tumor leads to selection of the appropriate studies to confirm its presence and to identify its precise site. Information from skull films, radioactive brain scan, electroencephalogram, and visual fields should be obtained and analyzed before proceeding to contrast studies. The electroencephalogram especially may provide the hint that additional studies are indicated when dealing with children with headache disorders or seizure problems. A well localized delta slow focus, not explained on the basis of previous head trauma, infection, or birth injury, raises immediate concern regarding the possibility of a mass lesion.

Carotid angiography is usually the most informative contrast procedure in children with cerebral hemisphere tumors. In some, both angiography and pneumography are desirable to obtain maximum information preoperatively. The majority of neoplastic cerebral lesions are evident on either or both of these procedures, but normal findings do not categorically exclude the possibility of tumor. The studies can be done too early, before significant enlargement has occurred to be identified by the contrast studies. Such "tumor suspects" are necessarily followed at periodic intervals with repetition of the examinations at the appropriate time.

THALAMIC TUMORS

Thalamic tumors are deep-seated neoplasms located within the thalamus, but often with extension into the internal capsule, the globus pallidus, or the corona radiata. Infiltration to the opposite side through the massa intermedia and to the upper brain stem may result in a complex array of neurologic signs in the late stages. Most are astrocytomas, some are mixed gliomas, and a few are glioblastomas.

McKissock and Paine studied 24 patients with thalamic tumors, including all age groups, and stressed the youthfulness of those involved. The mean age in this series was just under 20 years and three-quarters dated the onset of symptoms before the age of 25 years. Cheek and Tavaras reviewed a series of 51 patients and found two peaks in age of onset. The first peak was those in the first two decades of life and the second peak occurred in the fifth and sixth decades.

The duration of symptoms before diagnosis is extremely variable and may extend from a few weeks to several years. Headache, vomiting, and other manifestations of increased pressure are the most common initial symptoms. Lethargy, apathy, and mental deterioration become evident in some and cannot always be attributed to increased pressure.

Limb weakness opposite the side with the tumor may be the presenting complaint or may develop during the course of the illness. Slight hemiparesis recognized only on neurologic examination gradually evolves to complete hemiplegia. The muscle tone is often diminished in the hemiparetic arm and leg; deep reflexes may be either reduced or enhanced. Tremor, usually on intention, may be noted in the paretic extremities.

Sensory disturbances are less common than motor deficits even though the ventral posterior thalamic nuclear groups are implicated by the tumor. A subjective feeling of numbness may be described and may progress to marked loss of sensation to pin and touch on the hemiparetic side. Spontaneous thalamic pain, or the Dejerine-Roussy syndrome, is distinctly unusual with thalamic tumors and is more characteristic of infarction of the thalamus due to vascular occlusive disease.

Seizures are infrequent until the later stages of the disease, and in children, their absence is one of the features that suggests the deep-seated location of the tumor. Ocular signs are not specific and may be absent. Papilledema is present in patients with increased pressure, and a homonymous field defect indicates extension of the tumor into the adjacent white matter. Anisocoria and nystagmus are sometimes noted. In summary, one should suspect a thalamic tumor in a child with a progressive illness with pressure symptoms and signs, who exhibits hemiparesis and hemisensory deficits but without seizures.

Air encephalography is the most reliable method of establishing the diagnosis of a thalamic tumor. Ventriculography is preferred if significant papilledema is present; pneumography is chosen if the optic discs are flat. Elevation of the floor of the ipsilateral lateral ventricle involving the middle and posterior third of the body of the ventricle is demonstrable on the anteroposterior and lateral views. In cases with obstruction of the posterior third ventricle, both lateral ventricles are distended. In certain cases, only the lateral ventricle on the opposite side from the tumor is dilated. Displacement and bowing of the third ventricle on the anteroposterior view is another important roentgen sign. In some cases, a filling defect due to protrusion of the mass into the third ventricle adds additional localizing information. Ade-

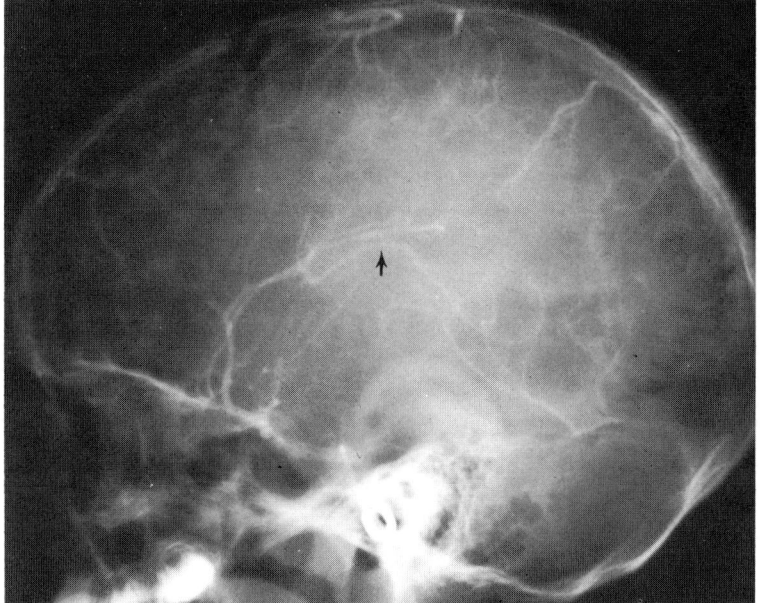

Figure 18–10. Thalamic glioma, five-year-old girl. Carotid angiogram, venous phase. Deep-seated neoplasm results in elevation and humping of the internal cerebral vein, which normally lies just above the third ventricle.

quate filling of the temporal horns may reveal lateral displacement of the horn on the same side as the tumor.

Carotid angiography is of less localizing value than air studies when dealing with tumors within the thalamus. The angiographic Sylvian point is displaced laterally on the frontal projection and the lenticulostriate vessels are moved outward and downward. On the lateral view, the middle cerebral complex may be elevated and the anterior choroidal artery depressed. On the venous phase, the internal cerebral vein is displaced superiorly on the lateral view and to the side opposite the tumor on the frontal projection (Fig. 18-10).

Treatment of gliomas in the thalamic region is largely limited to methods of relieving increased pressure, if present, and administering irradiation to the lesion. Surgery offers little in most cases and is best avoided if clinical symptoms and air studies localize the lesion well. Worsening of clinical signs may accompany the initiation of radiation therapy and can be alleviated by the temporary administration of corticosteroids. Prognosis in children with tumors in this region is generally considered to be poor.

REFERENCES

Batzdorf, V., and Malamud, N.: The problem of multicentric gliomas. *J. Neurosurg.*, **20**:122–136, 1963.

Baughman, F. A., Jr., List, C. F., Williams, J. R., Muldoon, J. P., Segarra, J. M., and Volkel, J. S.: The glioma-polyposis syndrome. *New Eng. J. Med.*, **281**:1345–1346, 1969.

Brand, M. M., and Marinkovich, V. A.: Primary malignant reticulosis of the brain in Wiscott-Aldrich syndrome. *Arch. Dis. Childh.*, **44**:536–542, 1969.

Cheek, W. R., and Taveras, J. M.: Thalamic tumors. *J. Neurosurg.*, **24**:505–513, 1966.

Courville, C. B.: Multiple primary tumors of the brain. Review of the literature and report of twenty-one cases. *Amer. J. Cancer*, **26**:703–731, 1936.

Elam, E. B., and McLaurin, R. L.: Multiple primary intracranial tumors. *J. Neurosurg.*, **18**:388–393, 1961.

Low, N. L., Correll, J. W., and Hammill, J. F.: Tumors of the cerebral hemispheres in children. *Arch. Neurol.*, **13**:547–554, 1965.

McKissock, W., and Paine, K. W. E.: Primary tumors of the thalamus. *Brain*, **81**:41–63, 1958.

Miller, R. H., Craig, W. M., and Kernohan, J. W.: Supratentorial tumors among children. *Arch. Neurol. Psychiat.*, **68**:797–814, 1952.

Oberman, B.: Intracranial teratoma replacing brain. *Arch. Neurol.*, **11**:423–426, 1964.

Page, L. K., Lombrosa, C. T., and Matson, D. D.: Childhood epilepsy and late detection of cerebral glioma. *J. Neurosurg.*, **31**:253–261, 1969.

Solomon, A., Perret, G. E., and McCormick, W. F.: Multicentric gliomas of the cerebral and cerebellar hemispheres. *J. Neurosurg.*, **31**:87–93, 1969.

ten Bensel, R. W., Stadlan, E. M., and Krivit, W.: The development of malignancy in the course of the Aldrich syndrome. *J. Pediat.*, **68**:761–767, 1966.

Turcot, J., Despres, J. P., and Pierre, F. S.: Malignant tumors of the central nervous system associated with familial polyposis of the colon. *Dis. Colon Rectum*, **2**:465–468, 1959.

van Der Horst, L.: Application of the field theory to gliomata. *J. Neuropath. Exper. Neurol.*, **14**:369–375, 1955.

Willis, R. A.: *Pathology of Tumors*. London, Butterworth and Co., 1953.

Chapter Nineteen

CONGENITAL TUMORS

Many of the neoplasms previously discussed have been considered to be congenital in that they may originate from embryonic rests present in the brain at birth. Craniopharyngiomas and medulloblastomas have received most attention in this regard, although the cellular origin of these tumors remains speculative. Teratomas appear more clearly in this class, as do the tumors to be discussed, including the chordoma, the nasal "glioma", and the cranial and intracranial cholesteatoma.

CHORDOMA AND ECCHORDOSIS

Intracranial chordomas are rare tumors at any age but especially in childhood. They develop from remnants of the embryonic notochord and therefore tend to be midline in location. The most common location is in the sacrococcygeal region; the intracranial chordoma usually originates along the clivus blumenbachii. In the clivus, small gelatinous hamartomas are more common than the larger, more aggressive chordomas (Wyatt et al.).

Gross observation of the chordoma reveals it to be composed of soft, gelatinous material with a gray or yellowish coloration, often with a thin capsule. Histologically, the structure varies in different areas. Solid portions contain tumors cells that are irregular in shape with round, hyperchromatic nuclei and indistinct cell boundaries. Cellular areas blend into regions containing physaliferous cells characterized by vacuolated cytoplasm with abundant mucinous material and with areas of cystic degeneration. Electron microscopic study has shown that much of the vacuolization observed by light microscopy is due to the interdigitation of cell processes forming intercellular spaces (Spjut and Luse, Wyatt et al.).

The tumor may grow from the region of the clivus in various directions, including caudally along the medulla, into the cerebellopontine angle, into the sphenoid sinus extending to the nasopharynx, and superiorly to the suprasellar region. This variable growth potential can result in a multiplicity of neurologic abnormalities rendering clinical localization exceedingly difficult.

Multiple cranial nerve palsies are common because the tumor may extend from the interpeduncular cistern to the anterior rim of the foramen magnum. Thus, any or all of the cranial nerves, from the optic to the hypoglossal, may be affected. Pontine compression from its ventral surface may lead to ataxia and long tract signs. Optic atrophy and loss of vision from chiasmal compression are on rare occasion the initial symptoms (Poppen and King), or may develop during the course of the illness.

Symptoms and signs of increased pressure, including headache, vomiting, and papilledema, precede signs of cranial nerve or brain stem compression in some cases. Occipital headaches are prominent in certain patients even without elevated pressure. A cerebellopontine angle syndrome with dysfunction of the fifth through eighth cranial nerves on one side may occur with the true nature of the tumor remaining unsuspected until surgical exploration.

Roentgenographic examination is of importance since bone destruction is common with chordomas. This may be evident on a basilar skull view, which may also reveal a soft tissue mass (Demir and Steegmann). Lateral skull films often demonstrate destruction of the dorsum sellae, posterior clinoid processes, and floor of the hypophyseal fossa. Mineral deposition occurs within the tumor in some cases but is not common. Pneumoencephalogram aids in localization of the lesion ventral to the pons or may reveal extension above the sella, producing a filling defect in the chiasmatic cistern or indentation of the anterior third ventricle.

Due to the relatively inaccessible location, complete surgical removal of an intracranial chordoma is unusual. Recurrence after partial resection can be anticipated. Irradiation therapy offers little hope and few cases will respond to this form of treatment.

NASAL "GLIOMAS"

This rare congenital tumor was termed a glioma by Schmidt in 1900 but it possesses few qualities of the intracranial gliomas. It is often referred to as a nasal neuroglial heterotopia, which is probably more accurate and descriptive. The origin of this tumor remains unclear. Postulations have included its development from the frontal process of the cerebral vesicle, from neuroglia surrounding the olfactory bulb, from displaced islands of glial tissue derived from neural ectoderm, and from remnants of an encephalocoele pinched off during fetal development.

The mass may be either extranasal or intranasal; the extranasal tumor is more common. The intranasal lesions resemble nasal polyps, with which they are readily confused (Strauss et al.). Symptoms include chronic nasal obstruction and nasal discharge. In some instances, there is an intracranial communication through a defect in the cribriform plate. Awareness of this possibility is of major importance because communication intracranially predisposes to rhinorrhea or recurrent meningitis, especially following operative removal of the intranasal portion (Ross).

Extranasal "gliomas" are smooth, incompressible mass lesions located at the bridge of the nose and covered by intact skin. The nasal bridge is broadened and the eyes appear wide-set. The mass characteristically does not pulsate, does not bulge significantly with crying or straining, and does not transilluminate. Lesions in the same area that must be differentiated from the nasal "glioma" include the nasal meningocoele or meningoencephalocoele, neurofibroma, dermoid cyst, and lipoma.

Histologically, these lesions are composed of nests of glial cells interlaced with fibrous tissue. The cells are largely astroglial; other neural cellular elements are not usually present. Multinucleated glial forms may be observed, but mitoses are not expected.

Although growth of these tumors is exceedingly slow, operative intervention is indicated to establish the diagnosis, to improve cosmetic appearance, and to exclude the hazard of cerebrospinal fluid rhinorrhea. Several authorities have proposed that frontal craniotomy precede removal of the nasal lesion (Walker and Resler, Ross). Careful search for a connecting stalk is made and is removed and disected to its exit if identified. At a subsequent date, the external portion of the tumor is then removed. In instances in which an intranasal "glioma" is identified unexpectedly on histologic examination after surgical removal, an explorative craniotomy should soon follow to eliminate the possibility of intracranial extension.

EPIDERMOID CYST (CHOLESTEATOMA)

The pearly appearance presented by these rare tumors was first mentioned by Cruveilheir in 1829 when he coined the term "tumor perlée." In 1854, Remak suggested that these tumors develop from displaced embryonic epithelial tissue; most authors now ascribe to this view. At approximately the fourth fetal week, the neural tube closes and the neural ectoderm becomes separated from the cutaneous ectoderm. Retention of fragments of the cutaneous ectoderm within the neural tube may result in midline epidermoid or dermoid tumors later in life.

A more advanced developmental disturbance with incomplete separation of the two ectodermal layers accounts for the sinus tracts sometimes noted with intracranial dermoids. The laterally placed epidermoids located in the skull or within the intracranial cavity are believed to be related to a similar process of ectodermal retention associated with the development of the optic and otic vesicles during the fifth and sixth weeks of intrauterine life.

It is important to distinguish the cholesteatoma due to the developmental defects already described from that better known in otolaryngology which appears secondary to chronic and recurrent middle ear infection. Although the two have histologic similarities, the general opinion is that the source of origin is different, with the middle ear lesion being a proliferative process stimulated by chronic inflammation.

Epidermoid tumors present a glistening white exterior with a thin, fibrous tissue capsule. It is a relatively avascular mass, the interior of which contains material that resembles cottage cheese (Fleming and Botterell). Those occurring within the diploe of the skull are often frontal or parietal in location. The lateral orbital region is also a common location. The intracranial tumors may occur in a variety of locations, including above the sella (Mark et al., Olivecrona), in the cerebellopontine angle (Olivecrona), in the paratrigeminal region (Baumann and Bucy), and in the posterior fossa (Rosenbluth and Lichtenstein).

Epidermoid cysts of the skull are occasionally found incidentally on skull x-rays taken for other purposes. In some instances, a nontender mass palpated in the scalp leads to its identification. Those of the lateral orbital region or roof of the orbit may produce proptosis, temporal pain, and loss of vision (Fleming and Botterell). On rare occasion, a cranial cholesteatoma invades the inner table of the skull, compressing structures sufficiently to displace the brain (Swisher and Tesluk).

The radiologic features of the epidermoid cyst of the skull are distinctive, usually allowing presumptive diagnosis before histologic examination. The tumor results in a round or oval radiolucent area located between the tables of the skull, with scalloped edges and sclerotic margins (Fig. 19-1). The rim of bone sclerosis margining this cranial tumor aids in differentiating it from the eosinophilic granuloma or cranial neurofibroma, which otherwise bears close resemblance. Surgical excision is advised in most cases since continued growth and bone destruction slowly occur over years (Greenberg).

The clinical manifestations of the intracranial cholesteatomas depend on the location. These tumors cause neurologic deficits by compression of adjacent structures; invasiveness is not characteristic. The most remarkable feature of these lesions is the extremely slow rate of growth, which may be measured over decades. This may account in part for the usual onset of symptoms being delayed to early or middle adulthood.

Radiologic abnormalities are also depend-

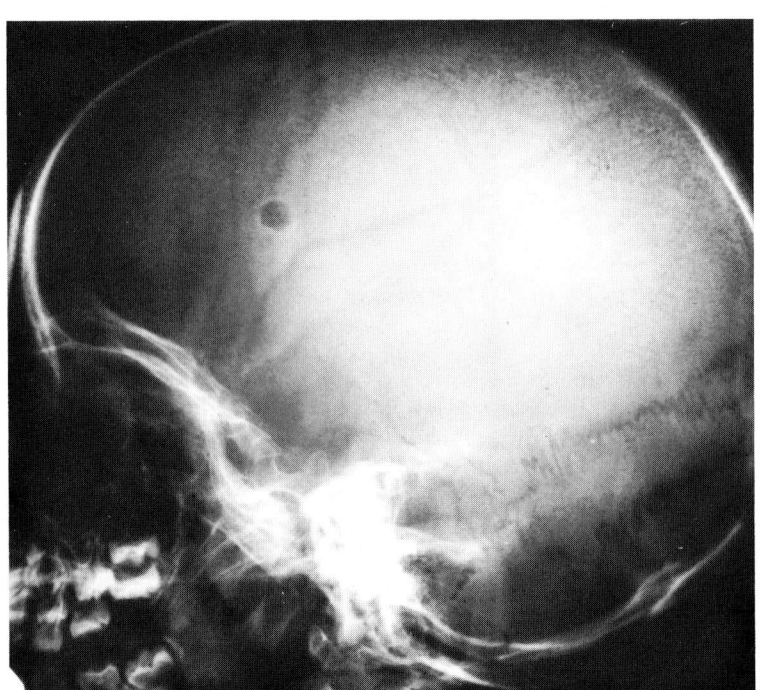

Figure 19-1. Cranial epidermoid cyst (cholesteatoma), three-year-old boy. Lesion was asymptomatic and was an incidental finding. Note circular defect in frontal bone with sclerotic margin.

ent on the intracranial location. Tumors at the base of the skull may produce erosion of the petrous tip, although there usually is little roentgen evidence that is specifically suggestive of this particular tumor. Spontaneous rupture of intracranial epidermoid or dermoid tumors (Manlapaz) is capable of inciting meningeal irritation resembling meningitis, or suddenly provoking coma or manifestations of increased intracranial pressure. Likewise, an aseptic meningitis syndrome may follow operative removal of these lesions if contents are spilled within the subarachnoid space.

Operative removal is indicated whenever possible, although the size of the tumor may preclude complete excision. The fibrous capsule in certain cases is densely adherent to vital areas, which also can prevent total removal. Even partial removal may allow considerable symptomatic improvement followed by years of good health.

POSTERIOR FOSSA DERMOID TUMORS WITH CONGENITAL DERMAL SINUS

Dermoid tumors may occur in the skull or within the intracranial space in a fashion analogous to the epidermoid tumors discussed previously. In addition, the pathogenesis of the dermoid cyst is believed to be similar to that of the epidermoid tumor with it resulting from retention of elements of cutaneous ectoderm beneath the surface during neural groove closure.

Dermoid tumors vary greatly in size and have heterogenous constituents, including thick, yellowish material secreted from sebaceous glands, mucinous substance, hair, sweat glands, and other debris. Dermoid tumors generally occur in a younger age group than do epidermoid tumors and thus are more common in childhood.

The most common site of the intracranial dermoid tumor in childhood is in the posterior fossa, either within the fourth ventricle or in the vermis of the cerebellum. A feature characteristic of many posterior fossa dermoid tumors is the presence of a congenital dermal sinus lined by squamous epithelium that connects the tumor with the skin surface. The surface opening may be surrounded by a tuft of hair or by a cutaneous hemangioma.

This lesion should be suspected in a child with recurrent bacterial meningitis due to an unusual bacterial organism in relation to the age of the child. Staphylococcal or streptococcal meningitis, proteus meningitis beyond the newborn period, or *Hemophilus influenzae* meningitis in a child over six years of age should warrant consideration of a possible dermal sinus. Thorough inspection of the occipital and suboccipital areas is important in such cases and may require shaving of the hair from this region (Altman). Neurologic examination may reveal truncal ataxia or papilledema, providing evidence of a mass lesion within the posterior fossa.

A small, circular defect in the occipital bone is evident on x-ray in some patients with a dermal sinus. The absence of a bony defect on x-ray, however, does not eliminate the possibility. Air encephalography is usually indicated in suspected cases to identify and localize the presumed posterior fossa mass. When the occipital dermal sinus becomes apparent during an episode of meningitis, appropriate antibiotics should be continued for several days after recovery. Air studies should be delayed for two to three weeks after recovery and antibiotics should be administered during and after the contrast procedure.

Surgical treatment consists of careful dissection and complete removal of the sinus tract from the surface to its intracranial termination. Removal of the intracranial dermoid tumor may be complete in many instances. In addition to the hazards of recurrent meningitis and intracranial abscess formation, the danger of spontaneous rupture of an intracranial dermoid is life-threatening, although rare.

REFERENCES

Altman, R. S.: Dermoid tumor of the posterior fossa associated with congenital dermal sinus. *J. Pediat.*, **62**:565–570, 1963.

Baumann, C. H. H., and Bucy, P. C.: Paratrigeminal epidermoid tumors. *J. Neurosurg.*, **13**:455–468, 1956.

Bloom, H. J. G., Wallace, E. N. K., and Henk, J. M.: The treatment and prognosis of medulloblastoma in children. *Amer. J. Roentgen.*, **105**:43–62, 1969.

Cruveilhier, J.: Anatomie pathologique du Corps humain. Vol. II. Paris, Bailliere, 1829.

Demir, R., and Steegmann, A. T.: Intracranial chordoma. *Neurology*, **9**:514–521, 1959.

Fleming, J. F. R., and Botterell, E. H.: Cranial dermoid and eipdermoid tumors. *Surg. Gynec. Obstet.*, **109**:403–411, 1959.

Greenberg, B. E.: Epidermoid cyst of the skull. *Radiology*, **76**:107–109, 1961.

Manlapez, J. S.: Ruptured intracranial dermoid. *Amer. J. Surg.,* **100**:723–730, 1960.

Mark, V. H., Smith, J. L., and Kjellberg, R. D.: Suprasellar epidermoid tumor. *Neurology,* **10**:81–83, 1960.

Olivecrona, H.: On suprasellar cholesteatomas. *Brain,* **55**:122–134, 1932.

Olivecrona, H.: Cholesteatomas of the cerebellopontine angle. *Acta. Psychiat.,* **24**:639–643, 1949.

Poppen, J. L., and King, A. B.: Chordoma: Experience with thirteen cases. *J. Neurosurg.,* **9**:139–163, 1952.

Rosenbluth, P. R., and Lichtenstein, B. W.: Pearly tumor (epidermoid cholesteatoma) of the brain. *J. Neurosurg.,* **17**:35–42, 1960.

Ross, E. E.: Nasal glioma. *Laryngoscope,* **76**:1602–1611, 1966.

Schmidt, M. B.: Uber seltene spaltibildungen in bereiche des mittleren spirnforsatzes. *Virchow Arch. Path. Anat.,* **162**:340–370, 1900.

Spjut, H. J., and Luse, S. A.: Chordoma: An electron microscopic study. *Cancer,* **17**:643–656, 1964.

Strauss, L., Callicott, J. H., Jr., and Hargett, I. R.: Intranasal neuroglial heterotopia. *Amer. J. Dis. Child.,* **111**:317–320, 1966.

Swisher, R. C., and Tesluk, H.: Epidermoid cyst of the skull causing displacement of brain. *J.A.M.A.,* **210**:1280–1281, 1969.

Walker, E. A., Jr., and Resler, D. R.: Nasal glioma. *Laryngoscope,* **73**:93–107, 1963.

Wyatt, R. B., Schochet, S. S., Jr., and McCormick, W. F.: Ecchordosis physaliphora. An electron microscopic study. *J. Neurosurg.,* **34**:672–677, 1971.

Chapter Twenty

MISCELLANEOUS TUMORS

CHOROID PLEXUS PAPILLOMA

Papilloma of the choroid plexus is an unusual type of intracranial tumor. It may occur at any age but is more common in children, especially infants. Of 408 intracranial tumors in children under 12 years of age, 16 (3.8 per cent) were this type (Matson and Crofton). In infants and children, these tumors occur more commonly in the lateral ventricles; in adults, they are more often within the fourth ventricle. Papillomas of the lateral ventricle usually are in the region of the trigone at the confluence of the temporal and posterior horns (Fig. 20-1). Microscopically, the tumor resembles normal choroid plexus with a single layer of cuboidal epithelium overlaying a stroma of highly vascular connective tissue. Seeding may rarely occur, with implantation of tumor cells in the meninges of the brain or spinal cord.

Symptoms and signs of a papilloma of the lateral ventricle in the infant may be those only of hydrocephalus with abnormal head enlargement and tenseness of the fontanel. Those occurring in the second year of life may be suspected by the development of hydrocephalus following a normal period in the first year. Papilledema in such a child would also suggest this type of tumor because nerve head edema is uncommon in babies with the more common types of congenital

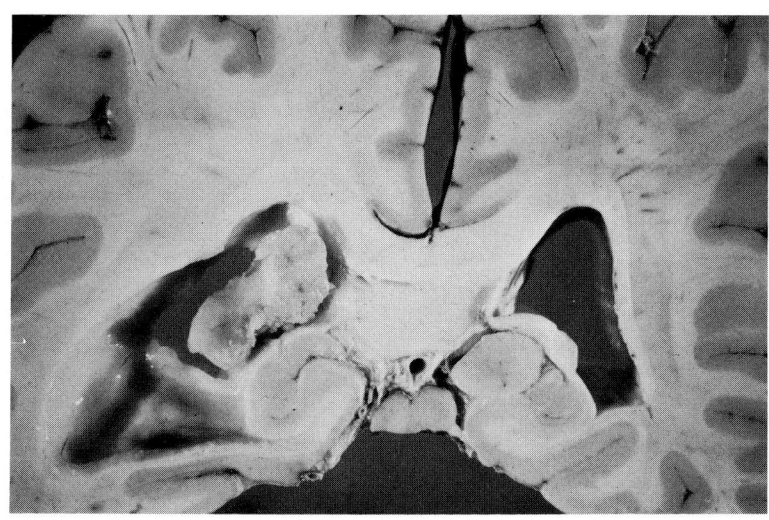

Figure 20-1. Choroid plexus papilloma. Tumor is entirely intraventricular and is located at the confluence of the posterior and temporal horns. Mild ventricular enlargment is present, presumably from hypersecretion of cerebrospinal fluid from the lesion.

hydrocephalus. Seizures may occur in addition to long tract signs, either bilaterally or opposite the side with the lesion. Children with papillomas of the fourth ventricle generally show manifestations of obstructive hydrocephalus usually with truncal ataxia.

Lumbar puncture is not indicated in children with symptoms previously described but ventricular fluid becomes available for examination when the ventriculogram is performed. The ventricular pressure is elevated, the protein content increased, and the fluid may be colorless or xanthochromic. Yellow discoloration and red cells are explained by the vascular nature of the lesion present within the ventricle. Cytologic examination of a properly prepared specimen may reveal tumor cells.

The mechanism of ventricular enlargement with lateral ventricle choroid plexus papillomas is of interest. In certain cases, the tumor extends to, or obstructs, the foramen of Monro, resulting in unilateral ventricular enlargement. In most cases, however, ventricular obstruction is not present, suggesting that communicating hydrocephalus results from excessive fluid secretion from the tumor. Matson and Crofton felt that the rapid regression of hydrocephalus after surgical removal of the tumor was compatible with this postulate. Hemorrhage from the tumor may cause extraventricular obstruction within the basilar cisterns. Some believe this may also contribute to the development of hydrocephalus in certain cases (Laurence et al.).

Ventriculography is the most satisfactory method of demonstrating a choroid plexus papilloma; however, sufficient air must be injected or the lesion can be missed. The "bubble" technique of ventriculography in which only a small quantity of air is used is unsatisfactory for this reason. Demonstration of communicating hydrocephalus with xanthochromic fluid and a mass within the lumen of one lateral ventricle is considered strong evidence of a choroid plexus papilloma.

Treatment is surgical removal of the tumor. Those in the lateral ventricle are usually approached by a posterior parietal cortical incision. Tenseness of the dura can be allieviated by cannulating the lateral ventricle. Matson and Crofton stated that at surgery the tumor may extend into the brain substance, resulting in porencephalic cyst formation in adjacent cerebral tissue. These authors found that if the arterial blood supply to the mass could be ligated, the tumor would shrink markedly, easing total removal. Postoperatively, the child should be observed for evidence of persisting communicating hydrocephalus. This appears to be uncommon but it would warrant a shunt procedure.

NEUROBLASTOMA (SYMPATHICOBLASTOMA)

Neuroblastoma is only rarely a primary intracranial tumor but is included here because it develops from primitive sympathetic cells of neural crest origin and because it has a tendency to spread to orbital tissue and the intracranial extradural space. Thus tumor has been of interest because of certain biochemical aspects and because of its occasional tendency toward spontaneous maturation to ganglioneuroblastoma and to the more highly differentiated ganglioneuroma.

Spontaneous maturation of neoplasms into more benign forms has been described with various tumors but has been discussed most often in regard to those of neural crest origin. Knowledge of biologic principles that stimulate transformation of this sort carries great importance in view of the potential therapeutic applications.

The most frequently quoted reference to spontaneous maturation of a neuroblastoma to a benign ganglioneuroma was that of Cushing and Wolbach in 1927. The patient described had been seen in 1911 at age 18 months with progressive weakness of the legs. A paravertebral tumor was biopsied and subsequently diagnosed as neuroblastoma. The patient was treated with Coley's toxin, and in 1921 laminectomy at the level of the previous biopsy revealed a sharply defined epidural mass that histologically proved to be a benign ganglioneuroma. The patient was again evaluated in 1947 at age 48 years and no evidence of tumor was found (Fox et al.).

Although several reports of complete maturation of neural crest tumors have appeared, the interest created has exceeded the occurrence of this rare phenomenon (Dyke and Mulkey, Haber and Bennington, Kissane and Ackerman). Differentiation within the tumor to a more benign form does not always indicate recovery. Aterman and Schueller described a case in which maturation to a ganglioneuroma was associated with death with diffuse metastases due to the neuroblastomatous component of the tumor. The reason certain neuroblastomas undergo this maturational change remains unknown. Some investigators have suggested that irradiation may provoke such alterations in growth characteristics within the tumor (Uhlmann and von Essen), although maturation has occurred in certain cases without irradiation therapy (Cushing and Wolbach).

Most neuroblastomas have their origin in the retroperitoneal space, either from the adrenal medulla or from ganglia of the sympathetic chain. Others develop in the cervical region or thoracic cavity along the sympathetic chain and less commonly, from the ciliary, otic sphenopalatine, nodose, and submaxillary ganglia. A rare type referred to as the olfactory neuroblastoma, or esthesioneuroblastoma, originates in the nasal fossa. Among 212 cases of neuroblastoma, deLorimier et al. found the primary site of origin to be retroperitoneal in 63 per cent, mediastinal in 16 per cent, sacral in 3 per cent and cervical in 2 per cent of cases. In 11 per cent, the tumor was so widespread when first seen that the primary site could not be determined. In this series, 32 per cent occurred in children under one year of age, 14 per cent were between one and two years, 37 per cent from two to seven years, and 17 per cent were seven to 19 years of age. Distant metastases were present in 76 per cent when the diagnosis was first made.

Symptoms and Signs

Clinical manifestations of a neuroblastoma are extremely variable and may be those of a localized lesion or secondary to metastatic involvement. A palpable abdominal mass may be identified incidentally or becomes apparent on examination of a child being assessed for fever of unknown origin, bone or joint pain, or anemia. Mediastinal neuroblastomas often become quite large before compression signs, such as cough or Horner's syndrome, are evident. Primary tumors in this location can extend medially into the spinal canal, producing signs of spinal cord compression.

Primary cervical neuroblastomas are unusual but present with a painless cervical mass, at times with a Horner's syndrome on the same side. Cervical adenopathy may also be due to metastatic spread from mediastinal or retroperitoneal lesions.

Neuroblastoma present in the newborn resembles that occurring later in infancy, although certain variations are apparent. Dissemination of the tumor from its primary site of origin results in a multiplicity of abnormalities, including hepatomegaly, palpable subcutaneous nodules, and spinal cord compression with paraplegia. The latter may be attributed to birth trauma unless a spinal block is demonstrated or an abdominal mass is palpated.

Subcutaneous metastatic lesions have been stated to be more common with neuroblastoma in the newborn than that developing later (Schneider et al.). Strauss and Driscoll reported two newborn infants with neuroblastoma with metastatic spread to the placenta. Anemia and generalized edema of these babies resembled that seen in hemolytic disease of the newborn due to blood group incompatibility.

Chronic diarrhea and hypertension have occasionally been described in children with neurogenic tumors, presumably secondary to catecholamine secretion from the lesion (Rosenstein and Engelman). The reason only certain patients with secreting tumors of neural crest origin exhibit these symptoms remains unclear. Although neuroblastomas are far more common than ganglioneuromas in the pediatric age group, ganglioneuromas have more often been associated with diarrhea or hypertension.

Another curious metabolic phenomenon rarely noted with neuroblastoma is the physical stigmas of Cushing's syndrome (Kogut and Donnell). Several nonadrenal tumors in adults have been associated with Cushing's syndrome, including carcinoma of the bronchus, thyroid, ovary, and pancreas. Secretion of ACTH-like material from the tumor has been proposed as the explanation for adrenal cortical hyperfunction in these patients (Meador et al.) although this remains to be demonstrated in those with neuroblastoma. Severe muscle weakness due to hypokalemia may represent the early clinical features in children with this odd symptomatic variation of neuroblastoma (Kenny et al.).

A relatively common mode of presentation of neuroblastoma in children results from metastatic spread to the orbital contents or to the intracranial extradural tissues (Fig. 20-2). Periorbital discoloration or ecchymosis may precede other findings or be associated with proptosis and swelling of the zygomatic or temporal region (Mortada). Necrotic changes within the metastatic deposits in the orbit induce local changes resembling an inflammatory process.

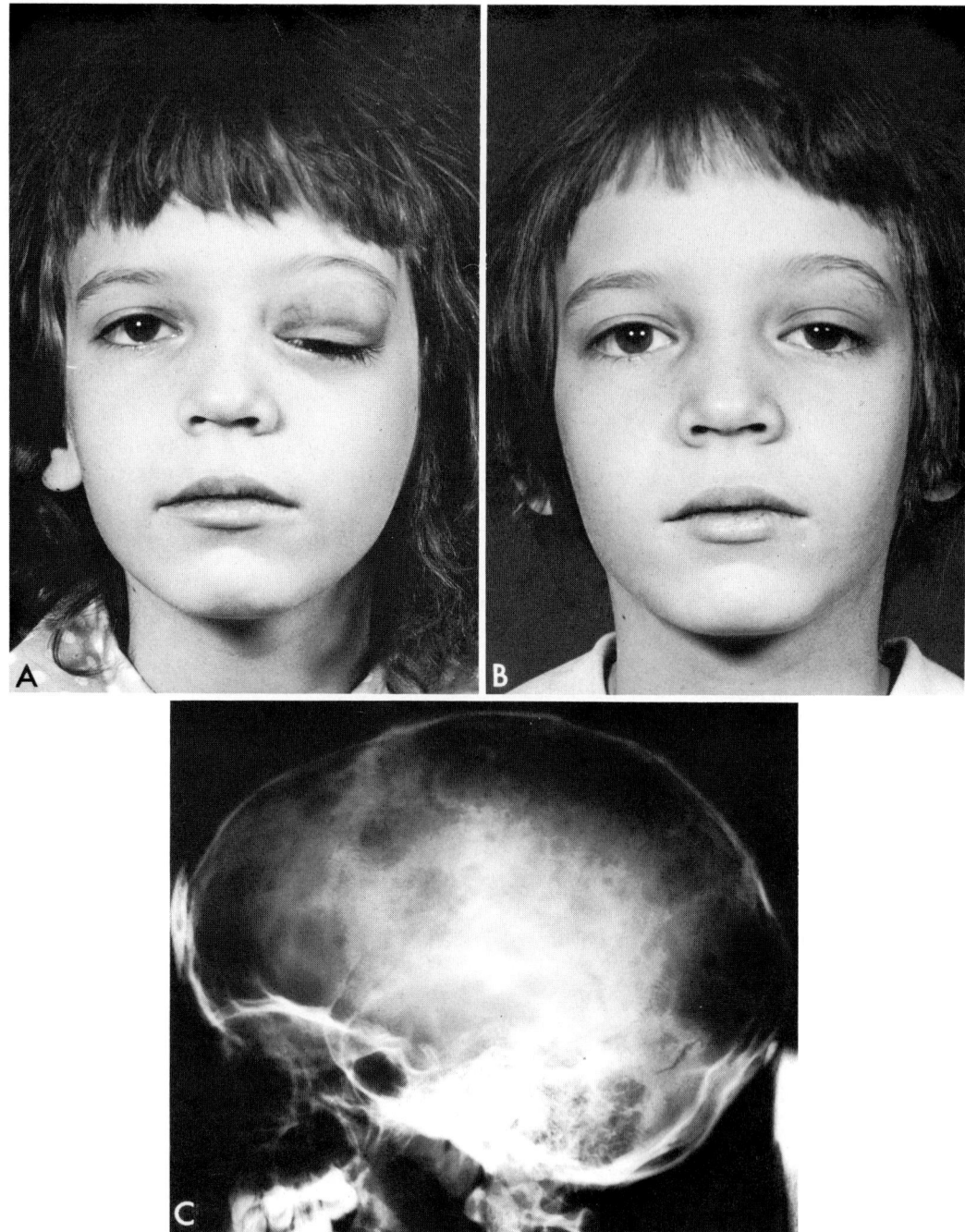

Figure 20-2. Mediastinal neuroblastoma with cranial and orbital metastases. A, Eight-year-old girl with three-week history of headache, vomiting, weight loss and pain in the left orbital region. B, Marked improvement with decrease in symptoms and reduction of proptosis after two weeks of irradiation therapy. C, Lateral skull x-ray shows diffuse osteolytic destructive lesions.

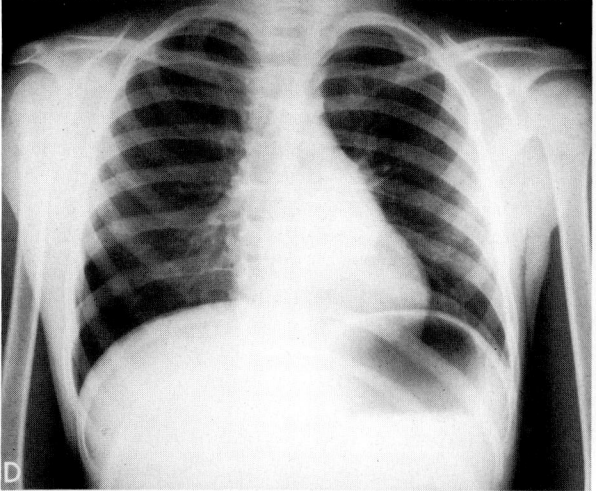
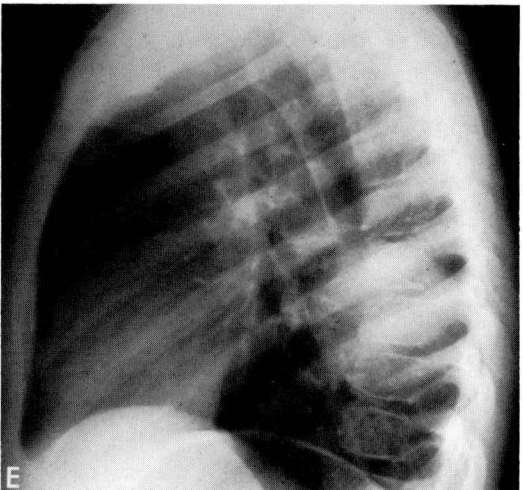
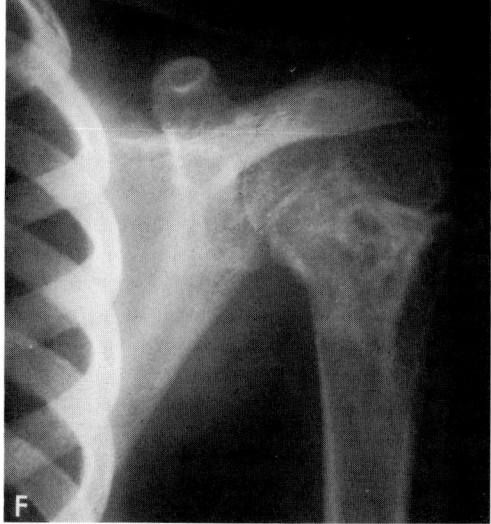

Figure 20-2. (Continued). D, Chest x-ray, posteroanterior view, reveals retrocardiac mass evident only on close inspection. E, Chest x-ray, lateral view, plainly shows the posterior mediastinal mass superimposed on the vertebral bodies. F, Metastatic lesions also present in right humerus. Child died six months after diagnosis was made.

Neuroblastoma only rarely spreads to the brain parenchyma but often is disseminated to the meninges and to the skull. Dural metastases favor the external surface of the dura mater and may be sufficiently thick to cause suture spread, signs of increased pressure, and rapid enlargement of the head. In infancy, the enlarged head resulting from meningeal infiltration with tumor is occasionally misdiagnosed as obstructive hydrocephalus until other signs indicate the more systemic nature of the process.

Metastatic spread of neuroblastoma to the skull and dural surface produces roentgen changes virtually diagnostic of this condition. Marked suture spread with indistinctness of serrations along the split sutures is associated with multiple, small osteolytic lesions with poorly defined margins and often with an associated periosteal reaction.

Neurologic complications of neuroblastoma unassociated with either metastases or compression by the primary tumor have recently been identified. The manifestations of this syndrome have received a variety of descriptive designations and have resembled those described by Kinsbourne in 1962 under the title of "myoclonic encephalopathy." Although the entity was unrecognized at the time, Cushing and Wolbach in 1927 recorded a case in which a severe cerebellar syndrome was associated with a paravertebral neuroblastoma.

Opsoclonus, cerebellar ataxia, and shock-like involuntary myoclonic jerks of limb and truncal muscles have now been noted in children with neuroblastoma but not on the basis of metastatic spread of tumor (Solomon and Chutorian, Bray et al., Moe and Nellhaus). Opsoclonus, or wildly chaotic and multidirectional eye movements, is sufficiently rare in childhood that its presence warrants a search for an occult neural crest tumor, either mediastinal or retroperitoneal.

Bray et al. preferred the term acute cerebellar encephalopathy for this constellation of findings and speculated on possible causes, including an effect on the cerebellum by substances liberated from the tumor, such as catecholamines or cystathionine. One case referred to as polymyoclonia-opsoclonus with a ganglioneuroblastoma responded favorably to ACTH even before the neoplasm was removed (Moe and Nellhaus).

Cerebral Neuroblastoma

Neuroblastoma developing primarily within the cerebrum has only rarely been documented (Hassin and Munch-Peterson, Kerohan et al., Miller and Ramsden) and is probably the same lesion referred to by some as the cerebral medulloblastoma. Histologically, the lesion resembles that within the adrenal medulla or along the sympathetic chain. Marked cellularity is present with cells showing a clear, vesicular nucleus and a prominent nucleolus. Mitoses are frequent and rosette formation is common. Differentiation to ganglion cells may be observed in certain areas of the tumor. Special histologic preparations, including Bielschowsky's silver method, help identify the neuroblastic origin of the neoplastic cells. Cerebral neuroblastomas are generally rapidly growing and have infiltrative and invasive qualities rendering a bad prognosis. In view of the radiosensitivity of neuroblastoma in the more common sites, radiation therapy subsequent to partial surgical removal is advisable for the primary cerebral neuroblastoma.

Olfactory Neuroblastoma

The olfactory neuroblastoma (esthesioneuroblastoma) is a rare lesion, which varies from the more common type of neuroblastoma by its occurrence in an older age group. Caballes stated that the youngest reported case was an eight-year-old child and the oldest was 79 years of age. Until 1969, 104 cases had been reported (Castro et al.). Berger et al. have been credited with the initial description of this tumor in 1924. These authors postulated the site of origin was from the olfactory placode, an entodermal structure believed to be an embryonic progenitor of the olfactory membrane. The precise site of origin has remained speculative, with recent authors suggesting an ectodermal origin, possibly from olfactory epithelium (Tingwald).

The olfactory neuroblastoma originates superiorly in the nasal cavity and may extend into the nasopharynx. The initial symptoms are nasal obstruction with a bloody nasal discharge and with recurrent epistaxis. A polypoid mass in the nasal cavity is evident and local invasion into the ethmoid sinus is common. Growth into the orbit may result in proptosis and diplopia; extension to the cribriform plate results in anosmia. The tumor may invade the frontal lobe (Robinson and Solitare) or may be disseminated through the meninges or to the spinal cord (Castro et al.). Erosion intracranially from the nasal cavity provides a route for serious infections, such as meningitis or brain abscess (Robinson and Solitare).

Although the chief tendency for olfactory neuroblastoma is local invasion, distant metastases to cervical lymph nodes, lung, and liver may occur. Treatment of the olfactory neuroblastoma includes local surgical resection followed by irradiation therapy. The tumor is markedly radiosensitive, although recurrences are well known. Prognosis is necessarily guarded. Hutter et al. described a 50 per cent five-year survival rate.

Diagnostic Studies

Certain diagnostic studies are of special value in evaluation of a child in whom mediastinal or retroperitoneal neuroblastoma is included in differential diagnosis. Chest and spine roentgenograms usually identify the lesion located in the posterior mediastinum and may suggest whether vertebral invasion has occurred. A flat plate of the abdomen should be inspected for evidence of calcification in the region of the adrenal gland. Intravenous pyelography is particularly useful because the adrenal neuroblastoma usually results in displacement of the adjacent kidney.

If reasonable evidence of a neuroblastoma is identified, skull and long bone films are ob-

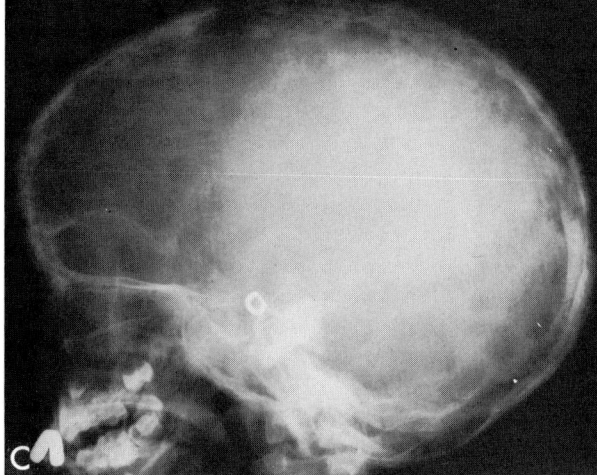

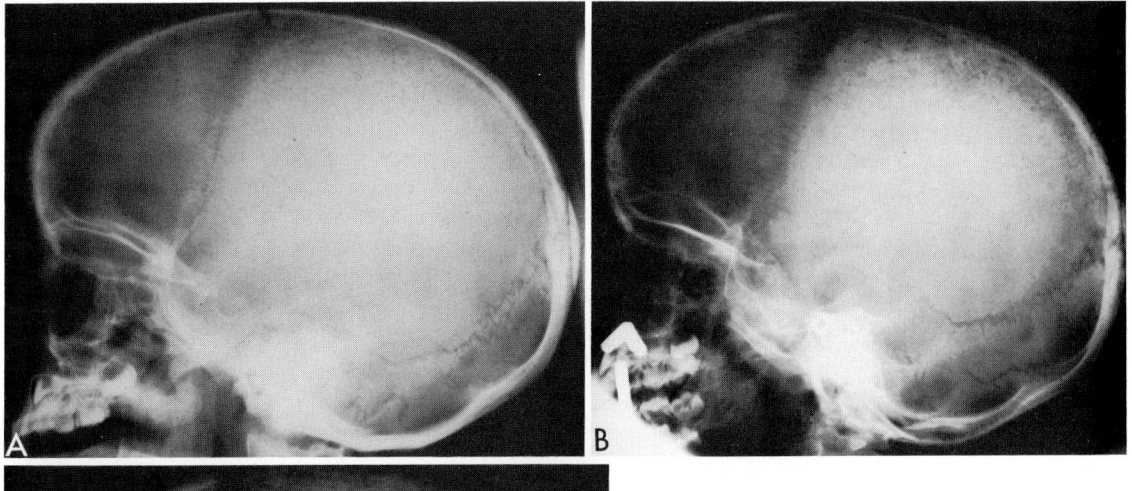

Figure 20-3. Neuroblastoma. Photographs demonstrate progressive metastatic involvement of the skull. Two and one-half year old child with six-week history of recurrent fever, joint pains, and weight loss. Adrenal neuroblastoma was identified by intravenous pyelography. A, Skull film on initial hospital admission shows minimal coronal suture spread and early destructive lesions in frontal and parietal regions. B, Four weeks later, suture separation is more apparent and osteolytic metastases more pronounced. C, Six months after initial admission, there is severe and diffuse bony destruction. At autopsy, the skull was invaded by tumor and a thick layer of neoplasm occupied the epidural space diffusely.

tained to search for metastatic lesions (Fig. 20-3). Bone marrow examination, likewise, is a valuable tool when looking for metastatic spread. Examination of 24-hour urine specimen for catecholamine level and the metabolite 3-methoxy-4-hydroxymandelic acid (VMA) has become an additional procedure in the diagnostic evaluation. This determination is more reliable if the urine is collected after a three-day period of abstention from salicylates, bananas, and vanilla. In one series of 40 patients with neural crest tumors, 39 had increased urinary excretion of catecholamines or the metabolites (de Gutierrez et al.).

Prognosis and Treatment

Prognosis is necessarily guarded in any child with a neuroblastoma, although possibility of cure exists, even in those with metastatic disease. Survival is related to the age of the child and the extent of the disease at the time the diagnosis is established. Possibility of cure is greater in children under one year of age than in older children. Priebe and Clatworthy found that 63 per cent of infants under one year of age survived for at least 14 months; deLorimier et al. found a 60 per cent survival, in the same group. By contrast, only 16 per cent of children over one year of age recovered (Priebe and Clatworthy).

Treatment of neuroblastoma must be individualized on the basis of site and size of the tumor and evidence of dissemination. Surgical removal or biopsy, irradiation therapy, and chemotherapy are used in various combinations, depending on the circumstances. The primary tumor is totally removed whenever possible and is followed by irradiation therapy to the tumor site. Chemotherapy is used for metastatic involvement, with cyclophosphamide and vincristine being the most popular drugs.

NASOPHARYNGEAL TUMORS

Tumors of the nasopharynx are of neurologic importance because of the tendency to infiltrate the base of the skull, resulting in multiple cranial nerve palsies. Neoplasms of this region are far more common in adults than in children. In the older person they are usually either epidermoid carcinoma or lymphoepithelioma. Woltman drew attention to the relatively high frequency of intracranial extension of tumors developing in this area

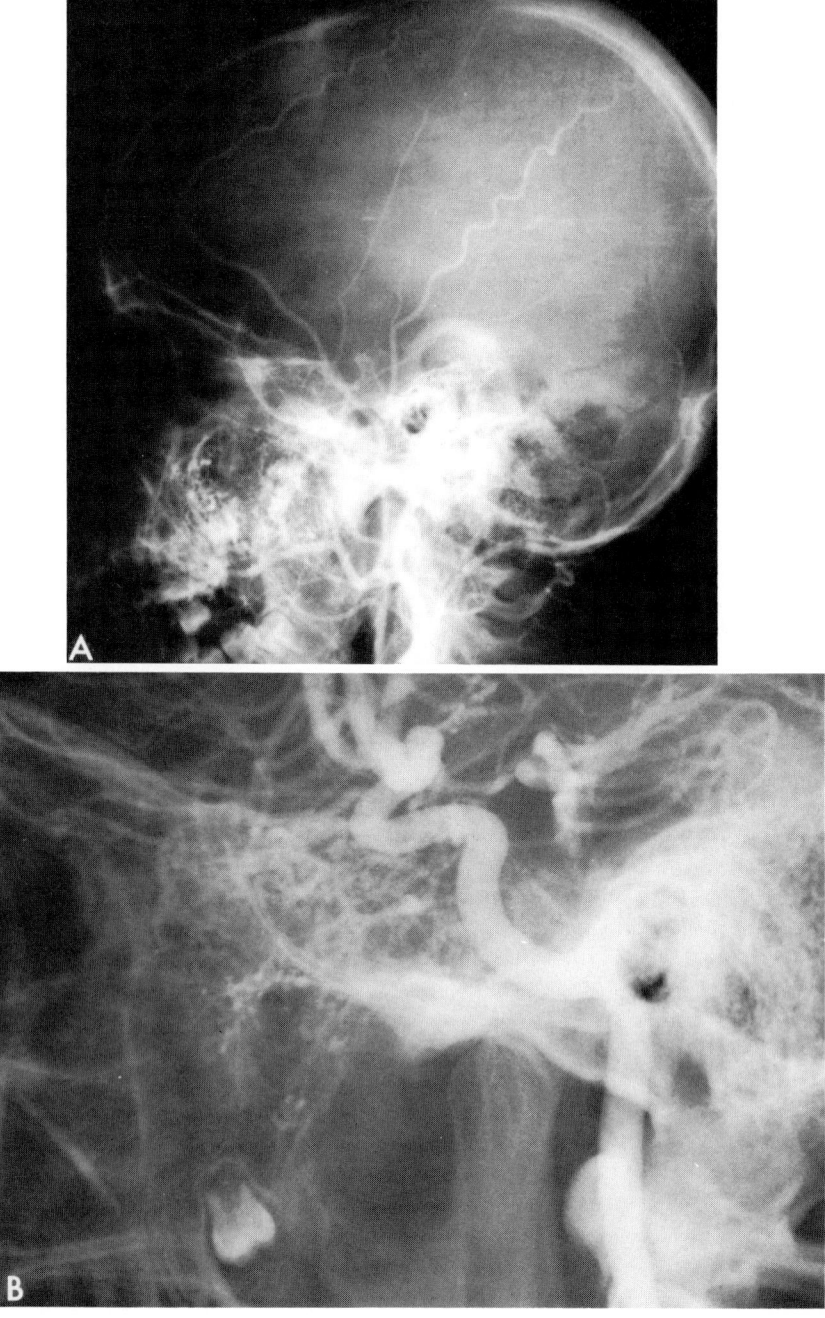

Figure 20-4. Nasopharyngeal angiofibroma. Sixteen-year-old boy with nasopharyngeal airway obstruction and recurrent nasal bleeding. Angiography demonstrates extensive neovascularity within the tumor. A, External carotid angiogram. B, Internal carotid angiogram.

and pointed out that neurologic deficits may precede other clinical manifestations.

Rosenbaum and Seaman stated that neurologic symptoms were the initial evidence of disease in 25 per cent of cases with nasopharyngeal tumors. Infiltration of tumor through the foramen lacerum or foramen ovale initially implicates the fifth and sixth cranial nerves, causing facial pain or numbness and diplopia. Further extension to the third and fourth nerves accentuates the ophthalmoparesis and extension posteriorly to the seventh nerves leads to facial paralysis. Horner's syndrome may also be evident and is ascribed to compression of sympathetic fibers entering the skull adjacent to the carotid artery.

Nasopharyngeal tumors in childhood differ from those in adults in several respects. Neoplasms in this region in children include the rhabdomyosarcoma, lymphoma, neuroblastoma, and the biologically peculiar juvenile nasopharyngeal angiofibroma.

The juvenile nasopharyngeal angiofibroma is a highly vascular, locally invasive lesion that is peculiar to the adolescent male (Fig. 20-4). Intracranial extension with cranial nerve deficits is uncommon (Henderson and Patterson). Nasal obstruction and epistaxis are the usual presenting symptoms of this tumor. Broadening of the bridge of the nose, facial swelling, and proptosis may also be present (Fitzpatrick). Spontaneous regression of this tumor has been claimed to occur after the attainment of sexual maturity, or at about 18 to 25 years of age (Henderson, and Patterson, Patterson). This tendency for regression after the patient has reached sexual maturation has led to the use of androgenic therapy, although most favor surgical resection with or without irradiation therapy.

Progressive involvement of cranial nerves in the middle fossa should raise suspicion of neoplastic extension from the nasopharynx, warranting consultation for inspection and perhaps biopsy of the nasopharynx (Fig. 20-5). Lateral skull x-rays may show the presence of a soft tissue mass in the nasopharynx and destruction of the floor of the sella turcica. The submental-vertex or basal view of the skull is the most valuable projection to demonstrate neoplastic invasion and bony destruction of the base of the skull. The absence of roentgen abnormalities, however, does not exclude the possibility of a nasopharyngeal tumor with intracranial extension.

MENINGIOMAS

The term meningioma was introduced by Cushing in 1922 to designate a group of neoplasms developing from the leptomeninges. Prior to that time, terms used to designate these lesions included dural endothelioma and meningeal fibroblastoma.

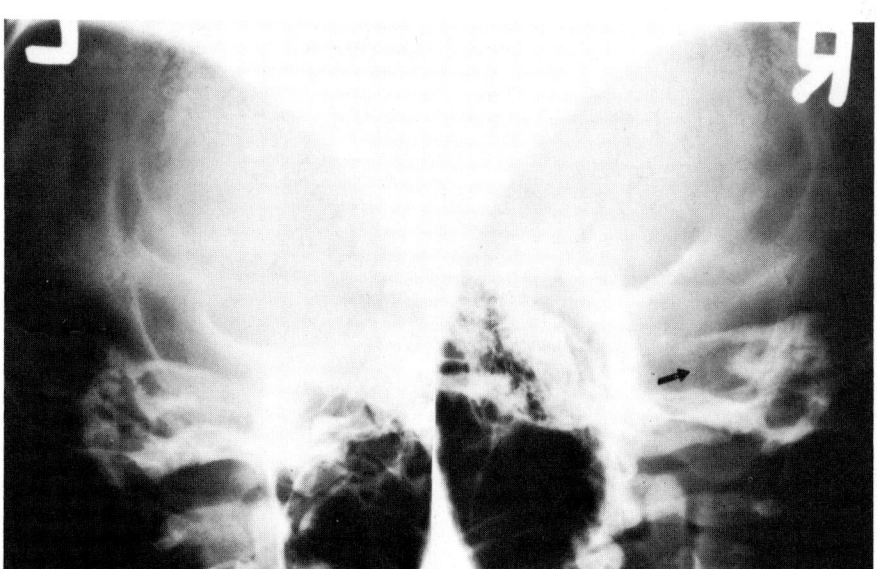

Figure 20-5. Nasopharyngeal rhabdomyosarcoma with intracranial extension. Sixteen-year-old girl with paralysis of the third, fifth, and sixth cranial nerves on the right. The x-rays of petrous ridges demonstrate a normal auditory canal on the left but bony destruction on the right (arrow).

Meningiomas are primarily tumors of adults and are more common in women. They occur only rarely in the childhood years. Kernohan and Sayre (1952) have stated that these tumors develop from arachnoid "cap cells" present on the outer surface of the arachnoid. Other possible sites of origin have been proposed in the past and the question remains open.

Many attempts at classification of these tumors have been made on the basis of the architectural characteristics or dominant cell form. Cushing and Eisenhardt described nine types and 20 subtypes in their monograph on this subject. Although histologic variations do exist, the biologic behavior of these tumors shows little relationship to the histologic pattern. Earle and Richany studied a series of 243 meningiomas subclassified into five groups. Histologic subclassification was not useful for predicting biological behavior. Location and surgical accessibility were more reliable prognostic indicators.

On gross examination, the meningioma is usually gray, firm, and well circumscribed. The brain is not invaded but more characteristically is distorted by extrinsic pressure from the tumor (Fig. 20-6). The size of the tumor is extremely variable; small, insignificant meningiomas are sometimes found incidentally at autopsy. Intracranial meningiomas may be multiple, especially when associated with generalized neurofibromatosis.

The meningiomas are often subdivided into different types, including meningotheliomatous, psammomatous, fibroblastic, angioblastic, and sarcomatous, depending on the morphology. The meningotheliomatous meningioma contains sheets of cells with

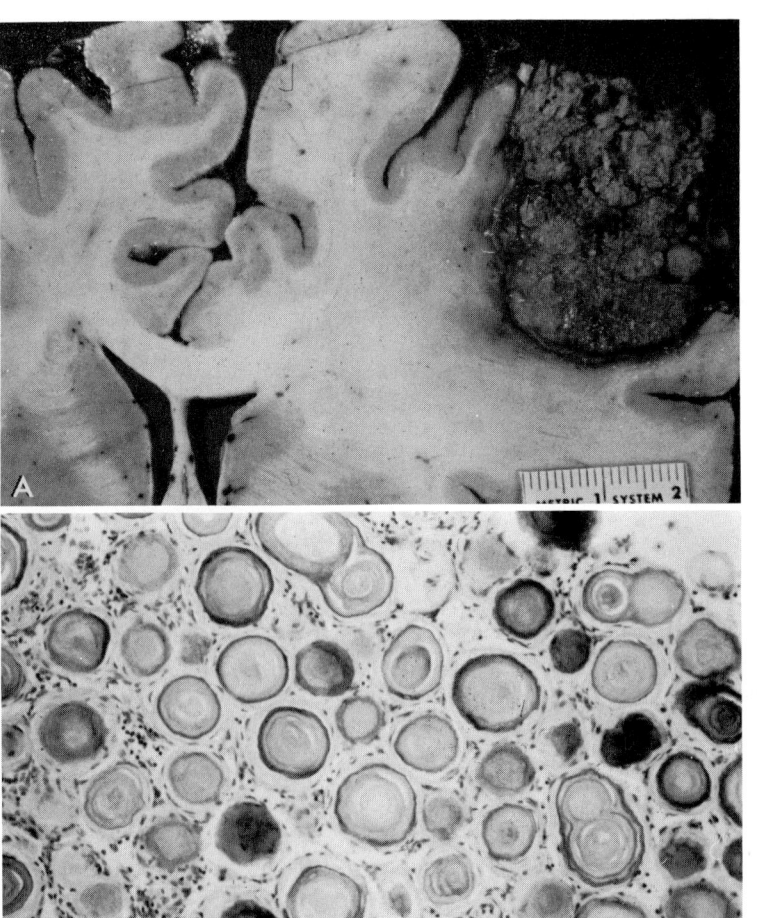

Figure 20-6. Meningioma of the cerebral convexity. A, Gross view shows cerebral compression without invasion by the neoplasm. B, Extensive psammoma body formation within the meningioma.

large, oval, vesicular nuclei. In some, the nuclei are pyknotic. The cytoplasm may appear homogenous or may be quite stringy. The psammomatous type does not deserve separation from the foregoing, because psammoma bodies only represent a progressive change from the whorl-formation seen in many meningiomas.

The position of the angioblastic meningioma within the meningioma group has been controversial. It is a richly cellular tumor with many capillary-sized vascular spaces but with wide variations in histologic pattern. Pitkethly and colleagues reviewed 81 angioblastic meningiomas, subdividing them into the hemangioblastic variant, the hemangiopericytoma variant, and transitional forms. Those resembling the hemangiopericytoma of soft tissue origin were associated with a more rapid evolution of clinical signs, and occasionally with extracranial metastases. They pointed out that the hemangioblastic types were histologically indistinguishable from the cerebellar hemangioblastoma.

Sites of Origin

Meningiomas occur in a variety of locations. The most common site is the parasagittal region. This is followed in frequency by occurrence over the convexity of the brain, at the sphenoid ridge, and on the olfactory groove (Earle and Richany). Other possible sites include the suprasellar area, the posterior fossa, and within the orbit. The symptoms and signs resulting are largely dependent on the size of the tumor and its location within the intracranial space. Signs of increased intracranial pressure are variable and may or may not be present.

Parasagittal meningiomas often become quite large before recognized clinically. The manifestations produced depend on the area involved along the midline of the brain and whether the tumor grows unilaterally or causes compression of both hemispheres. Tumors in the anterior frontal parasagittal region are often associated with headaches, memory disturbances, or progressive dementia. Parasagittal lesions in the posterior frontal region frequently cause a progressive spastic paresis of one or both lower extremities and thus may be confused with a spinal cord lesion. Focal motor seizures of either the leg or the arm may occur. Paramidline meningiomas in the parietal region result in sensory deficits, especially in the lower limbs, and recurrent focal sensory seizures.

Convexity meningiomas produce a multiplicity of clinical findings, depending on the function of the area involved. The history is usually prolonged and includes complaints secondary to increased pressure plus those due to focal cerebral involvement. Seizures, either focal or generalized, mental impairment, motor or sensory deficits, or visual disturbances are common.

Meningiomas of the medial (clinoidal) portion of the sphenoid ridge result in a group of clinical abnormalities referred to as the superior orbital fissure syndrome. Exophthalmos on the same side as the lesion is accompanied by diplopia and unilateral loss of vision with primary optic atrophy. Compression of the third, fourth, and sixth cranial nerves results in extraocular muscle paresis on the same side as the tumor. The first division of the trigeminal nerve is also involved as it enters the orbital fissure, causing sensory loss on the forehead and loss of the ipsilateral corneal reflex. As the tumor expands and increased intracranial pressure develops, papilledema may develop on the opposite side, resulting in the Foster Kennedy syndrome.

Meningiomas of the outer (pterion) portion of the sphenoid ridge grow to large size before recognizable signs are evident. The usual manifestations include symptoms of increased intracranial pressure and signs of extension of the tumor into the frontal or temporal regions. Seizures may be generalized, uncinate, or psychomotor in type. A central facial palsy is often observed.

Olfactory groove meningiomas grow on the surface of the anterior fossa beneath the frontal lobes and result in compression of the olfactory nerves and the basal surfaces of the frontal lobes. Usual clinical features include anosmia, memory and personality changes, and eventually, visual deficits from optic nerve or chiasm compression. Marked distortion of the frontal lobes may occur because of the enormous size the tumor may acquire.

Meningiomas of the tuberculum sellae are prone to expand asymmetrically. In the early stages, one optic nerve may be compressed or the pressure may be exerted at the junction of one optic nerve and the chiasm, producing the anterior chiasmal syndrome. This consists of marked unilateral loss of vision with a superior temporal or temporal hemianopsia of the other eye.

The quadrant defect in the visual field of the opposite eye is due to involvement of fibers from the contralateral optic nerve originating in the inferior nasal quadrant of the retina. These fibers loop across to the opposite side in the anterior part of the chiasm before turning posteriorly to enter the optic tract. In other cases, the visual field abnormality consists of an asymmetrical bitemporal hemianopsia. With growth of the lesion, both optic nerves become compressed with the outcome being progressive bilateral loss of vision and primary optic atrophy.

Congenital meningiomas are exceedingly rare and only a few have been reported. Seizures, head enlargement, abnormal transillumination, or identification of fluid in the subdural space has usually led to an erroneous preoperative diagnosis of subdural effusion or porencephaly in these cases (Mendiratta et al., Taptas).

Diagnostic Studies

Certain laboratory and ancillary procedures may be of diagnostic and localizing assistance in regard to intracranial meningiomas. The protein content of the cerebrospinal fluid is significantly elevated in most cases. Visual field determinations are of localizing value in the group of tumors in which there is direct compression of the optic nerves or chiasm. Electroencephalography is frequently not helpful in the presence of a large meningioma. The parasagittal group, especially, is very difficult to localize by electoencephalography. Convexity meningiomas are more commonly associated with focal slow activity; even here, exceptions exist.

Skull x-rays may provide evidence that both localizes the site of the tumor and suggests a meningioma as the histologic type. In some instances, the only abnormality noted on skull x-ray results from chronic increase of intracranial pressure. Cerebral convexity meningiomas may produce a shift of the pineal gland from the midline in the adult. More specific evidence suggesting a meningioma includes hyperostosis, increased vascularity, and calcification within the tumor (Taveras and Wood).

Hyperostosis secondary to a meningioma is due to a reactive change in the skull with new bone formation adjacent to the site of the tumor. Convexity meningiomas may cause localized bony hyperostosis with spicule formation in the same region. Sclerotic bony changes may be observed in the sphenoid wing with tumors in that area or in the planum sphenoidale with a tuberculum sellae meningioma.

The marked vascularity characteristic of the meningioma is often evidenced roentgenographically by enlargement of the middle meningeal artery with abnormal tortuosity and arborization of its channel on the lateral skull film. Calcification within the tumor is of help when present; however, the majority of meningiomas do not contain sufficient calcium to be visible on x-ray. When present, calcification may be either dustlike or dense and may accurately outline the tumor.

Further roentgenographic delineation of intracranial meningiomas is achieved by pneumoencephalography or angiography. The choice of procedure is dependent on the probable location of the lesion from the clinical data and the degree of elevation of the intracranial pressure. At times, both procedures may be necessary. Most meningiomas sufficiently large to produce symptoms or signs are well localized by radioactive brain scan examination. Treatment is surgical removal, which should be complete whenever possible.

DIFFUSE LEPTOMENINGEAL TUMORS

Several neoplasms already described are capable of dissemination from the primary site of origin to the leptomeninges. The medulloblastoma is best known for this tendency. The ependymoma, pinealoma, and choroid plexus papilloma, likewise, on rare occasion are associated with diffuse leptomeningeal spread. The most common neoplastic process with meningeal infiltration in children is lymphoblastic leukemia. Less frequently encountered disorders include leptomeningeal invasion with melanoma, lymphosarcoma, reticulum cell sarcoma, and other forms of sarcoma.

Meningeal Leukemia

Meningeal leukemia, or infiltration of the meninges with leukemic cells, has become a more common complication since the development of therapeutic methods that have prolonged the survival of leukemic victims. Nieri et al. stated that over the 70-year period from 1882 until 1951, only 31 patients with this syndrome had been reported. Many examples have subsequently been described, and it is now recognized as a common manifestation of acute lymphoblastic leukemia in its later stages. Meningeal leukemia is predominantly a disorder of children and is rarely observed in persons with myeloblastic or myelomonocytic leukemia.

Meningeal involvement is generally considered to occur more often in the late stages of the leukemic process but may develop at any time. On rare occasion, leukemic infiltration of the meninges precedes other more common systemic manifestations of the disease. Some cases become evident coincident with clinical and hematologic abnormalities of uncontrolled leukemia but many patients develop symptoms of meningeal involvement during complete peripheral and bone marrow remission. This is attributed to the lack of entrance of the antileukemic drugs into the subarachnoid space and central nervous tissue when given systemically. Thus, neoplastic cells deposited within the meninges during the active phase of the disease have a privileged environment regarding exposure to antileukemic drugs and remain to proliferate later.

The initial, and sometimes the only, symptoms and signs of meningeal leukemia are those of increased intracranial pressure. Headaches and vomiting are the most common early complaints, followed by diplopia, irritability, and lethargy. Papilledema is usually present, and in younger children, skull suture spread is apparent on x-ray examination. It is probable that the pathogenesis of increased pressure in these cases is largely the result of an absorptive defect due to leukemic cell invasion of the meninges. This is accompanied by brain swelling in some cases, which results in similar pressure symptoms and signs.

Although the pressure manifestations indicate meningeal infiltration, other signs may coexist that reflect the presence of leukemic deposits within the parenchyma of the brain or of the cranial nerves (Fig. 20-7). Facial paralysis is not uncommon, and seizures, either focal or generalized, may be the initial evidence of this type of neurologic involvement. Other patients with clinical evidence of meningeal infiltration abruptly develop profound hyperphagia and rapid weight gain, indicative of hypothalamic invasion by the leukemic process (Shaw et al., Hardisty and Norman).

In assessing the neurologic deficits in children suspected of having intracranial leukemic infiltration, it is important to distinguish signs due to chemotherapy rather than the disease. Vincristine, especially, is notable for its peripheral nerve toxicity resulting in weakness, sensory deficits, and reflex loss.

Cerebrospinal fluid examination in the majority of patients shows an increased pressure and a lymphocytic pleocytosis. With appropriate stains, the cell population in the spinal fluid can be shown to be leukemic blast cells. Cerebrospinal fluid sugar is usually normal but may be reduced. The protein content also is usually within the normal range; occasionally, it is mildly increased.

Treatment of meningeal leukemia may be approached by several methods. Irradiation to the skull is usually beneficial in alleviating symptoms, but improvement may be delayed and the remission may be short. Irradiation is probably best reserved for patients with cerebral infiltration rather than used on patients with evidence only of meningeal involvement.

Intrathecal methotrexate is the treatment of choice and usually results in prompt improvement of symptoms and signs of increased pressure. Methotrexate is injected via lumbar puncture in a dose of 0.25 mg. per kilogram of body weight and is repeated daily or every second day for three to five doses. Some determine the number of injections by continuing administration until the cell count in the spinal fluid has been reduced to less than 10 per cubic millimeter. Intrathecal methotrexate is tolerated well by the majority of children, although febrile reactions are occasionally observed (Naimann et al.). Back described a child who developed paraplegia that ended fatally following intrathecal methotrexate injection.

The performance of a lumbar puncture may temporarily relieve the pressure symptoms of meningeal leukemia. Hyman and colleagues showed that the spinal fluid pleocytosis was usually unchanged and the pressure measurements little altered by this procedure. Dexamethasone in oral dose of 0.2 mg. per kilogram of body weight per day also may dramatically improve the symptoms and signs in patients with meningeal leukemia (Mitus). The cellular response in spinal fluid is not significantly altered, however. Dexamethasone

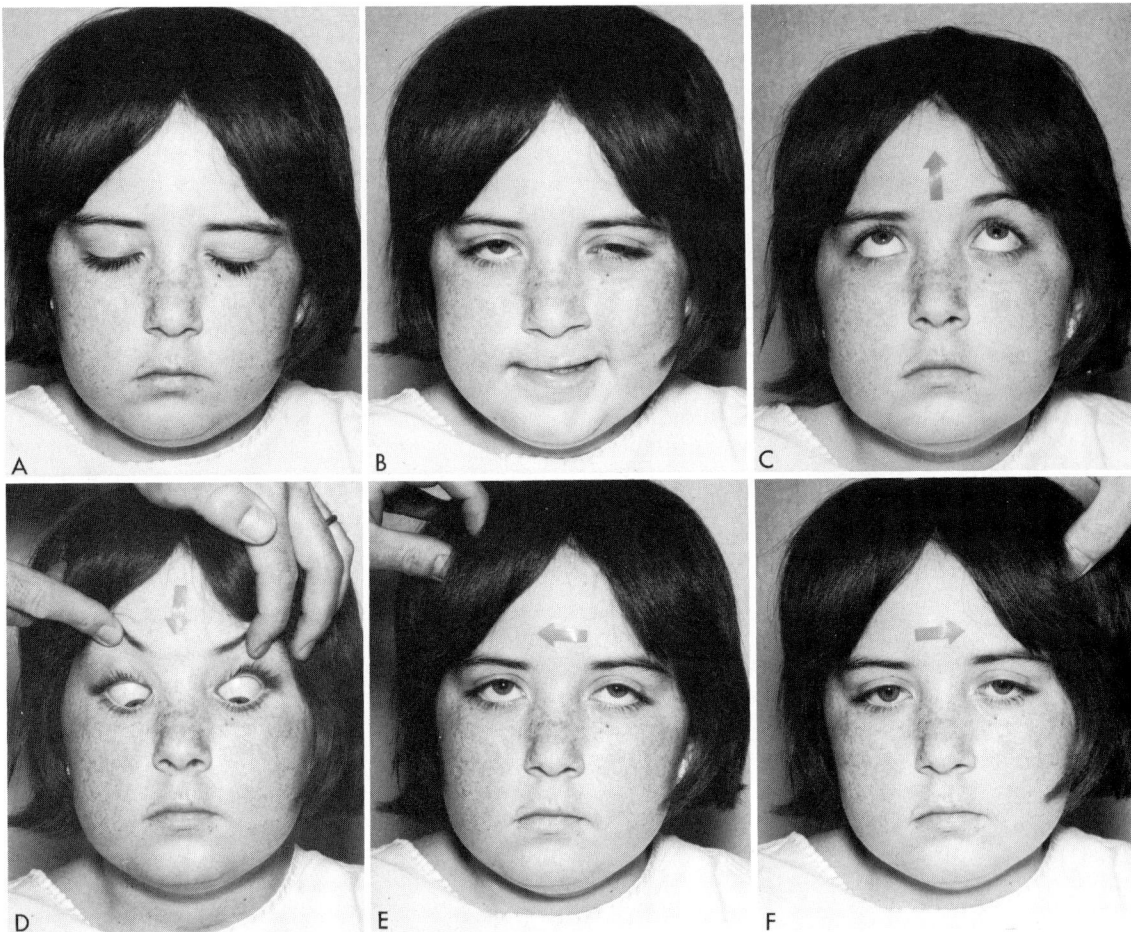

Figure 20-7. Meningeal and brain stem infiltration in a 12-year-old girl with acute lymphoblastic leukemia. Diagnosis of leukemia had been made one year before and remission occurred following antileukemic drug therapy. Three days before current admission she developed diplopia and bilateral facial paresis. Two days before admission, she experienced headache, vomiting, and ataxia. A, When patient is at rest with eyes closed, the bilateral facial weakness is not readily apparent because her face is symmetrical. When patient attempts to squeeze the eyelids closed, the lack of wrinkling of the right upper eyelid indicates a greater degree of weakness of the right orbicularis oculi muscle. B, When the patient tries to show teeth, the facial flattening becomes evident with greater weakness present on the right side. C and D, Vertical conjugate gaze up and down remains intact. E and F, Conjugate horizontal gaze to either side is virtually absent, although medial rectus function was present bilaterally on convergence. These ocular findings are of the type referred to as Foville's syndrome and indicate a dorsal pontine lesion. Postmortem examination revealed generalized meningeal invasion by leukemic cells. The brain stem, including the pons, was extensively infiltrated by blast cells and also showed a striking degree of gliosis.

has been recommended as a temporizing measure in patients with severe headaches and vomiting, in whom more definitive therapy with intrathecal methotrexate must be delayed for two or three days.

Recurrences of meningeal leukemia are common and subsequent episodes are often associated with signs pointing to cerebral or cranial nerve involvement. Some children respond favorably to several courses of intrathecal methotrexate from the symptomatic standpoint. Even though symptoms and spinal fluid pleocytosis may be completely controlled by such treatment, leukemic cells may be identified in the meninges at autopsy (Nies et al.).

Although the clinical symptoms produced by either meningeal or cerebral leukemic infiltration may promptly abate with treatment, this type of neurologic complication must be considered a poor prognostic sign. In the series studied by Shaw et al., median survival after onset of meningeal leukemia was three months.

MISCELLANEOUS TUMORS 253

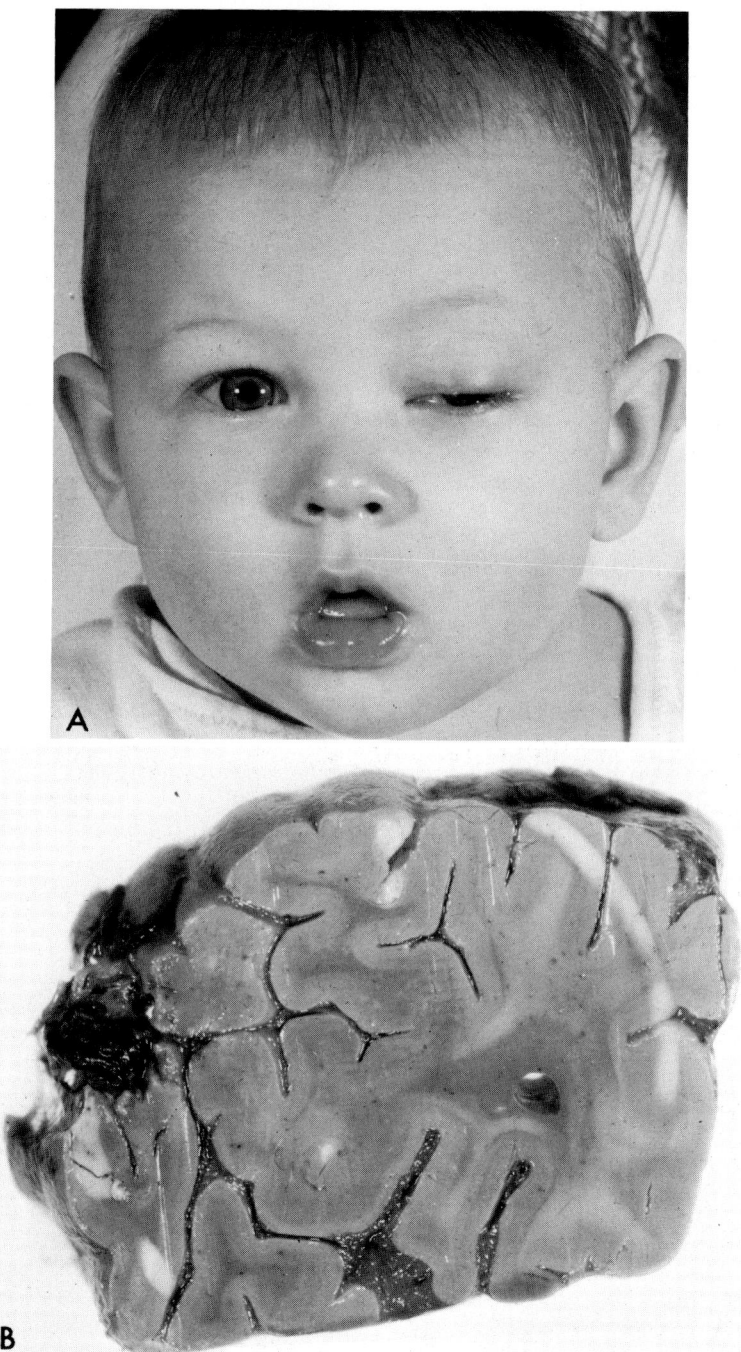

Figure 20-8. Meningeal sarcoma. One-year-old child with onset of left oculomotor paralysis one week before hospital admission. Subsequently, he developed multiple cranial nerve palsies and increased intracranial pressure. Death occurred four months after onset. A, Ptosis and slight lateral deviation of the left eye because of third nerve paralysis are evident. B, Anaplastic sarcoma is evident as a gelatinous infiltrate widening the cerebral sulci. Neoplastic invasion of the cerebrum is present over the lateral surface of the hemisphere.

Meningeal Sarcoma

Primary diffuse sarcoma of the meninges is a rare tumor but is noteworthy because most cases are found in children or young adults and because the clinical findings are usually extremely difficult to analyze (Fig. 20-8). Primary meningeal sarcomatosis (Martin and Moore) and meningeal meningiomatosis (Brown and Kernohan) are other designations used for these malignant lesions. Pathologic characteristics of the tumor may be that of a fibrosarcoma (Onofrio et al.), of a reticulum cell sarcoma (Burstein et al.), or of an anaplastic sarcoma that cannot be further categorized.

Symptoms and signs in these cases show remarkable variability, although manifestations of increased pressure are usually present early in the illness or are even presenting complaints. Some patients have abrupt onset of symptoms in a fashion suggestive of an infectious meningoencephalitis — a consideration further enhanced when mononuclear cells are observed in the cerebrospinal fluid. The underlying brain is often invaded by tumor cells, resulting in personality and mentation changes, recurrent seizures, speech disturbances, or long tract signs.

Ancillary diagnostic studies in patients with diffuse meningeal tumors may be of little assistance or even dissuade one from his working diagnosis of intracranial tumor. Spinal fluid pressure is usually elevated, the protein content is frequently increased, and neoplastic cells may be identified on cytologic examination of the fluid. The electroencephalogram is sometimes diffusely slow or may reveal multiple foci of slow activity on either side of the brain. Carotid angiography is not revealing in many cases, and air contrast studies are often normal or show mild, generalized ventricular dilatation. Leptomeningeal and cortical biopsy is the most rewarding procedure to establish the diagnosis of meningeal sarcoma. The possibility of this type of neoplastic process must be recognized, however, before surgical biopsy is considered as a helpful procedure.

Irradiation therapy is about all one has to offer in such cases and most are not expected to show more than a temporary response. When pressure signs persist and ventricular enlargment is evident, a ventriculovascular shunt deserves consideration.

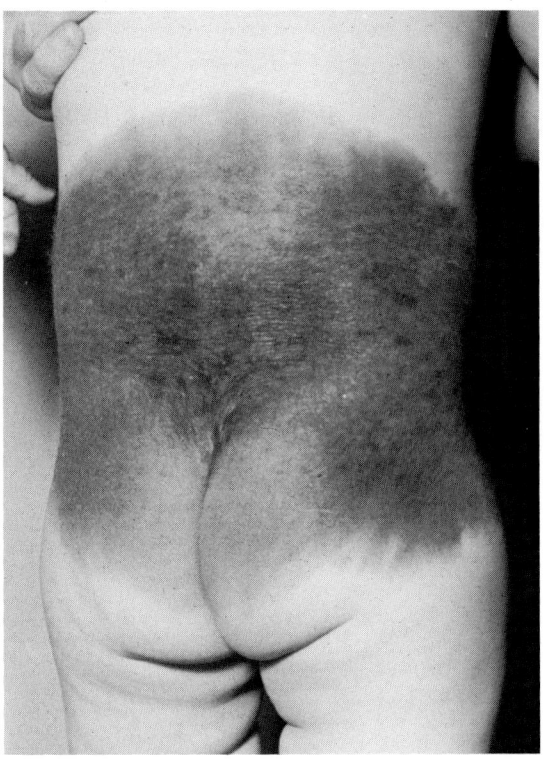

Figure 20-9. "Bathing suit" nevus often associated with leptomeningeal melanomatosis.

Leptomeningeal Melanomatosis

Primary intracranial melanin-containing tumors are rare lesions, the embryogenesis and pathogenesis of which have been the source of long—standing debate. Such tumors may primarily involve the meninges or may implicate both the meninges and the underlying brain tissue. Virchow has been credited with the first description of primary melanoma of the nervous system in 1859.

Melanin-containing cells are normally found in the meninges ventral to the brain stem. A neurocutaneous syndrome has been recognized in which diffuse melanosis at the base of the brain is associated with giant, hairy cutaneous nevi (Slaughter et al., Fox et al.) (Fig. 20-9). Such children may exhibit a variety of neurologic deficits including hydrocephalus, mental retardation, and seizures. Prognosis is poor for those with neoplastic change in the melanin-containing tissue within the nervous system. In other cases, leptomeningeal melanoma occurs without cutaneous lesions and is disseminated throughout the meninges of the brain and spinal cord.

REFERENCES

Aterman, K., and Schuller, E. F.: Maturation of neuroblastoma to ganglioneuroma. *Amer. J. Dis. Child.*, **120**:217–222, 1970.

Back, E. H.: Death after intrathecal methotrexate. *Lancet*, **2**:1005, 1969.

Berger, L., Luc, and Richard: L'esthesioneuroepitheliome olfactif. *Bull. Assoc. franc. etude cancer*, **13**:410–420, 1924.

Bray, P. F., Ziter, F. A., Lahey, M. E., and Myers, G. G.: The coincidence of neuroblastoma and acute cerebellar encephalopathy. *J. Pediat.*, **75**:983–990, 1969.

Brown, M. H., and Kernohan, J. W.: Diffuse meningiomatosis. *Arch. Path.*, **32**:651–658, 1941.

Burstein, S. D., Kernohan, J. W., and Uhlein, A.: Neoplasms of the reticuloendothelial system of the brain. *Cancer*, **16**:289–305, 1963.

Caballes, R. L.: Psammoma bodies in olfactory neuroblastoma. *Laryngoscope*, **75**:1749–1755, 1965.

Castro, L., de la Pava, S., and Webster, J. H.: Esthesioneuroblastoma. *Amer. J. Roentgen.*, **105**:7–13, 1969.

Cushing, H.: The meningiomas (dural endotheliomas): Their source and favored seats of origin. *Brain*, **45**:282–316, 1922.

Cushing, H., and Eisenhardt, L.: *Meningiomas: Their classification, Regional Behavior Life History, and Surgical End Results.* Springfield, Ill., Charles C. Thomas, 1938.

Cushing, H., and Wolbach, S. B.: Transformation of malignant paravertebral sympathicoblastoma into benign ganglioneuroma., *Amer. J. Path.*, 3:203–216, 1927.

de Gutierrez, M. B., Bergada, C., and Becu, L.: Cathecholamine excretion in forty children with sympathicoblastoma. *J. Pediat.*, **77**:239–244, 1970.

deLormier, A. A., Bragg, K. V., and Linden, G.: Neuroblastoma in childhood. *Amer. J. Dis. Child.*, **118**:441–450, 1969.

Dyke, P. C., and Mulkey, D. A.: Maturation of ganglioneuroblastoma to ganglioneuroma. *Cancer*, **20**:1343–1349, 1967.

Earle, K. M., and Richany, S. F.: Meningiomas. A study of the histology, incidence, and biologic behavior of 243 cases from the Frazier-Grant collection of brain tumors. *Med. Ann. Dis. Col.*, **38**:353–357, 1969.

Fitzpatrick, P. J.: The nasopharyngeal angiofibroma. *Clin. Radiol.*, **18**:62–68, 1967.

Fox, F., Davidson, J., and Thomas, L. B.: Maturation of sympathicoblastoma into ganglioneuroma. *Cancer*, **12**:108–116, 1959.

Fox, H., Emery, J. L., Goodbody, R. A., and Yates, P.O.: Neurocutaneous melanosis. *Arch. Dis. Childh.*, **39**:508–516, 1964.

Haber, S. L., and Bennington, J. L.: Maturation of congenital extra-adrenal neuroblastoma. *Arch. Path.*, **76**:121–125, 1963.

Hardisty, R. M., and Norman, P. M.: Meningeal leukemia. *Arch. Dis. Childh.*, **42**:441–447, 1967.

Hassin, G. B., and Munch-Peterson, C. J.: Central neurologic tumors. Neuroblastomas and gangioneuroma. *J. Neuropath. Clin. Neurol.*, **1**:63, 1951.

Henderson, G. P., Jr., and Patterson, C. N.: Further experience in treatment of juvenile nasopharyngeal angiofibroma. *Laryngoscope*, **79**:561–580, 1969.

Hutter, R. V.P., Lewis, J. S., Foote, F. W., Jr., and Tollasen, H. R.: Esthesioneuroblastoma: a clinical and pathological study. *Amer. J. Surg.*, **106**:748–753, 1963.

Hyman, C. B., Bogle, J. M., Brubaker, C. A., Williams, K., and Hammond, D.: Central nervous system involvement by leukemia in children. I. Relationship to systemic leukemia and description of clinical and laboratory manifestations. *Blood*, **25**:1–12, 1965.

Hyman, C. B., Bogle, J. M., Brubaker, C. A. Williams, K., and Hammond, D.: Cental nervous sytem involvement by leukemia in children. II, Therapy with intrathecal methotrexate. *Blood*, **25**:13–22, 1965.

Kenny, F. M., Iturzaeta, N. F., Mintz, D., Drash, A., Garces, L. Y., Susen, A., and Askari, H. A.: Iatrogenic hypopituitarism in craniopharyngioma: Unexplained catch'up growth in three children. *J. Pediat.*, **72**:766–775, 1968.

Kernohan, J. W., and Sayre, G. P.: *Tumors of the Central Nervous System.* Section 10, fascicles 35 and 37. Washington, D.C., Armed Forces Institute of Pathology, 1952.

Kernohan, J. W., Learmonth, J. R., and Doyle, J. B.: Neuroblastomas and gangliocytomas of the central nervous system. *Brain*, **55**:287–310, 1932.

Kinsbourne, M.: Myoclonic encephalopathy of infants. *J. Neurol. Neurosurg. Psychiat.*, **25**:271–276, 1962.

Kissane, J. M., and Ackerman, L. V.: Maturation of tumors of the sympathetic nervous system. *J. Facul. Radiol.*, **7**:109–114, 1955–1956.

Kogut, M. D., and Donnell, G. N.: Cushing's syndrome in association with renal ganglioneuroblastoma. *Pediatrics*, **28**:566–577, 1961.

Laurence, K. M., Hoare, R. D., and Till, K.: The diagnosis of the choroid plexus papilloma of the lateral ventricle. *Brain*, **84**:628–641, 1961.

Martin, B. F., and Moore, H. C.: Primary meningeal sarcomatosis. *Southern Med. J.*, **63**:419–422, 1970.

Matson, D. D., and Crofton, F. D. L.: Papilloma of the choroid plexus in childhood. *J. Neurosurg.*, **17**:1002–1027, 1960.

Meador, C. K., Liddle, G. W., Island, D. P., Nicholson, W. E., Lucas, C. P., Nuckton, J. G., and Luetscher, J. A.: Cause of Cushing's syndrome in patients with tumors arising from nonendocrine tissue. *J. Clin. Endocrinol.*, **22**:693–703, 1962.

Mendiratta, S. S., Rosenblum, J. A., and Strobos, R. J.: Congenital meningioma. *Neurology*, **17**:914–918, 1967.

Miller, A. A., and Ramsden, F.: A cerebral neuroblastoma with unusual fibrous tissue reaction. *J. Neuropath. Exper. Neurol.*, **25**:328–340, 1966.

Mitus, A.: Dexamethasone. Its effectiveness in the treatment of the acute symptoms of meningeal leukemia. *Amer. J. Dis. Child.*, **117**:307–312, 1969.

Moe, P. G., and Nellhaus, G.: Infantile polymyoclonia-opsoclonus syndrome and neural crest tumors. *Neurology*, **20**:756–764, 1970.

Mortada, A.: Clinical characteristics of early orbital metastatic neuroblastoma. *Amer. J. Ophth.*, **63**:1787–1793, 1967.

Naimann, J. L., Rupprecht, L. M., Tanyeri, G., and Philippidis, P.: Intrathecal methotrexate. *Lancet*, **1**:571, 1970.

Nieri, R. L., Burgert, E. O., Jr., and Groover, R. V.: Central nervous system complications of leukemia. A review. *Mayo Clin. Proc.*, **43**:70–79, 1968.

Nies, B., Thomas, L. B., and Freireich, E. J.: Meningeal leukemia. A follow-up study. *Cancer*, **18**:546–553, 1965.

Onofrio, B. M., Kernohan, J. W., and Uihlein, A.: Primary meningeal sarcomatosis. *Cancer,* **15**:1197–1208, 1962.

Patterson, C. N.: Juvenile nasopharyngeal angiofibroma. *Arch. Otolaryng.,* **81**:270–277, 1965.

Pitkethly, D. T., Hardman, J. M., Kempe, L. G., and Earle, K. M.: Angioblastic meningiomas. Clincopathologic study of 81 cases. *J. Neurosurg.,* **32**:539–544, 1970.

Priebe, C. J., Jr., and Clatworthy, H. W.: Neuroblastoma. *Arch. Surg.,* **95**:538–545, 1967.

Robinson, F., and Solitare, G. B.: Olfactory neuroblastoma. *J. Neurosurg.,* **25**:133–139, 1966.

Rosenbaum, H. E., and Seamen, W. B.: Neurologic manifestations of nasopharyngeal tumors. *Neurology,* **5**:868–874, 1955.

Rosenstein, B. J., and Engelman, K.: Diarrhea in a child with a catecholamine-secreting ganglioneuroma. *J. Pediat.,* **63**:217–226, 1963.

Schneider, K. M., Becker, J. M., and Krasna, I. H.: Neonatal neuroblastoma. *Pediatrics,* **36**:359–366, 1965.

Shaw, R. K., Moore, E. W., Freireich, E. J., and Thomas, L. B.: Meningeal leukemia. *Neurology,* **10**:823–833, 1960.

Slaughter, J. C., Hardman, J. M., Kempe, L. G., and Earle, K. M.: Neurocutaneous melanosis and leptomeningeal melanomatosis in children. *Amer. J. Dis. Child.,* **88**:298–304, 1969.

Solomon, G. E., and Chutorian, A. M.: Opsoclonus and occult neuroblastoma. *New Eng. J. Med.,* **279**:475–477, 1968.

Strauss, L., and Driscoll, S. G.: Congenital neuroblastoma involving the placenta. *Pediatrics,* **34**:23–31, 1964.

Taptas, J. N.: Intracranial meningioma in a four-month-old infant simulating subdural hematoma. *J. Neurosurg.,* **18**:120–121, 1961.

Taveras, M. M., and Wood, E. H.: *Diagnostic Neuroradiology.* Baltimore, The Williams and Wilkins Company, 1964.

Tingwald, F. R.: Olfactory placode tumors. *Laryngoscope,* **76**:196–211, 1966.

Uhlmann, E. M., and von Essen, C.: Neuroblastoma (neuroblastoma sympatheticum). *Pediatrics,* **15**:402–411, 1955.

Virchow, R.: Pigment and diffuse melanose der arachnoides. *Arch. Path. Anat.,* **16**:180, 1859.

Woltman, H. E.: Malignant tumors of the nasopharynx with involvement of the nervous system. *Arch. Neurol. Psychiat.,* **8**:412–429, 1922.

Index

Note: Page numbers in *italics* indicate illustrations.

Abscess, of brain, 147–153. See also *Brain abscess.*
Acetazolamide, in hydrocephalus, 102
Achondroplasia, 71, *73*
ACTH, pituitary tumors and, 222
Adenoma, acidophilic, 221
  pituitary, 219, *220*
Alexander's disease, 74
Amytal, in lead encephalopathy, 120
Angiography, in hydrocephalus, 83
Arachnoid cyst, intracranial, 181, *182*
Arachnoiditis, adhesive, 55
Arnold-Chiari malformation, definition of, 96
  manifestations of, 96, *97, 98*
  pathogenesis in, 99
Astroblastoma, 162
Astrocytoma, cerebellar, 189
  types of, 160, *161, 162*
Autonomic faciocephalagia, 19

"Battered child syndrome," 142, *142, 143, 144*
Benedikt's syndrome, 195
Blepharoplasts, in ependymoma, 166
Blood pressure, elevated, 5
"Bobble-head doll syndrome," 70, 203
Brain abscess, 147–153
  congenital heart disease and, 147, *148, 152*
  pathology of, 148, *150*
  symptoms of, 149
  tests for, 151
  treatment of, 152
Brain stem glioma, 193
Burns, intracranial pressure and, 55

Canavan's disease, 74
Carotid angiography, in intracranial tumor, 181
Cephalhematoma, 128, *129*
Cerebellar astrocytoma, 189, *190*
"Cerebral cry," 69
Cerebral edema, 58–61
  corticosteroids and, 60
  definition of, 58
  dexamethasone and, 61
  glycerol and, 61
  headache and, 24
  management of, 59
  manifestations of, 58, *58*
  mannitol and, 60

Cerebral edema (*Continued*)
  types of, 59
  urea and, 60
Cerebral gigantism, 74, *75*
Cerebral hemisphere, tumors of, 224–233
  diagnosis of, 231
  incidence of, 224, *225, 226*
Cerebrospinal fluid, absorption of, 64
  anatomy of, 63
  formation of, 64
Cerebrospinal fluid, hydrocephalus and, 63
  physiology of, 63
Chelating agents, in lead encephalopathy, 121
Cholesteatoma, 235, *236*
Chordoma, 234
Cisternography. See *Isotope encephalography.*
Cleidocranial dysostosis, 74
  in infants, 36
Concussion, cerebral, 124
Congenital tumor(s), 234–238. See also names of specific tumors.
Contusion, cerebral, 124, *125*
Corticosteroids, in cerebral edema, 60
  in craniopharyngioma, 210
Costen's syndrome, 26
Craniolacunia, in neonate, *37*
Craniopharyngioma, 205, *205, 207*
  corticosteroids and, 210
  symptoms of, 206, *206*
  treatment of, 208, *209*
Craniosynostosis, in childhood, *38*
Crouzon's syndrome, *50*
Cushing's disease, headaches and, 14
Cushing's syndrome, neuroblastoma and, 241
  pituitary tumors and, 222
Cyst(s), arachnoid, intracranial, 181, *182*

Dandy-Walker syndrome, 51
  hydromyelia and, 63
  manifestations of, 91, *92, 93*
  pathogenesis of, 91
  roentgen signs in, 34, 94, *94, 95*
  transillumination and, 77
  treatment of, 96
Dejerine-Roussy syndrome, 232
Dermoid tumor(s), 237
Dexamethasone, in cerebral edema, 61
Diabetes insipidus, hypothalamic tumors and, 217
  pituitary tumors and, 203, *204*, 210

"Diencephalic syndrome," 214, *215*
Disease, infectious, headache and, 24

Ecchordosis, 234
Edema, cerebral. See *Cerebral edema.*
Electroencephalography, headache and, 15
  in intracranial tumor, 173, *174*
Ependymoma, 166
  of fourth ventricle, 190, *191*
Epidermoid cyst, 235, *236*
Epidural hematoma, 140
Epileptic cephalea, headache and, 27
Ergotamine preparations, 20, 21
Erythrocytosis, hemangioblastoma and, 192
Eye, abnormalities of, 5-10

Faciocephalagia, autonomic, 19
Familial osteoectasia, 74
Fossa, posterior, tumors in, 184-197. See also names of specific tumors.
Foster Kennedy syndrome, 8
Foville's syndrome, *252*
Fractures, skull, 131, *132*
Frontal lobe, tumors of, 226, *227*
Fundus, ocular, abnormalities of, 5

Ganglioglioma, 166
Gigantism, 221
  cerebral, 74, *75*
Glioblastoma multiforme, 162, *163, 164, 165*
Glioma, brain stem, 193, *193, 196*
  nasal, 235
  of optic chiasm, 210, *211, 213*
  of optic nerve, 210, *211, 212*
Glomeruloids, *164*
Glycerol, in cerebral edema, 61
Goldmann perimetric examination, 6
Guillain-Barré syndrome, 56

Hakim valve system, in hydrocephalus, 103
Head trauma, 123-146. See also *Trauma, head.*
Headache(s), 11-30
  age distribution in, 11
  anxiety and, 22
  bacterial meningitis and, 25
  cerebral edema and, 24
  cluster, 19
  convulsive states and, 26
  dental disorders and, 26
  diagnosis of, 15
  ear infections and, 25
  electroencephalography in, 15
  facial structure disorders and, 26
  family discord and, 13
  febrile disorders and, 25
  hemorrhage and, 24
  historical aspects of, 12
  hypertension and, 28
  intracranial hypotension and, 28
  intracranial lesions and, 23-24
  location of, 11
  lumbar puncture and, 15

Headache(s) (*Continued*)
  migraine, 15-21
  physical examination in, 14
  postlumbar puncture and, 27
  psychogenic, 21
  rheumatoid arthritis and, 29
  sinusitis and, 25
  subarachnoid hemorrhage and, 24
  tumors and, 23
  vascular disorders and, 24
Hemangioblastoma, 192, *192*
Hematoma, epidural, 140
  subdural, 51. See also *Subdural hematoma.*
Hemorrhage, epidural, headache and, 24
  intracranial, in newborn, 130, *131*
  subarachnoid, headache and, 24
Herniation(s), cerebellar, *45*, 46
  tentorial, classification of, 41
    manifestations of, 41, 44
    pathogenesis of, 44
  transtentorial, 41-46, *42, 43, 44, 45*
Holter valve system, in hydrocephalus, 103
Horner's syndrome, 19
Hurler's disease, 74
"Hydranencephaly," 85, *86, 87*
  definition of, 85
  manifestations of, 88
  prognosis in, 88
Hydrocephalus, 62-110
  angiography and, *83*, 84
  cerebrospinal fluid and, 63
  classification of, 62
  clinical aspects of, 69-71
  definition of, 62
  differential diagnosis in, 71-76
  etiology of, 65
  head measurement and, 76, *78, 79*
  in early infancy, 51
  isotope encephalography and, 84, *85*
  manifestations of, 62
  occult, 88, *90*
  pathology of, 65
    aqueductal lesions and, 66, *67*
    encephalocoeles and, *66*
    meningomyelocoele and, 65
    viral infections and, 68
    white matter alterations and, 68
  pneumoencephalography and, *82*, 83
  roentgen studies and, 81, *81*
  transillumination and, 77
  treatment of, 101
  ventricular taps and, 77, *80*
"Hydrocephalus ex vacuo," 62
Hydroma, subepicranial, 134
Hypertension, headache and, 28
Hypertension, intracranial, benign, 111. See also *Pseudotumor Cerebri.*
Hypophosphatasia, in infants, 35
Hypotension, intracranial, headache and, 28
Hypothalamus, tumors of, 214-223
  in childhood, 217, *217*
  in infancy, 214, *215, 216*
  posterior, 217, *218*

Increased intracranial pressure, causes of, in childhood,
    adhesive arachnoiditis, 55
    burns, 55

Increased intracranial pressure, causes of,
   in childhood (*Continued*)
      Dandy-Walker syndrome, 55
      osteopetrosis, 56, *56*
      papilledema, 56
      pseudotumor cerebri, 54
      pulmonary disease, 55
      tumors, 54
   in infancy,
      craniosynostosis, 49, *50*
      head trauma, 52
      hydrocephalus, 51
      infections, 52
      subdural hematoma, 51
      tetracycline, 53
      tumors, 51
      vascular disorders, 52, *53*
      vitamin A intake abnormalities, 53
   clinical manifestations of, 3
   dangers in, 3
   false localizing signs in, 9
   personality changes in, 4
   roentgenographic signs in, 34–40
   symptoms of, 4
Infectious disease, headache and, 24
Isotope encephalography, hydrocephalus and, 84, *85*

Kernohan's notch, 43
Kleeblattschadel syndrome, definition of, 99, *100*

Lead encephalopathy, 116–122
   cerebral pathology in, 120
   diagnosis of, 118, *119*
   differential diagnosis in, 117
   symptoms of, 117
   treatment of, 120
Lead poisoning, 116
Leptomeningeal cysts, post-traumatic, 134, *135*
   melanomatosis, 254, *254*
Leptomeninges, tumor infiltration of, 250
Lesions, mass, in infants, 71, *72*
   of brain stem, traumatic, 125, *126*
Leukemia, meningeal, 250, *252*
Lumbar puncture, adverse effects of, 31
Lumbar puncture, headache and, 15
   increased intracranial pressure and, 31–33
   interpreting results of, 32
   precautions in, 31
   Queckenstedt test in, 32
   Tobey-Ayer test and, 33

Macewen's sign, 4
Mannitol, in cerebral edema, 60
Medulloblastoma, 184, *185, 187*
   prognosis in, 188
   symptoms of, 186
   treatment of, 187
Medulloepithelioma, 166
Megalencephaly, 71
Melanomatosis, leptomeningeal, 254
Meningioma(s), 247, *248*
   classification of, 248
   diagnosis of, 250
   location of, 249

Microglioma, 167, *167*
Migraine, 15
   abdominal, 17
   as familial tendency, 17
   cluster headaches and, 19
   electroencephalographic abnormalities in, 19
   hemiplegic, 17
   ophthalmoplegic, 17, *18*
   symptoms of, 16
   treatment of, 20

Nasopharynx, tumors of, 246, *246, 247*
Neoplasm. See names of specific neoplasms.
Neoplastic disease, 76, *76*
Neuroblastoma, 240, *242, 243, 245*
   cerebral, 244
   diagnosis of, 244
   olfactory, 244
   symptoms of, 241
   treatment of, 245
Neurofibromatosis, 169, *169, 225*
Nocardia asteroides, 149, *149*

Occipital lobe, tumors of, 231
Occult hydrocephalus, 88, *90*
   pneumography and, 89
Ocular fundus, abnormalities of, 5
Oligodendroglioma, 165
Osteoectasia, familial, 74
Osteopetrosis, 74

Panhypopituitarism, 204, *204*
Papilledema, 5–9, *7*
   blind spots and, 6
   chronic, 8
   differential diagnosis in, 8
   drusen and, 9
   indications of, 6
   in early infancy, 51
   ophthalmoscopic examination in, 5
   pathogenesis of, 8
   pseudopapilledema and, 9
   unilateral, 8
   visual acuity in, 6
Papilloma, in early infancy, 51
   of choroid plexus, 239, *239*
Paraldehyde, in lead encephalopathy, 120
Parietal lobe, tumors of, 226, *228, 229*
Pica, 116
Pickwickian syndrome, 55
Pineal gland region, tumors of, 198–202
   pinealoma, 199
   teratoma, 198
Pinealoma, 199, *200, 201*
   symptoms of, 199
   treatment of, 202
Pinealoma, ectopic, 218
Pituitary adenoma, 219, *220*
Pituitary gland, tumors of, 203–213. See also names of specific tumors.
   endocrinologic evaluation of, 203, *204*
Plumbism, 116
Pneumocephalus, 134
Pneumoencephalography, in hydrocephalus, 83
   in intracranial tumor, 178, *179*

Poisoning, lead, 116
Posterior fossa, tumors in, 184–197. See also names of specific tumors.
Pseudopapilledema, 9
Pseudotumor cerebri, 111–115
 definition of, 111
 diagnosis in, 113, *114*
 etiology of, 112
 prognosis in, 115
 symptoms of, 112
 treatment of, 114
Psychogenic headache, 21
 management of, 22
 manifestations of, 22
Pudenz-Heyer valve system, in hydrocephalus, 103
Pulmonary thromboembolism, shunting and, 105
Pycnodysostosis, 74
 symptoms of, 35

Queckenstedt test, in lumbar puncture, 32

Radioactive brain scan, in intracranial tumor, 177, *177, 178*
Rathke-pouch tumor, 205
Rheumatoid arthritis, headache and, 29
Roentgenography, abnormal suture spread in, 34
 convolutional markings in, 36, *36*
 increased intracranial pressure and, 34–40
 in pinealoma, 202
Russell dwarf, 74

Sarcoma, meningeal, *253*, 254
Seizures, intracranial tumor and, 170
Sella turcica, alterations of, 39, *39*
Septicemia, shunting and, 104
"Setting sun" sign, 69, *70*
Shunting procedures, in hydrocephalus, 102
Skull fractures, 131, *132*
 in neonate, 132, *133*
Skull, x-ray, in pinealoma, 202
Sphenopalatine neuralgia, 19
Spinal tap, in intracranial tumor, 172
Subarachnoid hemorrhage, headache and, 24
Subdural hematoma, in early infancy, 51
 in infants, 136, *138*
 in older children, 138, *139*
Suture spread, abnormal, in infants, 35
 roentgenographic signs in, *35*
Sympathicoblastoma, 240
Syndromes. See names of specific syndromes.

Tay-Sachs disease, 74
Temporal lobe, tumors of, 230, *230, 231*
Teratoma, 198
Tetracycline, as cause of intracranial pressure, 53
Tetralogy of Fallot, 147
Thalamus, tumors of, 232, *233*
Thromboembolism, pulmonary, shunting and, 105
Tobey-Ayer test, in lumbar puncture, 33
Toxoplasmosis, congenital, hydrocephalus and, 51
Transillumination, of the skull, 77
Trauma, head, 123–146
 blunt, 125, *126*
 clinical aspects of, 127
 in infancy, 52
 management in, 127
 pathology of, 124
 perinatal, 129
 prevention of, 123
 statistics on, 123
Tuberous sclerosis, *225*
Tumor(s), congenital, 234–238. See also names of specific tumors.
 dermoid, 237
 headache and, 23
 intracranial. See also names of specific tumors.
  classifications of, 158
  diagnosis of, 171
  differential diagnosis in, 181
  in childhood, 54
  in infancy, 51
  statistics on, 157
  symptoms of, 169
  types of, 158

Urea, in cerebral edema, 60

Valium, in lead encephalopathy, 120
Ventricular taps, in hydrocephalus, 77, *80*
Ventriculography, in intracranial tumor, 180, *180*
Vidian neuralgia, 19
Visual field testing, in intracranial tumor, 175
Vitamin A, abnormalities of intake in infants, 53
von Hippel-Lindau syndrome, hemangioblastoma and, 192

Weber's syndrome, 195
Wiskott-Aldrich syndrome, 56

X-ray, skull, in intracranial tumor, 172, *173*
 in pinealoma, 202